Minimally Invasive Urology: Past, Present, and Future

Editor

JOHN D. DENSTEDT

UROLOGIC CLINICS OF NORTH AMERICA

www.urologic.theclinics.com

Consulting Editor
KEVIN R. LOUGHLIN

February 2022 • Volume 49 • Number 1

ELSEVIER

1600 John F. Kennedy Boulevard • Suite 1800 • Philadelphia, Pennsylvania, 19103-2899

http://www.theclinics.com

UROLOGIC CLINICS OF NORTH AMERICA Volume 49, Number 1
February 2022 ISSN 0094-0143, ISBN-13: 978-0-323-84902-9

Editor: Kerry Holland
Developmental Editor: Diana Ang

Urologic Clinics of North America (ISSN 0094-0143) is published quarterly by Elsevier Inc., 360 Park Avenue South, New York, NY 10010-1710. Months of issue are February, May, August, and November. Business and Editorial Offices: 1600 John F. Kennedy Blvd., Suite 1800, Philadelphia, PA 19103-2899. Periodicals postage paid at New York, NY and additional mailing offices. Subscription prices are $403.00 per year (US individuals), $1054.00 per year (US institutions), $100.00 per year (US students and residents), $459.00 per year (Canadian individuals), $1075.00 per year (Canadian institutions), $100.00 per year (Canadian students/residents), $530.00 per year (foreign individuals), $1075.00 per year (foreign institutions), and $240.00 per year (foreign students/residents). Foreign air speed delivery is included in all *Clinics* subscription prices. All prices are subject to change without notice. **POSTMASTER:** Send address changes to *Urologic Clinics of North America*, Elsevier Health Sciences Division, Subscription Customer Service, 3251 Riverport Lane, Maryland Heights, MO 63043. **Customer Service: 1-800-654-2452 (US). From outside the United States, call 1-314-447-8871. Fax: 1-314-447-8029. E-mail: JournalsCustomerService-usa@elsevier.com (for print support)** and **JournalsOnlineSupport-usa@elsevier.com (for online support)**.

Reprints. For copies of 100 or more, of articles in this publication, please contact the Commercial Reprints Department, Elsevier Inc., 360 Park Avenue South, New York, New York 10010-1710. Tel.: 212-633-3874; Fax: 212-633-3820; E-mail: reprints@elsevier.com.

Urologic Clinics of North America is covered in MEDLINE/PubMed (*Index Medicus*), *Excerpta Medica, Current Contents/Clinical Medicine, Science Citation Index,* and *ISI/BIOMED*.

Contributors

CONSULTING EDITOR

KEVIN R. LOUGHLIN, MD, MBA
Emeritus Professor of Surgery (Urology), Harvard Medical School, Visiting Scientist, Vascular Biology Research Program at Boston Children's Hospital, Boston, Massachusetts, USA

EDITOR

JOHN D. DENSTEDT, MD, FRCSC, FACS, FCAHS
Professor of Urology, Schulich School of Medicine and Dentistry, Western University, London, Ontario, Canada

AUTHORS

HAIDER ABED, MD
Division of Urology, Department of Surgery, Western University, London, Ontario, Canada

PARWIZ ABRAHIMI, MD, PhD
Department of Urology, NewYork-Presbyterian Hospital, Weill Cornell Medical College, New York, New York, USA

SYLVIA L. ALIP, MD
Department of Urology, Yonsei University College of Medicine, Urological Science Institute, Seodaemun-ku Seoul, South Korea; Division of Urology, University of the Philippines, Philippine General Hospital, Manila, Philippines

ROHITH ARCOT, MD
Division of Urology, Duke University Medical Center, Duke University, Duke Cancer Center, Durham, North Carolina, USA

SARA L. BEST, MD
Associate Professor, Director of Simulation Education, Department of Urology, University of Wisconsin-Madison School of Medicine and Public Health, Madison, Wisconsin, USA

NAEEM BHOJANI, MD, FRCSC
Department of Surgery, University of Montreal (CHUM), Montreal, Quebec, Canada

ANDREW BREVIK, MS
Leadership and Innovation Fellowship Training Scholar, Department of Urology, University of California, Irvine, Orange, California, USA

GIOVANNI CACCIAMANI, MD
AI Center at USC Urology, USC Institute of Urology, Los Angeles, California, USA

JEFFREY D. CAMPBELL, MD, MPH
Assistant Professor, Division of Urology, Department of Surgery, Western University, London, Ontario, Canada

ANDREW B. CHEN, MD
USC Institute of Urology, Los Angeles, California, USA

BILAL CHUGHTAI, MD
Department of Urology, Weill Cornell Medical College, New York, New York, USA

RALPH V. CLAYMAN, MD
Distinguished Professor, Department of Urology, University of California, Irvine, Orange, California, USA

MARIELA CORRALES, MD
GRC Urolithiasis no. 20, Sorbonne University, Department of Urology AP-HP, Tenon Hospital, Paris, France

PROKAR DASGUPTA, MD
Faculty of Life Sciences and Medicine, King's College London, King's Health Partners, London, United Kingdom

JANAK DESAI, MS, MCh, FRCS
Department of Urology, Samved Hospital, Ahmedabad, India

ANDREW DI PIERDOMINICO, MD
Division of Urology, Department of Surgery, Western University, London, Ontario, Canada

DEAN ELTERMAN, MD, MSc, FRCSC
Division of Urology, Department of Surgery, University of Toronto, Toronto, Ontario

BRUCE GAO, MD
Division of Urology, Department of Surgery, University of Toronto, Toronto, Ontario

AHMED GHAZI, MD, FEBU, MHPE
Associate Professor of Urology, George W. Conner Deans Teaching Fellow, Endourology Fellowship Program Director, Department of Urology, Director, Simulation Innovation Laboratory, University of Rochester Medical Center, Rochester, New York, USA

WOONG KYU HAN, MD
Professor, Department of Urology, Yonsei University College of Medicine, Urological Science Institute, Seodaemun-ku Seoul, South Korea

TASEEN HAQUE, BA
Keck School of Medicine of USC, Los Angeles, California, USA

ANDREW J. HUNG, MD
AI Center at USC Urology, USC Institute of Urology, Los Angeles, California, USA

PIETER JANSSEN, MD
Department of Urology, University Hospital Ghent, Ghent, Belgium

PENGBO JIANG, MD
Fellow in Endourology, Department of Urology, University of California, Irvine, Orange, California, USA

JINU KIM, MD
Department of Urology, Yonsei University College of Medicine, Urological Science Institute, Seodaemun-ku Seoul, South Korea

MARGARET A. KNOEDLER, MD
Endourology Fellow, Department of Urology, University of Wisconsin-Madison School of Medicine and Public Health, Madison, Wisconsin, USA

STEVEN LU
Cumming School of Medicine, University of Calgary, Calgary, Alberta, Canada

DANNY MATTI
Division of Urology, Department of Surgery, Western University, London, Ontario, Canada

TIMOTHY McCLURE, MD
Departments of Urology and Radiology, NewYork-Presbyterian Hospital, Weill Cornell Medical College, New York, New York, USA

THOMAS J. POLASCIK, MD, FACS
Professor of Surgery, Division of Urology, Duke University Medical Center, Duke University, Duke Cancer Center, Durham, North Carolina, USA

SIRISHA RAMBHATLA, PhD
Viterbi School of Engineering at USC, Los Angeles, California, USA

KOON HO RHA, MD
Professor, Department of Urology, Yonsei University College of Medicine, Urological Science Institute, Seodaemun-ku Seoul, South Korea

SIDNEY ROBERTS, BA
Keck School of Medicine of USC, Los Angeles, California, USA

HEMENDRA N. SHAH, MD, MCh, MRCS
Associate Professor, Department of Urology, University of Miami Miller School of Medicine, Miami, Florida, USA

THOMAS TAILLY, MD, MSc, PhD
Department of Urology, University Hospital Ghent, Ghent, Belgium

OLIVIER TRAXER, MD
GRC Urolithiasis no. 20, Sorbonne University, Department of Urology AP-HP, Tenon Hospital, Paris, France

KEVIN C. ZORN, MD, FRCSC, FACS
Department of Surgery, University of Montreal (CHUM), Montreal, Quebec, Canada

Contents

Disposable Ureteroscopes in Urology: Current State and Future Prospects 153

Margaret A. Knoedler and Sara L. Best

Ureteroscopy is the most common surgical modality for stone treatment. Reusable flexible ureteroscopes are delicate instruments that require expensive maintenance and repairs. Multiple single use ureteroscopes have been developed recently to combat the expensive and time-intensive sterilization and repair of ureteroscopes. Although multiple studies have looked at different aspects of reusable and single use ureteroscopes, there is significant heterogeneity in performance measures and cost between the 2 categories, and neither has a clear advantage. Both can be used successfully, and individual and institution level factors should be considered when deciding which ureteroscope to use.

Mini Percutaneous Kidney Stone Removal: Applicable Technologies 161

Janak Desai and Hemendra N. Shah

Percutaneous nephrolithotomy (PCNL) remains the treatment of choice for large and complex renal stones. The technological advances over the past several decades gave birth to different varieties of minimally invasive PCNLs, including the mini-PCNL, ultra-mini PCNL, super mini-PCNL, and micro-PCNL, with indications being extended to stones even larger than 20 mm. This article provides an update of all these available techniques of miniaturized PCNL along with its anatomic and physiologic impact. This should assist urologists in providing a personalized approach to the patient based on various patient- and stone-related factors to provide the best of all available technology for treatment.

Technological Advancements for Treating Erectile Dysfunction and Peyronie's Disease 175

Jeffrey D. Campbell, Danny Matti, Haider Abed, and Andrew Di Pierdominico

Over the past decade, there have been several advancements in the technologies available to treatment erectile dysfunction and Peyronie's disease. Vacuum erection devices, penile traction devices, low-intensity extracorporeal shockwave therapy, and penile prosthesis surgery have evolved and are changing the way we treat men's health. Although significant improvements have been made, further work is needed to standardize treatment, create universal algorithms for technological applications, and simply their use.

New Stent Technologies 185

Pieter Janssen and Thomas Tailly

Ureteral stents are an indispensable part of any (endo-) urologic practice. Despite the widely demonstrated advantages of stents, they also carry a considerable risk of side effects and complications, such as urinary symptoms, pain, hematuria, decreased quality of life, stent-related infection, and encrustation. Multiple pathways in preventing or mitigating these side effects and complications and improving stent efficacy have been and are being investigated, including stent architecture and design, biomaterials, and coatings. This article provides an update on currently researched and available stents as well as future perspectives.

UROLOGIC CLINICS OF NORTH AMERICA

FORTHCOMING ISSUES

May 2022
Urologic Pharmacology
Craig Comiter, *Editor*

August 2022
Urologic Reconstructive Surgery
Jill Buckley, *Editor*

November 2022
Testosterone
Kevin R. Loughlin, *Editor*

RECENT ISSUES

November 2021
Sexual Dysfunction: A New Era
Alan W. Shindel and Tom F. Lue, *Editors*

August 2021
Prostate Cancer Genetics: Changing the Paradigm of Care
Leonard G. Gomella and Veda N. Giri, *Editors*

May 2021
The Changing Landscape of Urologic Practice
Deepak A. Kapoor, *Editor*

SERIES OF RELATED INTEREST
Surgical Clinics of North America
https://www.surgical.theclinics.com/

Foreword

One Small Step for a Urologist, One Giant Leap for Urologic Surgery

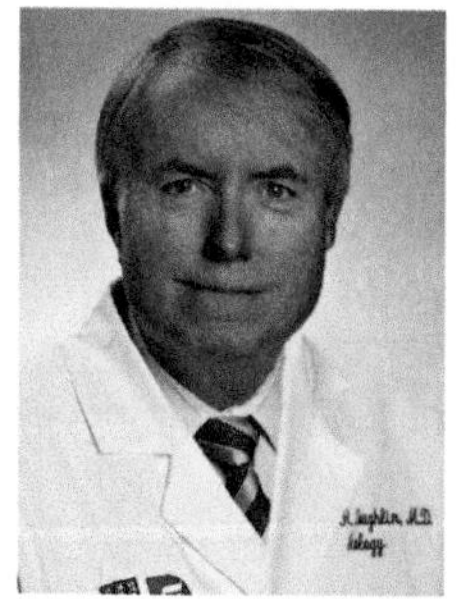

Kevin R. Loughlin, MD, MBA
Consulting Editor

To Americans of a certain age, the date of July 20, 1969 is etched forever in their memory. That is the day that Neil Armstrong stepped on the moon with the words, "That's one small step for a man, one giant leap for mankind." The "a" was lost in radio static. Accompanied by Buzz Aldrin, he changed the future of mankind.

Similarly, on June 25,1990, as Ralph Clayman walked into room 48 in Barnes Hospital in St. Louis, he didn't say, but could have said," That is one small step for a urologist, one giant leap for urologic surgery." Accompanied by Lou Kavoussi, he changed the future of urology.[1]

However, we all must acknowledge that the practice of urologic surgery is a continuum. We are all but temporary custodians of a very special profession. There have been other urologic astronauts prior to 1990.

In the early twentieth century, endoscopic prostatectomy was about in the same state as urologic laparoscopy was almost a century later. Hugh Hampton Young[2] at Johns Hopkins had championed the perineal prostatectomy and later the "punch" operation, where a tubular knife was passed down an endoscopic instrument to cut away pieces of the prostate by feel.

The underpinning that paved the way for transurethral resection of the prostate was provided by an eccentric inventor who was not even a physician. W.T. Bovie[3] held a doctorate in plant physiology and developed an innovative electrosurgical machine in 1920.[4] He worked at Peter Bent Brigham Hospital in Boston and showed it to Harvey Cushing, who introduced it into clinical practice.

The resectoscope was introduced by Maximilian Stern[5] in 1926. This instrument combined the ability to see as well as the ability to cut and coagulate the prostate using a loop of tungsten and electric current.[6] Further modifications of the technique and instruments continued, and in 1931, the Stern-McCarthy resectoscope was developed due to the continued efforts of the instrument maker, Frederick Wappler, and the urologist, Joseph McCarthy.[7]

Milestones in minimally invasive urologic surgery did not cease with the transurethral resection of the prostate. In 1955, Willard E. Goodwin and colleagues[8,9] at UCLA reported the first use of a percutaneous puncture of the kidney to relieve hydronephrosis. They noted that this advance was in large part serendipitous, as he inadvertently accessed the kidney while attempting a percutaneous arteriogram. Goodwin's discovery provided

Urol Clin N Am 49 (2022) xi–xii
https://doi.org/10.1016/j.ucl.2021.09.002

the foundation for the development of percutaneous renal procedures in subsequent decades.

As percutaneous renal procedures continued to proliferate, the next logical progression was transcutaneous procedures. In 1975, while a resident at the University of Munich, Christian G. Chaussy, together with Ferdinand Eisenberger and Bernd Forsmann,[10] began the preclinical and clinical research to investigate applications of the extracorporeal lithotripsy (ESWL) technology. In 1980, he performed the first ever ESWL treatment on a patient. In 1984, ESWL was introduced in the United States for evaluation at six institutions: Massachusetts General Hospital in Boston, Methodist Hospital in Indianapolis, Memorial Sloan Kettering in New York City, the University of Florida in Gainesville, the University of Virginia in Charlottesville, and Baylor Hospital in Houston.[11]

The first laparoscopic radical prostatectomy was performed by Clayman and his team in 1991.[12] This technique was soon embraced on both sides of the Atlantic as Guillonneau and Vallancien[13] popularized laparoscopic radical prostatectomy in Europe. As laparoscopic radical prostatectomy became more widely embraced, the transition to robotic surgery was a natural evolution.

The development of the AESOP and da Vinci robotic systems began in the 1990s, and the da Vinci system appeared in Europe in 1999 and received FDA approval in 2000.[14] In the ensuing two decades, robotic prostatectomy became the standard of care.

If Ralph Clayman is a urologic astronaut, then one of his former fellows, John Denstedt, is aptly noted to be a urologic ambassador. Since finishing his fellowship in St. Louis in 1989, John has served as a guest professor or invited lecturer over 400 times in 60 countries. He was the recipient of the prestigious AUA Gold Cystoscope Award in 1998 and currently serves as the AUA secretary, where he organizes the annual AUA meeting, the largest urology meeting in the world.

It should then come as no surprise that this issue of *Urologic Clinics of North America*, organized by John, contains contributions from authors from three continents and five countries. John has assembled experts in diverse fields and technologic applications, which are truly cutting edge. This issue reiterates that urologic practice is kinetic. Today's state-of-the-art is destined to become tomorrow's obsolete; it is just a question of how quickly. In 1969, man landed on the moon; a half-century later, a mission to Mars is within our grasp. In 1990, Clayman performed the first laparoscopic nephrectomy; one can only imagine what urologists will be doing in 2040.

Kevin R. Loughlin, MD, MBA
Vascular Biology Program at
Boston Children's Hospital
300 Longwood Avenue
Boston, MA 02115, USA

E-mail address:
kloughlin@partners.org

REFERENCES

1. Kerbl DC, McDougall em, Clayman RV, et al. A history and evolution of laparoscopic nephrectomy: perspectives from the past and future directions in the surgical management for renal tumors. J Urol 2011;185(3):1150–4.
2. Young HH. The "Punch" operation (transurethral resection of the prostate). In: Hugh Young: a surgeon's autobiography. New York: Harcourt, Brace and Company; 1940. p. 118–34.
3. Goldwyn RM. Bovie: the man and the machine. Ann Plast Surg 1979;2(2):135–53.
4. O'Connor JL, Bloom DA, William T. Bovie and electric surgery. Surgery 1996;119(4):390–6.
5. Stern M. Resection of obstruction at the vesical orifice. JAMA 1926;87:1726–30.
6. Wilde S. See one, do one, modify one: prostate surgery of the 1930s. Med Hist 2004;48:351–66.
7. McCarthy JF. A new apparatus for endoscopic plastic surgery of the prostate: diathermy and excision of vesical growths. J Urol 1931;26:695–6.
8. Goodwin WE, Casey WC, Woolf W. Percutaneous(-needle) nephrostomy in hydronephrosis. JAMA 1955;157(11):891–4.
9. Goodwin WE. A memoir of percutaneous access to the kidney (antegrade pyelography and percutaneous nephrostomy). J Endourol 1991;5(3):185–6.
10. Chaussy C, Schmied E, Joachim D, et al. Extracorporeal shock-wave lithotripsy (ESWL) for treatment of urolithiasis. Urology 1984;23(5):59–66.
11. Del Guercio G. Device destroys kidney stones without surgery. Washington, DC: United Press International; 1984.
12. Schuessler WW, Schulam PG, Clayman RV, et al. Laparoscopic radical nephrectomy: initial short-term experience. Urology 1997;50(6):854–7.
13. Guillonneau B, Vallancien G. Laparoscopic radical prostatectomy: the Montsouris experience. J Urol 2000;163(2):418–22.
14. Ballantyne GH, Moll F. The da Vinci telerobotic surgical system: the virtual operative field and telepresence surgery. Surg Clin North Amer 2003;83(6): 1293–304.

Preface

A Profound Past and a Very Bright Future: Minimally Invasive Urology

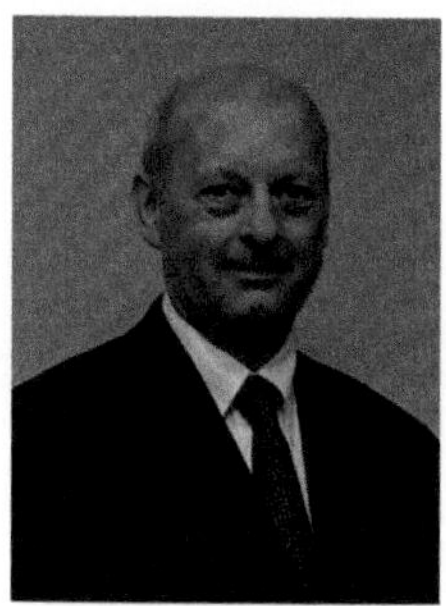

John D. Denstedt, MD, FRCSC, FACS, FCAHS
Editor

Since its inception as a subspecialty of surgery in the late 1800s, innovations in treatment in urology have been driven by the creative minds of urologic surgeons and by parallel advances in operative technology. Beginning with the first cystoscopes that enabled visualization of the human bladder for diagnostic purposes to resectoscopes, advances in kidney stone treatments that eliminated open surgery and more recently laparoscopy, robotics, and focal therapy, the march of advances in techniques and technologies continues. It is a fascination with minimally invasive surgery and urologic technology that often draws medical students to our specialty and inspires residents and fellows to become the next generation of innovators.

This issue of the *Urologic Clinics of North America* provides a tremendous overview of the scope of minimally invasive techniques across the wide breadth of our specialty. I am grateful to the authors, all of whom are well-recognized global experts in their respective fields of interest. From advanced imaging to robotics, energy sources, and prosthetics to the latest advances in 3D printing and artificial intelligence applications in urology, this issue covers the diverse aspects of minimally invasive diagnostic and therapeutic approaches to urologic disorders. At the same time, these excellent articles provide a wonderful historic perspective on the foundations for many of the techniques available today. I hope you enjoy reading these interesting and comprehensive articles as much as I have.

John D. Denstedt, MD, FRCSC, FACS, FCAHS
Schulich School of Medicine and Dentistry
Western University
St Joseph's Health Care
268 Grosvenor Street
London, Ontario N6A 4V2, Canada

E-mail address:
denstedt@uwo.ca

Urol Clin N Am 49 (2022) xiii
https://doi.org/10.1016/j.ucl.2021.09.001
0094-0143/22/© 2021 Published by Elsevier Inc.

New Lasers for Stone Treatment

Olivier Traxer, MD[a,b,*], Mariela Corrales, MD[a,b]

KEYWORDS

• Laser lithotripsy • Technology • Endourology • Urolithiasis • Thulium lasers

KEY POINTS

- Based on the current available clinical data, TFL represents a promising technology that could become the next gold standard for ELL.
- The main advantages of TFL are the great ablation efficiency, the reduced retropulsion, the smaller fibers, and the wide and flexible range of parameters, not seen before with the Ho:YAG laser technology.
- Tm:YAG is a new solid-state, diode-pumped, pulsed laser that can offer high frequencies (up to 200 Hz) and very low pulse energies (<0.1 J). Similar to the Ho:YAG laser, it performs EEL by a photothermal mechanism. Further clinical studies are needed to assess this new technology.
- Moses 2.0 offers an improved Moses technology in a high-power Ho:YAG with advantages yet to be confirmed in clinical practice.

INTRODUCTION

Since the term lithotomy was first cited by the Greeks in 276 BC,[1] the procedure evolved greatly over the years.[2] Almost 40 years ago the first minimally invasive technology for kidney stones was developed with the appearance of percutaneous nephrolithotomy (PCNL) using an ultrasonic lithotripter.[3] This development was followed by the introduction of the shockwave lithotripsy for urinary stones in the mid-1980s, and it was only in the 1990s, with the development of flexible fiberoptic ureteroscopes, that the true light activation by the stimulated emission of radiation (LASER) era for endoscopic lithotripsy began, exactly 33 years ago.[3–6]

Mid-2020 has been a crucial time for laser technology in urology, with the launch of novel laser devices approved by the US Food and Drug Administration. We aim to review the latest laser technology available in the market for endoscopic lithotripsy.

BACKGROUND AND HISTORY

When lasers made their first appearance in urology for lithotripsy in 1968, most of them worked in a continuous mode (ie, ruby, Nd:YAG, and CO_2 lasers). However, the results were not optimal, mainly because of excessive soft tissue thermal damage, turning them not suitable for endoscopic laser lithotripsy (ELL).[3,7–10] On the other hand, pulsed lasers are the only ones suited for this purpose because of the production of bursts of light spaced in time, which means that no light is produced between each emission (**Fig. 1**).[11]

Holmium:Yttrium-Aluminum Garnet Laser

The holmium:yttrium-aluminum garnet (Ho:YAG) laser has been and continues to be the gold standard for ELL since the 1990s.[3,10,12] The reason why this pulsed laser is still considered that way is because of its appropriate characteristics. For instance, it can ablate any type of urinary stone,

Funding sources: This is an independent study and is not funded by any external body.
[a] Sorbonne University, GRC Urolithiasis no. 20, Tenon Hospital, Paris F-75020, France; [b] Sorbonne University, Department of Urology AP-HP, Tenon Hospital, Paris F-75020, France
* Corresponding author. Sorbonne University GRC Urolithiasis no. 20 Tenon Hospital, Paris F-75020, France.
E-mail address: olivier.traxer@aphp.fr

Urol Clin N Am 49 (2022) 1–10
https://doi.org/10.1016/j.ucl.2021.07.006

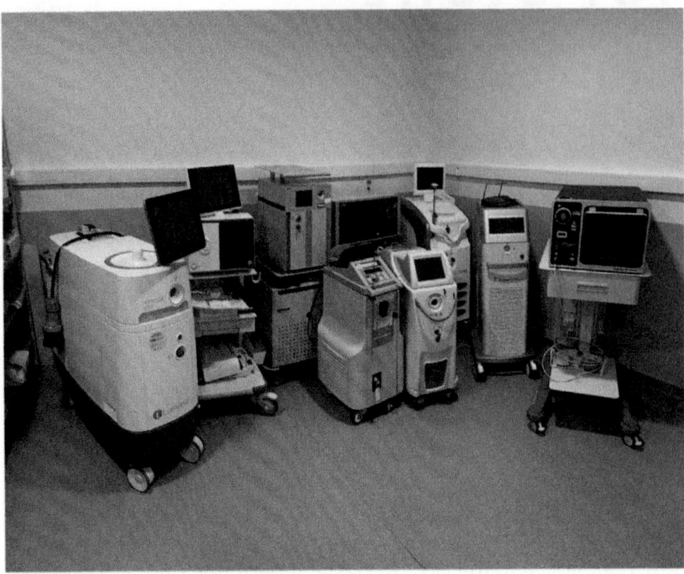

Fig. 1. Different laser machines. From left to right: The Lumenis Pulse 120H, the Soltive SuperPulsed Thulium Fiber Laser System for Olympus, different low-frequency Ho:YAG devices (30 W), and the Fiber dust from Quanta System (Milan, Italy).

unlike its predecessor (the pulsed-dye laser) that had difficulty in fragmenting cystine and “hard” stones (ie, calcium oxalate monohydrate [COM]).[3,9,13–15] Because the holmium infrared laser wavelength of 2100 nm is highly absorbed by water (water absorption coefficient of 3198 L/m),[3,16] the water absorbed energy results in the formation of a vapor microbubble at the tip of the laser that expands outwardly toward the target; once the microbubble reaches the target, the laser beam can pass through the vapor to the target with little attenuation because the density of the water molecules in the steam is much less than in the liquid state.[15,17] This phenomenon is known as the *Moses effect* (ME).[15,17,18] The bubble can be initiated with a very small amount of energy, and the threshold for bubble formation (100–200 μs) and expansion is independent of the duration or excess energy in the pulse.[15,19] In addition, this strong water absorption, at the mentioned wavelength, is responsible for an optical penetration depth of about 400 μm, a property that makes it suitable for incision/coagulation of soft tissues.[10,20] In terms of the laser machine specifications, it uses a sometimes loud water cooling system, the weight of the laser device can be between 245 and 300 kg (depending on the model), and it needs to be branched to a high-amperage power outlet due to its high energy consumption (9000 W).[21]

The Ho:YAG laser produces smaller stone fragments than the ones obtained with pulsed-dye lasers, pneumatic lithotripsy, or electrohydraulic lithotripsy, and it can be coupled to small flexible glass fibers.[3,10,22] Furthermore, the Ho:YAG laser has proved to be effective and safe in both ureteroscopy and PCNL, as long as we keep a safety distance.[23] In ureteroscopy, the safety distance for avoiding flexible ureteroscope tip damage is when the laser fiber tip reaches one-fourth of the screen because it is at that distance that the bubble generated by laser activation would never touch the camera of the ureteroscope.[24]

The first low-power (LP) Ho:YAG laser module (20 W), which contains one single laser cavity, had two parameters only: the pulse energy in Joules, up to 2 J, and the frequency in Hertz, up to 15 Hz; however, now we can find Ho:YAG LP lasers of 30 to 35 W, reaching up to 30 Hz. On the other side, the association of multiple synchronized Ho:YAG cavities to one single delivery fiber was developed to create the high-power (HP) Ho:YAG lasers (up to 140 W), which were developed mostly for benign prostate hypertrophy but can also be used for ELL, reaching up to 6 J and 100 Hz.[3,21,25–28]

Frequency-Doubled, Double-Pulse Nd:YAG Laser

The frequency-doubled, double-pulse Nd:YAG (FREDDY) laser is a short-pulsed laser that consists of a potassium titanyl phosphate crystal incorporated into an Nd:YAG laser, which enables 2 laser pulses at 532 nm (green light component) and 1064 nm wavelengths (infrared component).[3,29,30] The Ho:YAG laser produces stone fragmentation by vaporization, whereas the FREDDY laser generates a plasma bubble that will collapse, creating a mechanical shock wave that causes the fragmentation of the stone.[31,32]

Preclinical trials were performed to test its efficiency and safety and demonstrated that it could be used as an alternative to Ho:YAG laser and to ballistic lithotriptors (ie, LithoClast; EMS, Nyon, Switzerland) in selected patients[32,33]; it was also shown that even though stone fragmentation was significantly higher with the FREDDY laser,[32,34] stone retropulsion was also greater with the FREEDY laser when compared with the Ho:YAG laser.[32] The cost of this lithotriptor was also appealing; the purchase cost was substantially reduced, by about 30%, compared with the Ho:YAG laser.[33,34] After the promising results, clinical trials were done. Despite one report mentioning that it seemed that patients treated with Ho:YAG laser for ureteral stones had a higher stone-free rate (SFR) and lower complication rate than the ones treated with the FREDDY laser,[29] FREDDY laser lithotripsy was confirmed to be an effective and harmless method at a moderate cost for renal and ureteral stones.[29,35] However, it had 3 main limitations. FREDDY laser was ineffective for treating all types of stones, such as cystine or COM stones; it was not applicable for coagulation procedures; and it did not have soft tissue applications such as urinary tract stenosis and tumors.[29,31,35]

Moses Technology

Further advances in Ho:YAG lithotripsy have been related to the manipulation of the laser pulse. The ME is a physical phenomenon that occurs every time we activate an Ho:YAG laser in the operating room, independent of laser parameters, fiber dimension, and manufacturer.[17] Back in 1993, Trost had an idea about a pulse-shape modulation that would optimize the energy delivery through water to the target, an idea that was then patented in 1994 and, years later, marketed by Lumenis (Lumenis Ltd., Yokneam, Israel) as the "Moses technology" (MT) in 2017.[17,19,36] The purpose of MT is to modulate the laser pulse in 2 components, where the first one is used to separate the water between the laser tip and the target (tissue or stones) and the second one transmits the energy directly to it, without substantial energy loss.[19,36] Lumenis Pulse 120H Ho:YAG laser works at 2 different fiber-target distances: one being Moses A ("Contact") for operation at a close distance (around 1 mm) and the other being Moses B ("Distance") for lithotripsy at a distance (around 2 mm), sometimes needed in difficult scenarios (ie, anatomic restrictions).[36] In terms of laser specifications, this laser has a maximum power of 120 W, an energy rate of 0.2 to 6 J, and a frequency rate of 5 to 80 Hz.[37] In vitro studies have been done with its original laser fiber MOSES D/F/L (available in 200, 365, and 550 μm).[38] One report showed that "Moses A" did produce a more efficient ablation than long-pulse Ho:YAG and ever better if closer to the stone (0–1 mm); however, after in vitro classification of the stones into "hard" (ie, COM stones) or "soft" (ie, uric acid stones), pulse type did not have a significant impact on hard stone ablation at any distance from the surface of the stone but.[39] One adverse effect found at the laboratory was that MT seems to produce a more pronounced photothermal effect than the conventional Ho:YAG laser dusting, which translates into a stone dust that may not adequately reflect the true crystalline organization of the stone before ELL.[40] On the other side, clinical trials showed controversial results. Mullerad and colleagues[41] reaffirmed that MT demonstrates good stone fragmentation for kidney stones of similar volume (regular Ho:YAG: 422.5 mm^3 vs MT: 781 mm^3), but when compared with the regular Ho:YAG lithotripsy, MT did not achieve significantly less fragmentation time. In terms of cost analysis, Stern and colleagues[42] affirmed, after ureteroscopy of 40 patients with mean ureteral and renal stone size of 10.2 mm, that the decrease in lasing time achieved by the MT did not translate into sufficient cost savings due to the higher cost of the laser fiber and software. An initial experience in combined ultramini PCNL with this technology has shown promising results.[43]

RECENT MAJOR INNOVATIONS

We recapitulate the major innovations that were made last year. **Tables 1** and **2** summarize the main specifications of each new laser technology and each laser device, respectively.

Thulium Fiber Laser

Thulium fiber laser (TFL) has recently become available in urology as an alternative to the Ho:YAG laser, the current gold standard. TFL, as its name implies, is a silica fiber chemically doped with thulium ions, with the characteristic of being very thin (10–20 μm core diameter) and long (10–30 m long).[44,45] The mechanism of action is different from that of the Ho:YAG laser. In this case, multiple electronically modulated laser diodes are used to excite the thulium ions for laser pumping, instead of the flash lamps used in Ho:YAG lasers.[44,45] The emitted laser beam has a wavelength of 1940 nm, which can perform in a continuous or pulsed mode, is much more uniform and focused, and can be transmitted to smaller core diameter fibers (50–150 μm).[44,46,47] TFL has a 4- to 5-fold higher water absorption than that of Ho:YAG laser and

Table 1
Laser technology specifications

Technology Specifications	Ho:YAG Laser	TFL	Tm:YAG
Wavelength	2100 nm	1920–1960 nm	2013 nm
Water absorption coefficient	26 cm^{-1}	114 cm^{-1}	52 cm^{-1}
Mode of action	Pulsed	Pulsed	Pulsed
Gain medium	Bulk solid-state crystal (containing holmium ions)	Chemically doped silica optical fiber (10–20 μm thick)	Bulk solid-state crystal (containing thulium ions)
Generation of laser radiation	Flash lamp	Electronically controlled diode lasers	Flash lamp
Pulse profile	Irregular Several spikes	Symetrical and constant Square waves	Irregular Several spikes
Peak power	N.A	500 W	200 W

Abbreviations: N.A, not available; TFL, thulium-fiber laser; Tm:YAG, thulium:yttrium-aluminum garnet.

twice that of thulium:yttrium-aluminum garnet (Tm:YAG) laser.[3,44] These features, perhaps, can explain why this new laser has a great ablation efficiency for any type of urinary stones.[48,49] Furthermore, one of the greatest advantages of the TFL is that it offers the widest and flexible range of parameters among the laser's lithotripters in the urology market, working with low (as low as 0.025 J) to high pulse energies (6 J), high pulse frequencies (up to 2400 Hz for the latest TFL device), short to long pulse durations (200 μs–50 ms), peak power of 500 W, and average power of 2 to 60 W.[44,50,51] The low, constant, and prolonged peak power plus the longer pulse duration that the TFL offers makes it possible to deliver more energy to the target (stone) and may be the reason why this laser produces lesser retropulsion than the Ho:YAG laser.[45,52,53] Concerning the device itself, it is a 40-kg small device with a noiseless air cooling system (**Fig. 2**).[21,51]

Preclinical Studies

Several in vitro studies have demonstrated that TFL performs a more efficient lithotripsy than the Ho:YAG laser.[54,55] The 4 to 5 times higher

Table 2
Laser device specifications

Laser Device Specifications	Ho:YAG Laser	TFL	Tm:YAG
Average power	120–140 W	2–60 W	120 W
Pulse frequency	5–80 Hz (up to 120 Hz in Moses 2.0)	1–2400 Hz	1–200 Hz
Pulse energy	0.2–6.0 J	0.025–6.0 J	0.1 J – 3J
Pulse width	50–1300 μs -Moses 2.0: Adjustable (short, medium, and long)	200 μs–50 ms	Long (still need specifications)
Peak power	N.A	500 W	200 W
Silica fiber	≥200 μm	≥50 μm (technically feasible for some prototypes)	400 μm (in vitro studies)
Cooling system	Water	Air	Water
Weight	245–300 kg (260 kg in Moses 2.0)	40 kg	Not specified

Abbreviations: N.A, not available; TFL, thulium-fiber laser; Tm:YAG, thulium: yttrium-aluminum garnet.

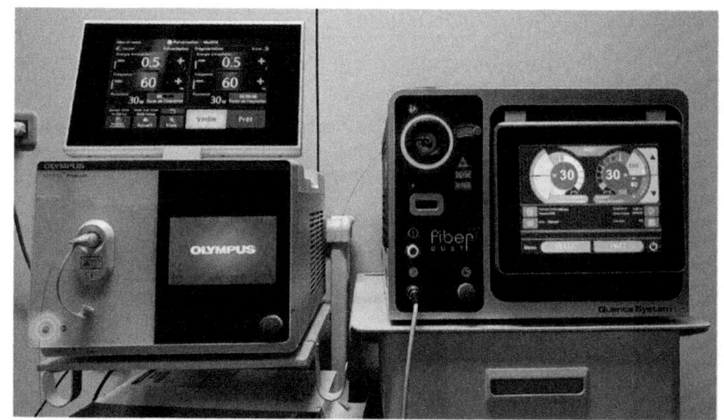

Fig. 2. Thulium fiber technology. To the left, the Soltive SuperPulsed Thulium Fiber Laser System for Olympus, and to the right, the Fiber dust from Quanta System.

dusting/fragmentation rate[56–58] is responsible for the "microdust" that TFL offers, a term that has been suggested for particles smaller than the 150 μm core diameter fiber.[59] This very fine dust is, at least, twice as much dust as the one produced by any Ho:YAG laser (including the MT).[60]

Another point that deserves attention is the flexibility, resistance, and less burnback of the TFL laser fibers, which overpasses the qualities offered by the Ho:YAG laser fibers,[56,61,62] including the new MOSES 200 laser fiber, recently released in the market.[63]

Clinical Outcomes

The first clinical trials come from Russia, where the first manufacturer (IRE-Polus, a Fryazino, Russia, subsidiary of IPG Photonics, Oxford, MA, USA) of this kind of promising technology possessed the clinical approval given by the Ministry of Health of Russian Federation.[64,65] TFL became available in the United States, Canada, and Europe and in selected countries of the Middle East and Africa, in June 2020, with the device name Soltive Premium (manufactured by IPG Photonics for Olympus, Japan).[51,66] Clinical trials have shown that TFL is a safe and effective modality for lithotripsy, resulting in less retropulsion and minimal complication rates.[57,59,67–73] The wide range of settings modalities allows disintegrating stones of different diameters and densities in both fragmentation and dusting modes[74,75]; using a low pulse energy it can achieve effective dusting for urinary stones.[59,67,73,76–79] Lately, it has been documented that the ablation speed for renal stones is 2 times faster than the average documented by the Ho:YAG laser,[59] confirming what had been seen in preclinical trials.[50]

Controversies

One of the current discussions about the novel thulium laser technology is if it produces less retropulsion than the MT. A study that compared both lasers in vitro concluded that the retropulsion effect given by the TFL was 1.8 times lower than the one given by the Ho:YAG with MT,[80] whereas another study affirms that both technologies give equivalent retropulsion.[61]

As expected, the search for optimal settings continues. Settings using higher-frequency regimens (100–200 Hz) for renal stones during Retrograde intrarrenal surgery have been related to higher efficacy and ablation speed without increased complication rates.[59,73] Even if high-frequency regimes have been related to poor visibility, it seems that TFL can achieve a proper visibility even when using a high-frequency mode.[73] It is the urologist's duty to continue to look for the best combination settings in the clinical practice.

Furthermore, there are controversies around the increase in temperature during TFL lithotripsy, especially around the idea that perhaps this technology may overheat the water, due to its higher water absorption, being responsible for possible tissue damage.[81,82] However, it has been proved that at equivalent settings, TFL produces equivalent water temperature elevation as the Ho:YAG laser, for all lithotripsy settings.[50,83,84] To avoid heat damage, it is vital to assure proper irrigation during the intervention.[85] Even a 3-month follow-up report, after TFL lithotripsy, shows no cases of strictures or stenosis.[67] Perhaps this subject will be better explained in further publications, in the follow-up of the first clinical experiences performed around the world.

Thulium:Yttrium-Aluminum Garnet

The Tm: YAG is a solid-state laser that was first introduced in urology, as a constant wave technology, to treat bladder outlet obstruction and bladder tumors[86–88] but not suitable for ELL owing to its low peak power (maximum 200 W).[89]

However, new developments have appeared in the market. Dornier MedTech Laser GmbH (Wessling, Germany) evaluated a novel diode-pumped, pulsed Tm:YAG laser that should not be confused with the TFL.[3,16] This novel device differs from the TFL and from the Tm:YAG constant wave technology, offering 120 W of power with frequencies of 1 to 200 Hz and possible pulse energies as low as 0.1 J upto 3 J.[90,91] As well as Ho:YAG, it performs Endocorporeal laser lithotripsy (EEL) by a photothermal mechanism with a higher water absorption coefficient[34] and at a different wavelength (2013 nm).[3,16,90,92]

Preclinical Studies

Petzold and colleagues[16] showed in an in vitro study that Tm:YAG and Ho:YAG lasers shared a similar temperature variation risk profile, which was also similar to the one of TFL. Recently, the same group of investigators compared, in vitro, the dusting performance of this novel solid-state Tm:YAG device with that of the standard Ho:YAG device and concluded that both have similar dusting performance at similar settings. However, the Tm:YAG device significantly outperformed the Ho:YAG device by giving longer pulse durations with similar settings, and additionally, it was related to an increased ablation effectiveness due to its higher fiber movement.[90] Some investigators have affirmed that the rapid laser gas bubble expansion may cause damage in the surrounding ureteral mucosa in ELL with both Ho:YAG and Tm:YAG; it is recommended to use low energies (<1 J) in the ureter. However, Tm:YAG would have the advantage of having a reduced lateral bubble expansion, possibly leading to less collateral damage.[93]

Retropulsion has also been assessed, and Tm:YAG generated lower energy pulses and longer pulse durations to produce even lower retropulsion than the Ho:YAG laser at similar settings.[91] This novel technology needs to be analyzed in clinical trials to corroborate those promising results.

MOSES 2.0

The latest release of Lumenis is the MOSES 2.0, introduced in July 2020.[94] Manufacturer data mention 50% less retropulsion, 20% faster procedures, 33% more efficient fragmentation, and high frequency (120 Hz) with ultraspeed stone dusting.[95–97] In addition, the manufacturer has improved the laser fiber; the new MOSES 200 D/F/L is a more flexible fiber designed with a smooth fiber tip, a property that enables smooth initial fiber insertion through the deflected scope.[38,95,96]

Preclinical Studies

As mentioned, in the older version, when Moses A was used the closer it was to the stone, the greater was the stone ablation achieved; with this newest version, the ablation rate is higher when both Moses modes are used very close to the stone (0–1 mm).[55] These findings are based on sponsored studies by the manufacturer in vitro[98–100] and in vivo.[96] However, large clinical trials are lacking because of its novelty. Further larger comparative studies are needed.

SUMMARY

The development of new lasers for urinary stone treatment is undeniable. The Ho:YAG laser is the current gold standard for ELL. However, given the promising results of newer technologies, in the near future we could have a new gold standard. It is important to focus not only on the pulse frequency parameter but also on all the benefits that each new laser offers, such as the wider parameter range, the retropulsion effect, the laser fiber characteristics (ie, flexibility), and the laser machine itself. Let us not forget that a high-pulse-frequency device only increases the ablation efficacy when delivered directly on the surface of the target, which does not always happen in the real life.

FUTURE DIRECTIONS

Owing to the recently accepted new technologies for clinical use, clinical trials still remain limited. Further clinical trials are undoubtedly needed. Nonetheless, for what we have seen, encouraging clinical results are ahead to come.

CLINICS CARE POINTS

- Patients that are selected for ELL may benefit from TFL, due to its benefits and safety seen in recent clinical trials. The safety in terms of radiation and temperature is similar to the one given by the current gold standard laser.
- The new laser technologies (TFL, Moses 2.0 and Tm:YAG) need long-term outcome data for future changes in the endourology practice.

DISCLOSURE

Prof. O. Traxer is a consultant for Coloplast, Rocamed, Olympus, EMS, Boston Scientific, and IPG.

CONFLICT OF INTEREST

The authors declare that they have no conflict of interest.

REFERENCES

1. Herr HW. "Cutting for the stone": The ancient art of lithotomy. BJU Int 2008;101(10):1214–6.
2. Khan SR, Pearle MS, Robertson WG, et al. Kidney stones. Nat Rev Dis Prim 2016;2. https://doi.org/10.1038/nrdp.2016.8.
3. Fried NM, Irby PB. Advances in laser technology and fibre-optic delivery systems in lithotripsy. Nat Rev Urol 2018;15(9):563–73.
4. Grasso M, Bagley D. A 7.5/8.2 F actively deflectable, flexible ureteroscope: A new device for both diagnostic and therapeutic upper urinary tract endoscopy. Urology 1994;43(4):435–41.
5. COPTCOAT MJ, ISON KT, WATSON G, et al. Lasertripsy for Ureteric Stones in 120 Cases: Lessons Learned. Br J Urol 1988;61(6):487–9.
6. Use of pulsed Nd:YAG laser in the ureter - PubMed. Available at: https://pubmed.ncbi.nlm.nih.gov/2900567/. Accessed April 29, 2021.
7. Kronenberg P, Somani B. Advances in Lasers for the Treatment of Stones—a Systematic Review. Curr Urol Rep 2018;19(6). https://doi.org/10.1007/s11934-018-0807-y.
8. Pal D, Ghosh A, Sen R, et al. Continuous-wave and quasi-continuous wave thulium-doped all-fiber laser: implementation on kidney stone fragmentations. Appl Opt 2016;55(23):6151.
9. Dretler SP. Laser lithotripsy: A review of 20 years of research and clinical applications. Lasers Surg Med 1988;8(4):341–56.
10. Terry RS, Whelan PS, Lipkin ME. New devices for kidney stone management. Curr Opin Urol 2020;30(2):144–8.
11. Panthier F, Doizi S, Corrales M, et al. Pulsed lasers and endocorporeal laser lithotripsy. Prog en Urol 2021. https://doi.org/10.1016/j.purol.2020.11.008.
12. Denstedt JD, Razvi HA, Sales JL, et al. Preliminary Experience with Holmium:YAG Laser Lithotripsy. J Endourol 1995;9(3):255–8.
13. Chan KF, Vassar GJ, Pfefer TJ, et al. Holmium:YAG laser lithotripsy: A dominant photothermal ablative mechanism with chemical decomposition of urinary calculi. Lasers Surg Med 1999;25(1):22–37.
14. Floratos DL, De la Rosette JJMCH. Lasers in urology. BJU Int 1999;84(2):204–11.
15. van Leeuwen TGJM, Jansen ED, Motamedi M, et al. Bubble formation during pulsed laser ablation: mechanism and implications. In: Jacques SL, Katzir A, editors. Laser-tissue interaction IV, vol. 1882. Los Angeles, CA, USA: SPIE; 1993. p. 13. https://doi.org/10.1117/12.147658.
16. Petzold R, Suarez-Ibarrola R, Miernik A. Temperature assessment of a novel pulsed Thulium solid-state laser compared to a Holmium:YAG laser. J Endourol 2020. https://doi.org/10.1089/end.2020.0803.
17. Ventimiglia E, Traxer O. What Is Moses Effect: A Historical Perspective. J Endourol 2019;33(5):353–7.
18. Isner J, Clarke R, Katzir A, et al. Transmission characteristics of individual wavelengths in blood do not predict ability to accomplish laser ablation in a blood field: Inferential evidence for the "Moses effect. Circulation 1986;74(II):361.
19. Trost D. Laser pulse format for penetrating an absorbingfluid. United Statets Pat; 1994.
20. Hale GM, Querry MR. Optical Constants of Water in the 200-nm to 200-μm Wavelength Region. Appl Opt 1973;12(3):555.
21. Kronenberg P, Traxer O. The laser of the future: reality and expectations about the new thulium fiber laser-a systematic review. Transl Androl Urol 2019;8(4). https://doi.org/10.21037/tau.2019.08.01.
22. Gu Z, Qi J, Shen H, et al. Percutaneous nephroscopic with holmium laser and ultrasound lithotripsy for complicated renal calculi. Lasers Med Sci 2010;25(4):577–80.
23. Bader MJ, Gratzke C, Hecht V, et al. Impact of collateral damage to endourologic tools during laser lithotripsy-in vitro comparison of three different clinical laser systems. J Endourol 2011;25(4):667–72.
24. Talso M, Emiliani E, Haddad M, et al. Laser fiber and flexible ureterorenoscopy: The safety distance concept. J Endourol 2016;30(12):1269–74.
25. Matlaga BR, Chew B, Eisner B, et al. Ureteroscopic Laser Lithotripsy: A Review of Dusting *vs* Fragmentation with Extraction. J Endourol 2018;32(1):1–6.
26. Aldoukhi AH, Roberts WW, Hall TL, et al. Holmium Laser Lithotripsy In the New Stone Age: Dust or Bust? Front Surg 2017;4(September):1–6.
27. Santiago JE, Hollander AB, Soni SD, et al. To Dust or Not To Dust: a Systematic Review of Ureteroscopic Laser Lithotripsy Techniques. Curr Urol Rep 2017;18(4). https://doi.org/10.1007/s11934-017-0677-8.
28. De Coninck V, Hente R, Claessens M, et al. High-power, High-frequency Ho:YAG Lasers Are Not Essential for Retrograde Intrarenal Surgery. Eur Urol Focus 2021;7(1):5–6.
29. Yates J, Zabbo A, Pareek G. A comparison of the FREDDY and holmium lasers during ureteroscopic lithotripsy. Lasers Surg Med 2007;39(8):637–40.
30. Zarrabi A, Gross AJ. The evolution of lasers in urology. Ther Adv Urol 2011;3(2):81–9.
31. Papatsoris AG, Skolarikos A, Buchholz N. Intracorporeal laser lithotripsy. Arab J Urol 2012;10(3):301–6.
32. Marguet CG, Sung JC, Springhart WP, et al. In vitro comparison of stone retropulsion and

fragmentation of the frequency doubled, double pulse Nd:YAG laser and the holmium:YAG laser. J Urol 2005;173(5):1797–800.

33. Z örcher T, Hochberger J, Schrott K-M, et al. In vitro study concerning the efficiency of the frequency-doubled double-pulse Neodymium:YAG laser (FREDDY) for lithotripsy of calculi in the urinary tract. Lasers Surg Med 1999;25(1):38–42.
34. Delvecchio FC, Auge BK, Brizuela RM, et al. In vitro analysis of stone fragmentation ability of the FREDDY laser. J Endourology 2003;17:177–9.
35. Dubosq F, Pasqui F, Girard F, et al. Endoscopic lithotripsy and the FREDDY laser: Initial experience. J Endourol 2006;20(5):296–9.
36. Elhilali MM, Badaan S, Ibrahim A, et al. Use of the Moses Technology to Improve Holmium Laser Lithotripsy Outcomes: A Preclinical Study. J Endourol 2017. https://doi.org/10.1089/end.2017.0050.
37. Lumenis® PulseTM 120H - Lithotripsy Products - Boston Scientific. Available at: https://www.bostonscientific.com/en-US/products/lithotripsy/Lumenis-PulseTM-120H.html. Accessed May 7, 2021.
38. Laser Fibers & Accessories for Holmium Lasers | Lumenis. Available at: https://lumenis.com/medical/holmium-products/holmium-accessories/. Accessed May 7, 2021.
39. Winship B, Wollin D, Carlos E, et al. Dusting Efficiency of the Moses Holmium Laser: An Automated in Vitro Assessment. J Endourol 2018;32(12):1131–5.
40. Keller E, De Coninck V, Audouin M, et al. Fragments and dust after Holmium laser lithotripsy with or without "Moses technology": How are they different? J Biophotonics 2019;12(4). https://doi.org/10.1002/jbio.201800227ï.
41. Mullerad M, Aguinaga JRA, Aro T, et al. Initial Clinical Experience with a Modulated Holmium Laser Pulse—Moses Technology: Does It Enhance Laser Lithotripsy Efficacy? Rambam Maimonides Med J 2017;8(4):e0038.
42. Stern KL, Monga M. The Moses holmium system - time is money. an J Urol. 2018 Jun;25(3):9313-16.
43. Leotsakos I, Katafigiotis I, Lorber A, et al. Initial experience in combined ultra-mini percutaneous nephrolithotomy with the use of 120-W laser and the anti-retropulsion "Moses effect": the future of percutaneous nephrolithotomy? Lasers Med Sci 2020;35(9):1961–6.
44. Traxer O, Keller EX. Thulium fiber laser: the new player for kidney stone treatment? A comparison with Holmium:YAG laser. World J Urol 2020;38(8):1883–94.
45. Kronenberg P, Hameed BZ, Somani B. Outcomes of thulium fibre laser for treatment of urinary tract stones: results of a systematic review. Curr Opin Urol 2021;31(2):80–6.
46. Scott NJ, Cilip CM, Fried NM. Thulium fiber laser ablation of urinary Stones through small-core Optical fibers. IEEE J Sel Top Quan Electron 2009;15(2):435–40.
47. Blackmon RL, Hutchens TC, Hardy LA, et al. Thulium fiber laser ablation of kidney stones using a 50-μm-core silica optical fiber. Opt Eng 2014;54(1):011004.
48. Taratkin M, Laukhtina E, Singla N, et al. How Lasers Ablate Stones: In Vitro Study of Laser Lithotripsy (Ho:YAG and Tm-Fiber Lasers) in Different Environments. J Endourol 2021. https://doi.org/10.1089/end.2019.0441.
49. Keller EX, De Coninck V, Doizi S, et al. Thulium fiber laser: ready to dust all urinary stone composition types? World J Urol 2020. https://doi.org/10.1007/s00345-020-03217-9.
50. Andreeva V, Vinarov A, Yaroslavsky I, et al. Preclinical comparison of superpulse thulium fiber laser and a holmium:YAG laser for lithotripsy. World J Urol 2020;38(2):497–503.
51. Olympus. SuperPulsed Laser System SOLTIVE Premium: Sell Sheet; S00316EN . 10/20 OEKG. 2020. Available at: https://d3a0ilwurc1bhm.-cloudfront.net/asset/084438885177/c947cc763044fc953bb2253b056edf7b. Accessed October 25, 2020.
52. Enikeev D, Shariat SF, Taratkin M, et al. The changing role of lasers in urologic surgery. Curr Opin Urol 2020;30(1):24–9.
53. Ventimiglia E, Doizi S, Kovalenko A, et al. Effect of temporal pulse shape on urinary stone phantom retropulsion rate and ablation efficiency using holmium:YAG and super-pulse thulium fibre lasers. BJU Int 2020;126(1):159–67.
54. Gao B, Bobrowski A, Lee J. A scoping review of the clinical efficacy and safety of the novel thulium fiber laser: The rising star of laser lithotripsy. Can Urol Assoc J 2020;15(2). https://doi.org/10.5489/CUAJ.6804.
55. Schembri M, Sahu J, Aboumarzouk O, et al. Thulium fiber laser: The new kid on the block. Turkish J Urol 2020;46(Supp. 1):S1–10.
56. Panthier F, Doizi S, Lapouge P, et al. Comparison of the ablation rates, fissures and fragments produced with 150 μm and 272 μm laser fibers with superpulsed thulium fiber laser: an in vitro study. World J Urol 2020. https://doi.org/10.1007/s00345-020-03186-z.
57. Pattnaik P, Pattnaik S, Pattnaik M. MP21-16 Holmium Laser versus thulium fiber laser for treatment of urinary calculus disease. J Endourol 2019;33:A237.
58. Panthier* F, Doizi S, Berthe L, et al. PD04-12 In vitro comparison of ablation rates between superpulsed thulium fiber laser and ho:Yag laser for endocorporeal lithotripsy. J Urol 2020;203(Supplement 4):e83.

59. Corrales M, Traxer O. Initial clinical experience with the new thulium fiber laser: first 50 cases. World J Urol 2021. https://doi.org/10.1007/s00345-021-03616-6.
60. De Coninck VMJ, Keller EX, Kovalenko A, et al. Dusting efficiency comparison between Moses technology of Ho: YAG laser and superpulse thulium fiber laser. Eur Urol Suppl 2019;18(1): e1757–8.
61. Knudsen* B, Chew B, Molina W. MP79-16 super pulse thulium fiber laser compared to 120w holmium:yag laser: impact on retropulsion and laser fiber burn back. J Urol 2019;201(Supplement 4). https://doi.org/10.1097/01.ju.0000557395.71689.0d.
62. Chiron PHL, Doizi S, De Coninck V, et al. Impact of SuperPulse Thulium Fiber Laser settings and curve diameter on optical fiber fracture during intracorporeal lithotripsy. Eur Urol Suppl 2019;18(1): e1756.
63. Knudsen B, Molina W, City K, et al. PD30-01 comparison of small core diameter laser fibers used for lithotripsy with a 120w ho:yag laser and the soltive superpulsed thulium fiber laser. The Journal of Urology. Vol. 203, No. 4S, 2020.
64. Ali S, Rapoport L, Tsarichenko D, et al. VS1-3 Clinical study on Superpulse Thulium Fiber Laser for Lithotripsy. J Endourol 2018;32:A496.
65. Traxer O, Rapoport L, Tsarichenko D, et al. V03-02 First clinical study on superpulse thulium fiber laser for lithotripsy. J Urol 2018;199(4S):e321–2.
66. Olympus Launches the Soltive SuperPulsed Thulium Fiber Laser System for Urology. Launched June 17. 2020. Available at: https://medical.olympusamerica.com/articles/olympus-launches-soltive-superpulsed-thulium-fiber-laser-system-urology.
67. Enikeev D, Taratkin M, Klimov R, et al. Thulium-fiber laser for lithotripsy: first clinical experience in percutaneous nephrolithotomy. World J Urol 2020; 38(12):3069–74.
68. Korolev D, Akopyan G, Tsarichenko D, et al. Minimally invasive percutaneous nephrolithotomy with SuperPulsed Thulium-fiber laser. Urolithiasis 2021. https://doi.org/10.1007/s00240-021-01258-2.
69. Martov AG, Ergakov DV, Guseinov MA, et al. Initial experience in clinical application of thulium laser contact lithotripsy for transurethral treatment of urolithiasis. Urologiia 2018;1:112–20.
70. Dymov* A, Rapoport L, Tsarichenko D, et al. PD01-06 prospective clinical study on superpulse thulium fiber laser: initial analysis of optimal laser settings. J Urol 2019;201(Supplement 4). https://doi.org/10.1097/01.ju.0000555018.13063.41.
71. Traxer* O, Martov A, Ergakov D, et al. V01-01 prospective transurethral lithotripsy study with superpulse tm fiber laser. J Urol 2019;201(Supplement 4). https://doi.org/10.1097/01.ju.0000555073.09285.09.
72. Martov A, Ergakov D, Guseynov M, et al. VS1-2 SuperPulse Thulium Fiber Laser for UreteroscopicLithotripsy: 1 Year Experience. J Endourol 2018; 32:A495.
73. Enikeev D, Taratkin M, Klimov R, et al. Superpulsed Thulium Fiber Laser for Stone Dusting: In Search of a Perfect Ablation Regimen—A Prospective Single-Center Study. J Endourol 2020;XX(Xx):1–5. https://doi.org/10.1089/end.2020.0519.
74. Korolev D, Klimov R, Tsarichenko D, et al. Rirs for kidney stones with novel superpulse thulium (TM) fiber laser: First clinical experience. Eur Urol Open Sci 2020;19:e14.
75. Dymov* A, Rapoport L, Enikeev D, et al. MP17-12 OPTIMIZING STONE FREE RATE EVALUATION TIME POINT FOR LASER LITHOTRIPSY IN DUSTING MODE. J Urol 2019;201(Supplement 4). https://doi.org/10.1097/01.ju.0000555437.99672.2f.
76. Keller* EX, De Coninck V, Vinnichenko V, et al. V01-09 SUPERPULSE THULIUM FIBER LASER FOR LITHOTRIPSY OF LARGE RENAL STONES: INITIAL EXPERIENCE. J Urol 2019;201(Supplement 4). https://doi.org/10.1097/01.ju.0000555081.47403.44.
77. Martov A, Ergakov D, Andronov A, et al. MP12-3 First Ultra-mini-percutaneous Nephrolithotripsy(UM-PCNL) with the New Thulium SuperPulse Fiber Laser(TSPFL). J Endourol 2018;32:A:111.
78. Martov* A, Andronov A, Moscow SD, et al. V01-11 THULIUM SUPERPULSE FIBER LASER (TSPFL) MICRO-PCNL: HOW TO IMPROVE STONE-FREE RATE (SFR). J Urol 2019;201(Supplement 4). https://doi.org/10.1097/01.ju.0000555083.32156.03.
79. Martov AG, Dutov SV, Popov SV, et al. Micropercutaneous laser nephrolithotripsy. Urologiia 2019; 2019(3):72–9.
80. Traxer* O, De Coninck V, Keller EX, et al. MP17-03 comparing short, long, and moses regimes of HO: YAG laser vs super pulse tm fiber laser in vitro: ablation speed and retropulsion effect. J Urol 2019;201(Supplement 4). https://doi.org/10.1097/01.ju.0000555428.84425.1d.
81. Secker A, Rassweiler J, Neisius A. Future perspectives of flexible ureteroscopy. Curr Opin Urol 2019; 29(2):113–7.
82. Peng Y, Liu M, Ming S, et al. Safety of a Novel Thulium Fiber Laser for Lithotripsy: An in Vitro Study on the Thermal Effect and Its Impact Factor. J Endourol 2020;34(1):88–92.
83. Dragoş LB, Somani B, Keller E, et al. Super-pulse thulium fiber versus high power holmium lasers. What about temperature? Eur Urol Suppl 2019; 18(1):e505–8.
84. Taratkin M, Laukhtina E, Singla N, et al. Temperature changes during laser lithotripsy with Ho:YAG laser and novel Tm-fiber laser: a comparative in-vitro study. World J Urol 2020;38(12). https://doi.org/10.1007/s00345-020-03122-1.

85. Khusid JA, Khargi R, Seiden B, et al. Thulium fiber laser utilization in urological surgery: A narrative review. Investig Clin Urol 2021;62(2):136–47.
86. Kamal W, Kallidonis P, Koukiou G, et al. Stone Retropulsion with Ho: YAG and Tm: YAG Lasers: A Clinical Practice-Oriented Experimental Study. J Endourol 2016;30(11):1145–9.
87. Zhu Y, Zhuo J, Xu D, et al. Thulium laser versus standard transurethral resection of the prostate for benign prostatic obstruction: a systematic review and meta-analysis. World J Urol 2015;33(4): 509–15.
88. Gao X, Ren S, Xu C, et al. Thulium laser resection via a flexible cystoscope for recurrent non-muscle-invasive bladder cancer: Initial clinical experience. BJU Int 2008;102(9):1115–8.
89. Proietti S, Rodríguez-Socarrás ME, Eisner BH, et al. Thulium:YAG Versus Holmium:YAG Laser Effect on Upper Urinary Tract Soft Tissue: Evidence from an Ex Vivo Experimental Study. J Endourol 2021;35(4): 544–51.
90. Petzold R, Miernik A, Suarez-Ibarrola R. In Vitro Dusting Performance of a New Solid State Thulium Laser Compared to Holmium Laser Lithotripsy. J Endourol 2020. https://doi.org/10.1089/end.2020.0525.
91. Petzold R, Miernik A, Suarez-Ibarrola R. Retropulsion force in laser lithotripsy—an in vitro study comparing a Holmium device to a novel pulsed solid-state Thulium laser. World J Urol 2021;1–6. https://doi.org/10.1007/s00345-021-03668-8.
92. Vassar GJ, Chan KF, Teichman JMH, et al. Holmium:YAG lithotripsy: Photothermal mechanism. J Endourol 1999;13(3):181–90.
93. Petzold R, Suarez-Ibarrola R, Miernik A. Gas bubble anatomy during laser lithotripsy – an experimental in-vitro study of a pulsed solid-state Tm: YAG and a Ho:YAG device. J Endourol 2020. https://doi.org/10.1089/end.2020.0526.
94. Lumenis Launches Next-Generation MOSESTM 2.0 Holmium Laser Technology - Lumenis. Available at: https://lumenis.com/medical/specialties/urology/resource-hub/lumenis-launches-next-generation-moses-2-0-holmium-laser-technology/. Accessed May 9, 2021.
95. Moses Laser: Holmium Laser Lithotripsy & Enucleation Machine. Available at: https://lumenis.com/medical/holmium-products/lumenis-moses-pulse-120h/. Accessed May 7, 2021.
96. Ibrahim A, Elhilali MM, Fahmy N, et al. Double-Blinded Prospective Randomized Clinical Trial Comparing Regular and Moses Modes of Holmium Laser Lithotripsy. J Endourol 2020;34(5):624–8.
97. Aldoukhi AH, Roberts WW, Hall TL, et al. Watch Your Distance: The Role of Laser Fiber Working Distance on Fragmentation When Altering Pulse Width or Modulation. J Endourol 2019;33(2):120–6.
98. King J, Katta N, McElroy A, et al. MP15-13 MECHANISM OF PULSE MODULATED HOLMIUM:YAG LITHOTRIPSY. J Urol 2020;203(Supplement 4). https://doi.org/10.1097/ju.0000000000000840.013.
99. Black KM, Aldoukhi AH, Teichman JMH, et al. Pulse modulation with Moses technology improves popcorn laser lithotripsy. World J Urol 2020;1–7. https://doi.org/10.1007/s00345-020-03282-0.
100. Ibrahim A, Badaan S, Elhilali MM, et al. Moses technology in a stone simulator. Can Urol Assoc J 2018;12(4):127–30.

New Technologies for Treatment of Benign Prostatic Hyperplasia

Dean Elterman, MD, MSc, FRCSC[a,*], Bruce Gao, MD[a], Steven Lu[b], Naeem Bhojani, MD, FRCSC[c], Kevin C. Zorn, MD, FRCSC[c], Bilal Chughtai, MD[d]

KEYWORDS

• Prostate • BPH • LUTS • Voiding • Technology • Minimally invasive

KEY POINTS

- Benign prostatic hyperplasia (BPH) is a common disease in aging men, which significantly impacts quality of life.
- Through shared decision-making, an individualized treatment plan considers factors including prostate anatomy, severity of symptoms, patient medical status, treatment efficacy, procedure safety, side effects, and costs. Ideally, a decision aid can and should be utilized.
- Novel BPH technologies including Rezūm, UroLift, Aquablation, iTind, Zenflow, Optilume, XFLO, and Butterfly show promising short-term functional outcomes while possibly minimizing side effects such as bleeding and sexual dysfunction
- True minimally invasive surgical therapy (TMIST) is an off-the-shelf BPH solution requiring only a standard flexible cystoscope that can be performed in a urology office without sedation or general anesthesia. iTind (Food and Drug Administration (FDA) approved), Zenflow, Optilume, and XFLO are TMISTs currently in development.

INTRODUCTION

Benign prostatic hyperplasia (BPH) is a ubiquitous disease that affects 50% of men at age 60 years and 90% of men aged older than 80 years.[1,2] Bothersome lower urinary tract symptoms (LUTSs) secondary to BPH are responsible for a significant health care system burden, incurring approximately 4 billion dollars annually in the United States.[3] Furthermore, LUTSs contribute to a significant reduction in patient quality of life (QoL) with more than 35 million men aged older than 30 years having at least mild LUTSs.[4] In an aging society with rising rates of BPH, there is a significant need for safe, effective, reliable, and universally available (both to the patient and urology community with access and a short learning curve) therapeutic options.

BPH is a urologic disease managed by a stepwise approach involving lifestyle alteration, medical therapy, and surgery. Through shared-decision making and ideally the use of a BPH decision aid, an individualized treatment plan takes into account factors including prostate anatomy, treatment efficacy, severity of symptoms, safety, side effects, and costs.[5] Medical therapy in the form of alpha-blockers or 5-alpha-reductase inhibitors, although effective, may be complicated by unwanted sexual side effects such as erectile dysfunction (ED), decreased libido, and ejaculatory problems, along with the burden of taking lifelong medications.[6] Recent studies have also shown that some of these

[a] Division of Urology, Department of Surgery, University of Toronto, 399 Bathurst Street, MP-8-317, Toronto, Ontario M5T 2S8, Canada; [b] Cumming School of Medicine, University of Calgary, 3330 Hospital Drive Northwest, Calgary, Alberta T2N 4N1, Canada; [c] Department of Surgery, University of Montreal (CHUM), 2900 Edouard Montpetit Boulevard, Montreal, Quebec H3T 1J4, Canada; [d] Department of Urology, Weill Cornell Medical College, 25 East 68th Street, Starr 9, New York, NY 10065, USA
* Corresponding author.
E-mail address: dean.elterman@uhn.ca

Urol Clin N Am 49 (2022) 11–22
https://doi.org/10.1016/j.ucl.2021.07.007
0094-0143/22/

medications can have significant neurocognitive and psychiatric effects, including dementia and depression.[7]

Indications for surgery may include LUTSs refractory to medical therapy, patient preference, or certain medical situations such as recurrent Urinary tract infections, bladder stones, gross hematuria, renal insufficiency, or urinary retention. In these cases, transurethral resection of the prostate (TURP) remains the gold standard. Although efficacious, TURP requires the use of general or spinal anesthesia as well as runs the risk of bleeding, urinary incontinence, retrograde ejaculation, and ED.[8] Sexual health surveys indicate that maintenance of sexual function is significantly prioritized by patients who underwent BPH surgery, with postoperative erections and ejaculatory function important to 95% and 92% of men, respectively, regardless of age.[9]

To address these treatment shortcomings, innovative new technologies for the treatment of BPH have been developed. These technologies target rapid recovery and symptom relief, low complication rates, sexual preservation, and the ability to perform the procedure in an outpatient setting with local anesthesia.

In this review, we provide an update on techniques and outcomes of seven novel technologies for BPH including Aquablation, Rezūm, UroLift, iTind, Zenflow, Optilume, and XFLO.

AQUABLATION

Technique

The AquaBeam Robotic System (PROCEPT BioRobotics, Redwood City, Ca, USA) is an ultrasound-guided surgical technique that uses a heat-free, high-velocity waterjet (Aquablation) to endoscopically resect obstructing prostatic tissue.[10,11] The AquaBeam system consists of three main components: the robotic handpiece, the surgeon console, and the conformal planning unit (CPU).[10] The patient is prepped and positioned in the dorsal lithotomy position under general or spinal anesthesia. A bi-plane transrectal ultrasound transducer (TRUS) is inserted and positioned to visualize the prostate in real time. The 24-Fr robotic handpiece with an integrated flexible scope is inserted into the bladder, and the scope is retracted back to visualize the bladder neck. Once the TRUS and the handpiece are successfully positioned and locked in place to robotic arms, the surgeon defines the length, depth, and angle of resection in the CPU using the transverse and sagittal ultrasound views of the prostate.[10] The maximum angle of resection is 225°, and the maximum cut depth is 25 mm, allowing the surgeon to tailor the procedure to the specific prostate.[10] In a "windshield wiper" motion, high-velocity saline follows the outlined plan and resects the obstructing prostatic tissue while sparing the bladder neck and verumontanum. Reported average resection times are around 5 minutes.[12] Lastly, hemostasis may be achieved through focal bladder neck cautery (FBNC) via a standard resectoscope, and a three-way catheter is inserted afterward for bladder irrigation.[13] (**Fig. 1**).

Efficacy and Safety

Since US FDA approval in 2017, two separate clinical trials (WATER and WATER II) have investigated the safety and efficacy of Aquablation. The first pivotal trial, the WATER study, was a prospective, multicenter, randomized double-blinded study that compared the safety and efficacy of Aquablation to TURP for the treatment of LUTSs due to BPH.[14] A total of 181 men aged between 45 and 80 years were randomized 2:1 to Aquablation (116 men) and TURP (65 men), respectively. Notable inclusion criteria included moderate-to-severe symptomatic BPH (IPSS $\geq$12), a prostate volume of 30 cm^3 to 80 cm^3, and a Qmax <15 mL/s. The mean prostate size was 53 cm^3, and 81% of them were sexually active. Initial 6-month results showed Aquablation to be noninferior in efficacy (reduction in IPSS) and superior in safety (development of persistent grade 1, or $\geq$ 2 Clavien-Dindo surgical complications) compared with TURP.[14] The rate of anejaculation was lower after Aquablation than after TURP for sexually active men with prior normal ejaculation (10% vs 36%, P = .0003). Furthermore, the superior safety profile was more pronounced in the subgroup analysis of larger prostates ($\geq$50 cm^3). Final 3-year outcomes published in 2020 showed sustained treatment outcomes.[15] There was no statistically significant difference in IPSS reduction, IPSS QoL reduction, and Qmax increase across groups or across time. Comparing Aquablation with TURP, IPSS decreased by 64% (22.9–8.5) versus 61% (22.2–8.3), both IPSS QoL decreased by 67% (4.8–1.6) and Qmax increased by 55% (9.4 mL/s to 21 mL/s) versus 47% (9.1 mL/s to 17.3 mL/s), respectively. Moreover, anejaculation rates remained lower in the Aquablation group than in the TURP group (11% vs 29%, P = .0039). The superior anejaculation rates after Aquablation are likely due to increased precision from ultrasound guidance and robotic assistance, effectively avoiding ejaculatory structures close to the verumontanum.[10,16,17]. Other adverse events showed similar rates across treatment groups. There was no reported ED in either group. The

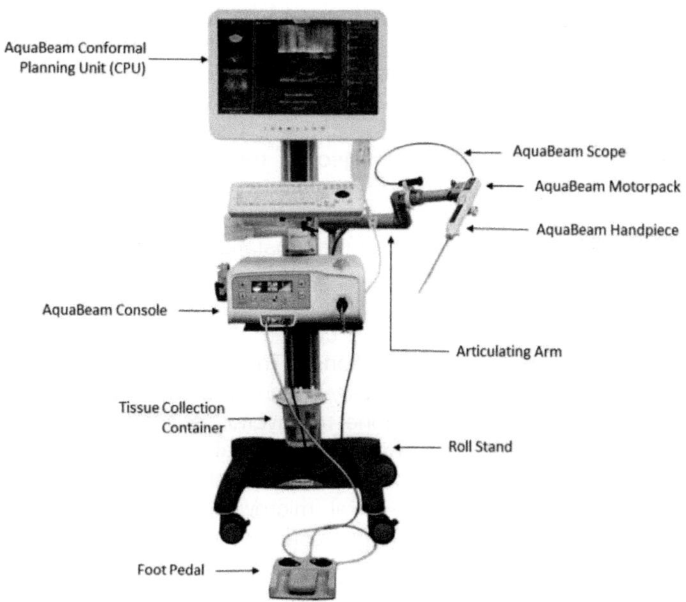

Fig. 1. AQUABEAM system. (*From* public open access FDA approval https://www.accessdata.fda.gov/cdrh_docs/reviews/DEN170024.pdf.)

surgical retreatment rate was low for both Aquablation and TURP (4.3% and 1.5%, respectively). Medical retreatment rate at 3 years was 9% for Aquablation and 14% for TURP. The mean total operative time was similar for Aquablation and TURP (33 vs 36 minutes, $P = .2752$), but resection time was lower for Aquablation (4 vs 27 minutes, $P<.0001$).

The second clinical trial, the WATER II study, is a prospective, single-arm, multicenter trial that enrolled men with a large prostate size (80 cm^3 to 150 cm^3) that is usually deemed ineligible for TURP.[18] The study is currently following patients to 5 years with 2-year outcomes published in 2020.[19] Inclusion and exclusion criteria were nearly identical to the WATER study. However, unlike WATER, the WATER II study included men with larger prostates, men with prior prostate surgery, and men with catheter use for less than 90 days.[18] The mean prostate size was 107 cm^3, and 76.2% of them were sexually active. Initial 3-month results met the efficacy (mean IPSS reduction of 16.5 points, $P < .001$) and safety (45.5% of men developed persistent grade 1 or $\geq$2 Clavien-Dindo surgical complications) endpoints. Anejaculation occurred in 19% of sexually active men. At 2 years, IPSS decreased by 75% (23.2–5.8), IPSS QoL decreased by 76% (4.6–1.1), and Qmax increased by 52% (8.7 mL/s to 18.2 mL/s). The surgical retreatment rate was 2%, and medical retreatment rate was 7.9%.[19] Current results are similar to those of the WATER trial of smaller prostates and suggest Aquablation is an effective surgical technique for large prostates $\geq$80 cm^3. The mean total operative time was 37 minutes, and resection time was 8 minutes, suggesting that resection times are consistent regardless of prostate size and anatomy.

Like other surgical BPH technologies, Aquablation is associated with the risk of blood loss and possible transfusion. It is not an approved treatment of BPH for men on anticoagulation. One key difference between TURP and Aquablation is that the latter lacks a direct method of achieving postresection hemostasis.[10] However, recent publications have highlighted the most optimal methods of achieving post-Aquablation hemostasis. Elterman and colleagues[20] published in 2020 an analysis of transfusion rates in 801 men who underwent Aquablation between 2014 and 2019 in both clinical trials and commercial settings. Altogether, the transfusion rate was 3.9%, and larger prostates (>77 cm^3) had the highest rates. Moreover, nonresective FBNC combined with standard traction showed the lowest transfusion rates over other methods including balloon tamponade.[20] Starting in late 2019, FBNC became a mainstay in postresection hemostasis for Aquablation. Following Aquablation, the surgeon introduces a standard resectoscope to first remove the “fluffy” tissue remnants and then cauterize the deeper bleeding vessels.[13] Importantly, this cautery is nonresective. Recently, Elterman and colleagues[13] published an analysis of transfusion rates in 2089 men who underwent Aquablation, as well as received FBNC, and observed an overall transfusion rate of 0.8%, further strengthening the efficacy of FBNC for postresection hemostasis.[13]

WATER VAPOR THERMAL THERAPY (REZŪM)

Technique

Rezūm (Boston Scientific Corp, Marlborough, MA, USA) water vapor therapy is a type of thermal ablative technique that achieves heat transfer via convection.[21–23] (**Fig. 2**). The key components of the system include a radiofrequency (RF) generator, a single-use transurethral delivery device with an integrated 30° cystoscopic lens for direct visualization, a retractable 18-gauge polyetheretherketone (PEEK) needle, and a saline flush.[21] Once the patient is prepped and positioned in a dorsal lithotomy position, coupled with patient anesthesia (local block or sedation), the surgeon guides the delivery device into the prostatic urethra under direct cystoscopic visualization. The RF generator converts sterile water into steam that is then delivered and injected into prostatic adenomatous tissue by the delivery device and PEEK needle, respectively.[21] The needle is designed to circumferentially disperse steam through its 3 rows of 4 holes spaced at 120° intervals.[22] When the steam travels through the prostatic adenoma, it immediately phase shifts from vapor back to liquid, releasing and transferring 208 cal of thermal energy to the target tissue.[22] This release of stored thermal energy causes irreversible cell membrane damage and cell death. Furthermore, because the vapor is physically less dense than the zonal boundaries of the prostate, the necrosis is contained within the zone of prostatic adenomatous tissue.[22] Postprocedural MRI imaging at 6 months showed a mean reduction of total prostate volume of 15%; however, the patient sample size was small.[21] Each injection travels a fixed depth of ~10 mm and takes 9 seconds on average.[23] The number of injections a patient requires depends on the length of the prostatic urethra, the amount of prostatic tissue, and the presence of a median lobe.[23] The saline flush is responsible for both visualization and cooling of the prostatic urethra between injections. The procedure can be completed quickly in an office-based setting and is typically done using oral sedation (~70%).[23] Compared with other thermal ablative techniques that use conduction (Transurethral needle ablation and Transurethral microwave therapy), Rezūm causes tissue necrosis at a lower temperature in a shorter amount of time.[23]

Efficacy and Safety

Since US FDA approval in 2015, multiple Rezūm studies have been published, most notably the pivotal Rezūm II randomized controlled trial with final 5-year data published in 2021.[24,25] In Rezūm II, a total of 196 patients were enrolled with a 2:1 split between treatment (135 patients) and sham control arms (61 patients). Notable inclusion criteria

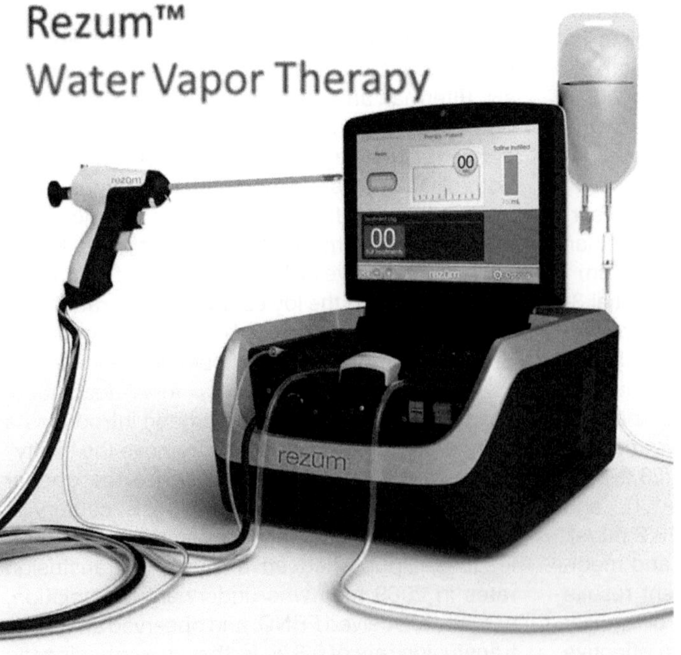

Fig. 2. Rezūm delivery device and vapor needle. (*Courtesy of* Boston Scientific https://www.bostonscientific.com/)

included moderate-to-severe symptoms (IPSS ≥13) and a prostate volume of 30 cm^3 to 80 cm^3 with no restrictions on the presence of a middle lobe.[24] Final study data show sustained improvements over 5 years with decrease in IPSS by ~48% (22.0–11.1), decrease in IPSS QoL by ~45% (4.4–2.2), and increase in Qmax by ~49% (9.9 mL/s to 14 mL/s).[25] Treatment arm patients had a medical retreatment rate of 11.1% and surgical retreatment rate of 4.4%.[25] Notably, none of the treatment arm patients experienced ED or retrograde ejaculation at the conclusion of the study. The authors of Rezum II consider Rezūm a first-line treatment for BPH.

Dixon and colleagues[26] published a nonrandomized pilot study on 65 patients with similar inclusion criteria as Rezūm II but included larger prostate volumes (20 cm^3 to 120 cm^3). Improvements in IPSS (21.7–9.6), IPSS QoL (4.4–1.8), and Qmax (8.3 mL/s to 12 mL/s) from baseline were seen at 2 years. Darson and colleagues25 in 2017, Mollengarden and colleagues26 in 2019, and Alegorides and colleagues27 in 2020 conducted three retrospective studies which also demonstrate comparable functional improvements, low retreatment rates, and minimal sexual dysfunction at 1 year, 6 months, and 1 year, respectively.[27–29]

Rezūm viability is further supported by two recent multicenter prospective cohort studies. Both studies included men with urinary retention and larger prostates (≥80 cm^3). The first UK-based study was published in 2020.[30] Two hundred ten patients were enrolled (25 of which were in urinary retention) with an average prostate volume of 56.9 cm^3. Outcomes at 1 year showed a ~79% reduction in IPSS (20.4–4.3), a ~72% reduction in IPSS QoL (4.3–1.2), and a ~50% increase in Qmax (9.2–18.1). Zero cases of de novo ED were reported, and two patients underwent retreatment within 1 year. The second Italy-based prospective study consisting of 135 patients with an average prostate volume of 60 cm^3 was published in 2021.[31] Early results from this study at 6 months indicate a reduction in IPSS scores (21.5–4.4) consistent with previous studies.

Current evidence suggests that water vapor therapy does not have a significant negative impact on sexual function.[24] McVary and colleagues[32] compared two large randomized controlled trials: medical therapy in Medical Therapy of Prostatic Symptoms study versus Rezum. The analysis investigated the impact of medical therapy and water vapor therapy on sexual function over 3 years.[32] Patients in the drug treatment groups showed worsening sexual desire and ejaculatory function over 3 years. By contrast, patients who underwent water vapor therapy showed no worsening ejaculatory function and exhibited slight improvements in sexual desire. All studies have reported no de novo ED.

Rezūm appears to be safe with most reported complications minor in nature (Clavien I-II). In Rezūm II, the most common issues were dysuria (16.9%), hematuria (11.8%), frequency or urgency (5.9%), acute urinary retention (3.7%), and suspected UTI (3.7%).[25] All of these complications were resolved within 30 days.

UroLift (PROSTATIC URETHRAL LIFT)

Technique

UroLift (NeoTract/Teleflex Inc, Pleasanton, CA, USA) or prostatic urethral lift (PUL) uses permanent implants which are cystoscopically deployed through obstructing prostatic tissue.[33] (**Fig. 3**). This mechanical solution is similar in theory to window curtain tie backs that retract the obstructed prostatic urethra to the prostatic capsule. The UroLift system consists of two main components: a transurethral delivery device with an integrated cystoscope and permanent nitinol and stainless steel implants.[33] Once the surgeon positions the transurethral delivery device at the desired location, the implants are inserted and subsequently compress and retract the prostatic adenomatous tissue. Similar to Rezūm, the number of implants a patient requires depends on the length of the prostatic urethra and the amount of prostatic tissue and presence of a median lobe. The procedure typically takes less than 1 hour and can be done in the office using local anesthesia.[34]

Efficacy and Safety

UroLift gained US FDA approval in 2013 and received an expanded indication in 2020 to include prostates between 80 cm^3 and 100 cm^3. The LIFT study was a multicenter, prospective, double-blinded randomized control trial (RCT) involving prostates less than 80 cm^3, whereby 140 men were assigned to the UroLift procedure and 66 men to sham rigid cystoscopy.[35] Five-year outcomes published in 2017 indicated a ~35% reduction in IPSS (22.3–14.5), ~50% reduction in IPSS QoL (4.62–2.54), ~50% increase in Qmax (7.88–11.1), and a surgical retreatment rate of 13.6% for the treatment arm.[36] The incidence of medical retreatment after UroLift was 3.6% after 1 year and 10.7% at 5 years. Importantly, there were no de novo, sustained ejaculatory or ED. Fifty-three patients crossed over from the sham group, and their 2-year outcomes matched the treatment group. The MedLift study published in 2018 acted as an extension of the

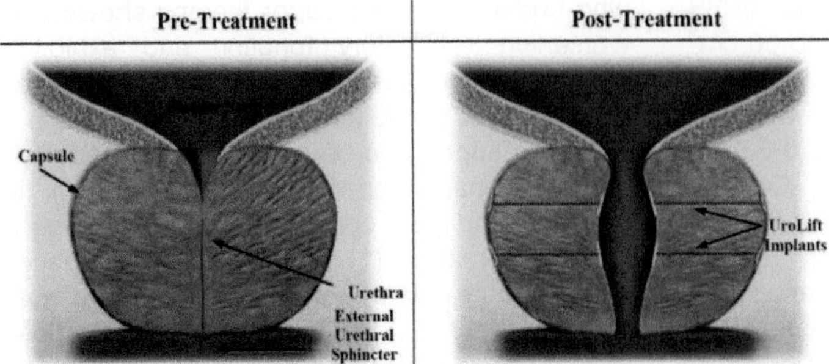

Fig. 3. Illustrations showing UroLift implants retracting the obstructing prostatic tissue. (*From* public open access FDA approval https://www.accessdata.fda.gov/cdrh_docs/reviews/K130651.pdf.)

LIFT study by including patients with an obstructive middle lobe (OML) that were excluded from the original study.[37] Forty-five patients with OML were all successfully treated with UroLift. Moreover, at 1 year follow-up, improvements in IPSS, IPSS QoL, and Qmax were comparable with the patients with lateral lobe enlargement only. The retreatment rate for the OML arm was 2% at 1 year. The American Urological Association guidelines currently exclude men with an obstructive median lobe for UroLift due to MedLift being a randomized cohort study rather than an RCT.

The surgical reintervention rate for UroLift is still being determined but has been estimated at 2% to 3% per year. A recent systematic review and meta-analysis involving 2016 patients from 11 studies suggests a higher retreatment rate at 6% per annum. The annual rate of surgical intervention appeared to be affected by the mean duration of follow-up with 1 year or less mean follow-up at 4.3% per year, 1 to 3 years mean follow-up at 10.7% per year, and more than 3 years mean follow-up in a single study at 5.8% per year.[38]

A majority (>95%) of complications in UroLift are minor in nature (Clavien grade 1).[39] In a recent retrospective observational cohort study out of England, the most common adverse events were urinary retention (1.4%), followed by bleeding (0.9%).[40] Sexual function appears to be preserved in PUL. The LIFT and crossover study both reported 0% de novo sustained ejaculatory or ED.[36]

True Minimally Invasive Surgical Therapies

True minimally invasive surgical therapy (TMIST) is a novel concept within minimally invasive surgical therapies for BPH that bridges medical therapy and more aggressive surgical therapy. TMIST is an off-the-shelf BPH therapy requiring only a standard flexible cystoscope that can be performed in a urology office without sedation or general anesthesia.[41] This paradigm shift in BPH management allows flexible cystoscopy to become both diagnostic and therapeutic. Durability is not necessarily the primary target for TMISTs but rather an effective and cost-effective bridge between conservative medical therapy and more invasive surgical therapy that may decrease health care system costs, operating room burden, and need for added equipment.[41]

The following novel technologies below are considered by these authors to be TMISTs. iTind is currently the only TMIST with FDA approval. The Optilume BPH Catheter System, Prodeon XFLO Expander System, Zenflow Spring System, and Butterfly Prostatic Retraction device are currently in phase 3 clinical trials.

iTind (TEMPORARILY IMPLANTED NITINOL DEVICE)

Technique

The second-generation iTind system (Medi-Tate, Hadera, Israel) is a temporarily implanted nitinol device that is deployed in the prostatic urethra and bladder neck.[42,43] (**Fig. 4**). The device is made up of three elongated nitinol struts connected at the distal end, an antimigration anchoring leaflet, and a polyester retrieval suture.[42] In the lithotomy position, using a standard 19 to 22 Fr cystoscope, the surgeon inserts the enclosed device through the cystoscope sheath and into the bladder. The device is then deployed and retracted so that the anchoring leaflet is under the bladder neck at the 6 o'clock position and the 3 struts are in the 12, 5, and 7 o'clock positions within the prostatic urethra.[42] Once inserted, the bladder is drained, and the patient is discharged with simple analgesia. The total procedure time is less than 10 minutes, and the most cases are done in the office-based setting using local anesthesia. Over the next 5 to 7 days, the 3 struts apply continuous pressure on the prostatic urethra and cause ischemic incisions at the contact points.[43] This process expands and reshapes the bladder neck and prostatic urethra, creating an open channel for the flow of urine. After a week, the patient has the device removed by using the retrieval

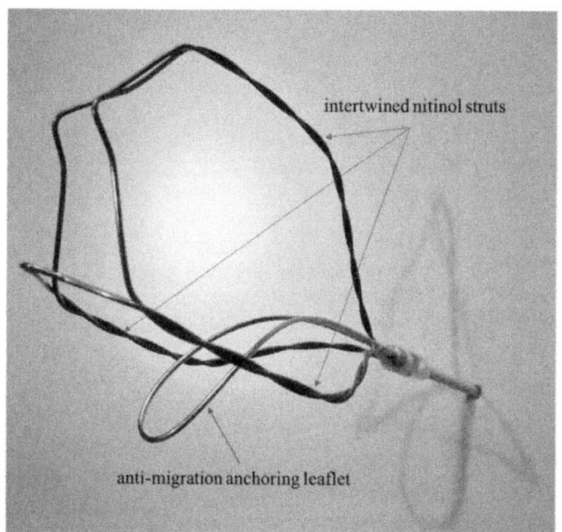

Fig. 4. Second-generation iTIND device with three struts and one anchoring leaflet. (*From* Amparore D, Fiori C, Valerio M, et al. 3-Year results following treatment with the second generation of the temporary implantable nitinol device in men with LUTS secondary to benign prostatic obstruction. Prostate Cancer Prostatic Dis. 2021 Jun;24(2):349-357. doi:10.1038/s41391-020-00281-5.)

suture and a special open-ended silicone catheter that allows the device to be collapsed and removed safely without a cystoscope or anesthesia.[43] Catheterization is not necessary after placement and removal of the device. Patients are discharged on the same day. The first-generation iTind system differed from the second-generation iTind system by the use of 4 elongated struts and a tip that was pointed and covered in soft plastic material.[43]

Efficacy and Safety

iTind (second generation) gained FDA approval in 2020. Current literature consists of 3 trials and 1 early RCT. Porpiglia and colleagues[44] enrolled 32 patients into a single center, single-arm, prospective study of the first-generation device and published their 3-year results in 2018. Improvements in IPSS, IPSS QoL, and Qmax were sustained through 3 years. Additionally, no patients required retreatment nor experienced reduced sexual function.

Following this trial, two prospective, single-arm, multicenter studies were carried out for the second-generation device. Amparone and colleagues[45] published their 3-year results in 2020. Eighty-one men with prostate volumes less than 75 cm^3 reported sustained improvements in IPSS (20.7–8.55), IPSS QoL (3.96–1.76), and Qmax (7.71 mL/s to 15.2 mL/s) over 3 years. De Nunzio and colleagues[46] published their 6-month results soon after which enrolled 70 men with expanded inclusion criteria (prostate volumes <120 cm^3). Similar to the study by Amparone and colleagues,[45] the iTIND device showed significant improvements in IPSS (21.2–8.3), IPSS QoL (4.1–2.0), and Qmax (7.3–12.0) at 6 month follow-up.

Notably and most recently, the first multicenter, prospective, sham-controlled, single-blinded RCT was published at the end of 2020.[47] A total of 185 men were randomized 2:1 and split among iTind (128 men) and sham control (57 men). Notable inclusion criteria included a prostate volume of 25 cm^3 to 75 cm^3 and moderate-to-severe symptomatic BPH (IPSS $\geq$10). The sham control consisted of the insertion and removal of an 18F silicone Foley catheter to mimic the experience of treatment arm patients. There was a 40.1% reduction in IPSS at 3 months (22.4–12.6) that sustained through 12 months (21.6–12.7). Similar improvements were seen in IPSS QoL at 3 months (4.55–2.54) and 12 months (4.51–2.45), as well as in Qmax at 3 months (8.63–13.6) and 12 months (8.42–11.9). In line with the 3-year prospective studies, there were no reported de novo retrograde ejaculation or ED. The retreatment rate within 1 year was 4.7%.

Current studies on iTind have reported perioperative minor self-limiting complications (Clavien grade 1 and 2). Common complications included transient hematuria, urgency, and dysuria (**Table 1**).

OPTILUME BPH CATHETER SYSTEM

Technique

The Optilume BPH Catheter System (Urotronic Inc, Plymouth, Minnesota, USA) Is a mechanical solution (balloon dilation) that also delivers a localized antiproliferative drug to achieve immediate and long-term urethral patency.[48] (**Fig. 5**). Previous clinical studies in the 1990s demonstrated that transurethral balloon dilation techniques were safe but lacked long-term durability.[48] The novelty of the Optilume system revolves around the use of two balloon catheters: a predilation balloon and a drug-coated balloon. The drug-coated balloon delivers paclitaxel, a chemotherapy drug that is widely used in coronary and peripheral stents to prevent restenosis. Under the visualization of a standard flexible cystoscope, the predilation balloon catheter is advanced until the proximal end is at the level of the external sphincter. The balloon is inflated for a short amount of time and removed. Next the drug-coated balloon repeats the same steps, further dilating the prostatic urethra as well as delivering paclitaxel to the prostatic urethral surface. The second inflation lasts for a minimum of 5 minutes

Table 1
Published randomized control trial (RCT) results for Aquablation, Rezūm, UroLift, and iTIND

Technology	FDA Approval	Pivotal RCTs (Follow-up Months)	Prostate Size Range (cc)	Middle Lobe (Yes/no)	Δ IPSS (% Decrease)	Δ IPSS QoL (% Decrease)	Δ Qmax (% Increase)	Surgical Retreatment Rate (%)	Sexual Side Effects
Aquablation	2017	WATER (36) and WATER II (24)	30–150 cc	Yes	64%–75%	67%–76%	52%–55%	2%–4.3%/ 24–36 mo	Anejaculation rates lower in Aquablation compared with TURP (11% vs 29%)
Rezūm	2015	Rezūm II (60)	30–80 cc	Yes	48%	45%	49%	4.4%/60 mo	Minimal sustained ED or retrograde ejaculation
UroLift	2013, 2020	LIFT (60)	Up to 100 cc	No[a]	35%	50%	50%	Variable (2%–3% per year)	Minimal sustained ED or retrograde ejaculation
iTind	2020	MT-06 (12)	25–75 cc	Yes	41%	46%	41%	4.7%/12 mo	Minimal sustained ED or retrograde ejaculation

Aquablation is the only technology with an RCT for prostates >80 cc. There are ongoing RCTs for the newer TMISTs.
Optilume BPH Catheter System, XFLO Expander System, Zenflow Spring System, and Butterfly Prostatic Retraction device are newer TMISTs with ongoing RCTs.
[a] The AUA guidelines currently exclude men with an obstructive median lobe for UroLift due to MedLift being a randomized cohort study rather than an RCT.

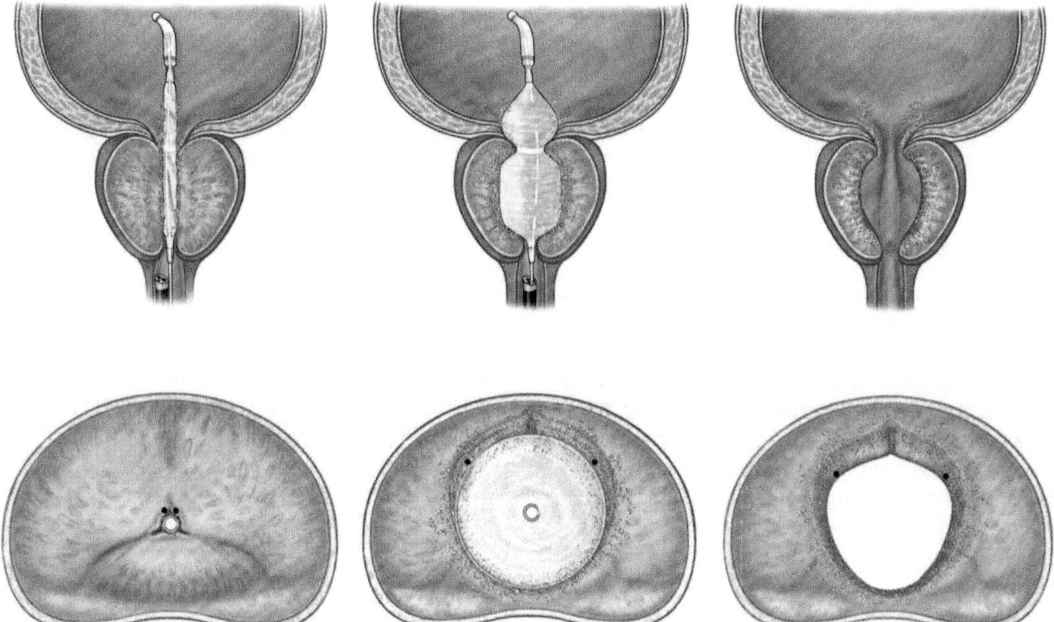

Fig. 5. Illustration of the Optilume BPH Catheter System balloon expansion and drug delivery from sagittal (*top*) and transverse (*bottom*) planes. (*From* Kaplan SA, Pichardo M, Rijo E, Espino G, Lay RR, Estrella R. One-year outcomes after treatment with a drug-coated balloon catheter system for lower urinary tract symptoms related to benign prostatic hyperplasia. Prostate Cancer Prostatic Dis. 2021;10.1038/s41391-021-00362-z. https://doi.org/10.1038/s41391-021-00362-z.)

before the balloon is removed.[48] The balloons are locked in place by a proprietary balloon design. In both balloon dilations, the intent is to only apply dilating force to the prostatic adenomatous tissue while sparing the bladder neck. Moreover, the balloon size, diameter, and length used are specific to the prostate size and length. Initial clinical trials are performed under general anesthesia or spinal block; however, the hope is that Optilume can be deployed in an office-based setting. A Foley catheter is placed postprocedurally.

Efficacy and Safety

First-year results evaluating the safety and efficacy of Optilume were published in 2021 under the EVEREST-I study.[48] A total of 80 men were enrolled in this prospective, single-arm, nonrandomized, open-label, multicenter study. Key inclusion criteria included prostate volume of 20 cm^3 to 80 cm^3 and IPSS $\geq$13. The primary endpoint of a $\geq$40% reduction in IPSS from baseline was met at 3 months (22.3–8.1) with 81.3% (65/80) of patients reaching this target. At 1-year follow-up, improvements appeared durable in IPSS (22.3%–7.9%, 64.9% reduction), IPSS QoL (4.6%–1.3%, 70.7% reduction), and Qmax (10.9 mL/s to 18.4 mL/s). There were no reported de novo ejaculatory or ED. Furthermore, adverse events were minor and self-limiting and comparable with established MISTs such as UroLift. A 500-participant prospective, double-blinded, randomized controlled trial is currently being conducted to more thoroughly evaluate the safety and efficacy of Optilume.

XFLO EXPANDER SYSTEM

Technique

The XFLO Expander System (Medeon Biodesign, Inc, Taiwan) is another mechanical solution for BPH. Based on currently available information, the XFLO system consists of a reversible nitinol tissue expander that is delivered to the prostatic urethra using a standard flexible cystoscope.[49] The device is left inside the prostatic urethra but is designed to be removable using a standard flexible cystoscope and the XPRO Retrieval Sheath in an office setting. Exact device specifications, technique details, and implant durations are still in development and not fully available to the public.

Efficacy and Safety

An ongoing, First-in-Human/Feasibility, open-label, prospective trial recently released interim results of 32 patients in 2021.[49] Key inclusion criteria included prostate volume of 30 cm^3 to

80 cm^3 and IPSS ≥13. The EXPANDER-1 study demonstrated a 40% reduction in IPSS at 2 weeks that appeared durable through 6 months (N = 14). Preliminary reports suggest safety with preservation of sexual function. Long-term follow-up data are currently being obtained and will provide additional efficacy and safety outcome measures.

ZENFLOW SPRING SYSTEM

Technique

The Zenflow Spring System (Zenflow, South San Francisco, CA, USA) uses a nitinol implant that is delivered through a proprietary flexible cystoscope to the prostatic urethra.[16] Unlike the XFLO system, the spring is designed to be a permanent device that is embedded into the wall of the prostatic urethra through internal tension. Exact device specifications, technique details, and implant durations are still in development and not fully available to the public.

Safety and Efficacy

Currently, interim results are available from a small first-in-man study with 24 months of follow-up. Although exact numbers are still being determined, it appears that significant IPSS improvements were seen at 12 months. Adverse events appeared to be few and minor in nature. Further results are currently being gathered in a larger, prospective, single-arm study in Canada.[16]

BUTTERFLY PROSTATIC RETRACTION DEVICE

Technique

The Butterfly Prostatic Retraction device (Butterfly, Medical Ltd, Yokneam, Yilit, Israel) is a nitinol implant shaped like a butterfly designed to reside in the prostatic urethra and unobstruct lateral prostate lobes. The single-use device is folded into a thin and flexible unit and can be placed with a flexible cystoscope. The Butterfly is designed to be a permanent solution but can also be removed easily under local anesthesia.[16]

Safety and Efficacy

A multicentre trial to assess safety and efficacy is currently in progress.[16]

SUMMARY

BPH is a common, progressive disease affecting aging men which has a significant impact on patient QoL. In an effort to address a rising demand for BPH therapy that is both effective and safe, innovative technologies promise rapid recovery and symptom relief, low complication rates (especially lower rates of sexual dysfunction), and, ideally, the ability to perform the procedure in an outpatient setting with local anesthesia. Such technologies will also help expand global patient access and democratize urologic BPH care. Current results, especially for TMISTs, will require long-term data to properly assess safety and durability of outcome.

CLINICS CARE POINTS

- An individualized treatment plan requires shared decision-making and considers factors including prostate anatomy, treatment efficacy, severity of symptoms, safety, side effects, and costs. Ideally, a decision aid can and should be utilized.
- Aquablation is an effective surgical technique that can be used for large prostates beyond 80 cm^3 with durable improvements in IPSS (75%) with sexual preservation (retrograde ejaculation: 11%–19%). Nonresective focal bladder neck cautery is recommended for postresection hemostasis.
- Rezūm is an office-based benign prostatic hyperplasia (BPH) procedure that is FDA approved for prostates between 30 cm^3 and 80 cm^3 which results in durable IPSS improvements (45%–79%) and low reported cases of erectile or ejaculatory dysfunction. It is also highly effective for the treatment of median lobes. Beneficial results have been reported for large prostates beyond 80 cm^3 as well.
- UroLift is an office-based BPH procedure that can be used for prostates up to 100 cm^3 which results in IPSS improvement (35%) and no erectile or ejaculatory dysfunction. It may also be effective for prostates with obstructive median lobes.
- iTind, Optilume BPH, XFLO, Zenflow, and Butterfly are true minimally invasive surgical therapies which are an off-the-shelf BPH solution requiring only a standard flexible cystoscope that can be performed in a urology office without sedation or general anesthetic. Current studies are investigating prostates less than 80 cm^3. Long-term data are currently being obtained regarding safety and efficacy.

DISCLOSURE

Dr Elterman is a consultant for Boston Scientific, Procept Biorobotics, Olympus, Urotronic and Prodeon; Dr. Chughtai is a consultant for Boston

Scientific and Olympus; Dr. Zorn is a consultant for Boston Scientific and Procept Biorobotics; Dr. Bhojani is a consultant for Boston Scientific, Olympus and Procept Biorobotics. Drs Gao and Mr Lu have no conflicts to disclose.

REFERENCES

1. Lim KB. Epidemiology of clinical benign prostatic hyperplasia. Asian J Urol 2017;4(3):148–51.
2. Berry SJ, Coffey DS, Walsh PC, et al. The development of human benign prostatic hyperplasia with age. J Urol 1984;132:474–9.
3. Taub DA, Wei JT. The economics of benign prostatic hyperplasia and lower urinary tract symptoms in the United States. Curr Urol Rep 2006;7(4):272–81.
4. Ulchaker JC, Martinson MS. Cost-effectiveness analysis of six therapies for the treatment of lower urinary tract symptoms due to benign prostatic hyperplasia. Clinicoecon Outcomes Res 2017;10: 29–43.
5. Bouhadana D, Nguyen DD, Schwarcz J, et al. Development of a patient decision aid for the surgical management of lower urinary tract symptoms secondary to benign prostatic hyperplasia. BJU Int 2021;127(1):131–5.
6. Zabkowski T, Saracyn M. Drug adherence and drug-related problems in pharmacotherapy for lower urinary tract symptoms related to benign prostatic hyperplasia. J Physiol Pharmacol 2018;69(4). https://doi.org/10.26402/jpp.2018.4.14.
7. Nguyen DD, Marchese M, Cone EB, et al. Investigation of suicidality and psychological adverse events in patients treated with finasteride. JAMA Dermatol 2021;157(1):35–42.
8. Rassweiler J, Teber D, Kuntz R, et al. Complications of transurethral resection of the prostate (TURP)–incidence, management, and prevention. Eur Urol 2006;50(5):969–80.
9. Bouhadana D, Nguyen DD, Zorn KC, et al. Patient perspectives on benign prostatic hyperplasia surgery: a focus on sexual health. J Sex Med 2020; 17(10):2108–12.
10. MacRae C, Gilling P. How I do it: aquablation of the prostate using the AQUABEAM system. Can J Urol 2016;23(6):8590–3.
11. Gilling P, Reuther R, Kahokehr A, et al. Aquablation - image-guided robot-assisted waterjet ablation of the prostate: initial clinical experience. BJU Int 2016; 117(6):923–9.
12. Gilling P, Anderson P, Tan A. Aquablation of the prostate for symptomatic benign prostatic hyperplasia: 1-year results. J Urol 2017;197(6):1565–72.
13. Elterman DS, Foller S, Ubrig B, et al. Focal bladder neck cautery associated with low rate of post-Aquablation bleeding. Can J Urol 2021;28(2): 10610–3.
14. Gilling P, Barber N, Bidair M, et al. WATER: a double-blind, randomized, controlled trial of Aquablation® vs transurethral resection of the prostate in benign prostatic hyperplasia. J Urol 2018;199(5):1252–61.
15. Gilling P, Barber N, Bidair M, et al. Three-year outcomes after aquablation therapy compared to TURP: results from a blinded randomized trial. Can J Urol 2020;27(1):10072–9.
16. Sountoulides P, Karatzas A, Gravas S. Current and emerging mechanical minimally invasive therapies for benign prostatic obstruction. Ther Adv Urol 2019;11. 1756287219828971.
17. Nguyen DD, Mantri SS, Zorn KC, et al. Which anatomic structures should be preserved during aquablation contour planning to optimize ejaculatory function? a case-control study using ultrasound video recordings to identify surgical predictors of postoperative anejaculation. Urology 2021. https://doi.org/10.1016/j.urology.2021.01.023.
18. Desai M, Bidair M, Bhojani N, et al. WATER II (80-150 mL) procedural outcomes. BJU Int 2019;123(1): 106–12.
19. Desai M, Bidair M, Bhojani N, et al. Aquablation for benign prostatic hyperplasia in large prostates (80-150 cc): 2-year results. Can J Urol 2020;27(2): 10147–53.
20. Elterman D, Bach T, Rijo E, et al. Transfusion rates after 800 Aquablation procedures using various haemostasis methods. BJU Int 2020;125(4):568–72.
21. Mynderse LA, Hanson D, Robb RA, et al. Rezum system water vapor treatment for lower urinary tract symptoms/benign prostatic hyperplasia: validation of convective thermal energy transfer and characterization with magnetic resonance imaging and 3-dimensional renderings. Urology 2015;86:122.
22. Woo HH, Gonzalez RR. Perspective on the Rezūm® System: a minimally invasive treatment strategy for benign prostatic hyperplasia using convective radiofrequency water vapor thermal therapy. Med Devices (Auckl) 2017;10:71–80.
23. Westwood J, Geraghty R, Jones P, et al. Rezum: a new transurethral water vapour therapy for benign prostatic hyperplasia. Ther Adv Urol 2018;10(11): 327–33.
24. McVary KT, Gange SN, Gittelman MC, et al. Minimally invasive prostate convective water vapor energy ablation: a multicenter, randomized, controlled study for the treatment of lower urinary tract symptoms secondary to benign prostatic hyperplasia. J Urol 2016;195:1529.
25. McVary KT, Gittelman MC, Goldberg KA, et al. Final 5-year outcomes of the multicenter randomized sham-controlled trial of rezūm water vapor thermal therapy for treatment of moderate-to-severe lower urinary tract symptoms secondary to benign prostatic hyperplasia. J Urol 2021. https://doi.org/10.1097/JU.0000000000001778.

26. Dixon C, Cedano ER, Pacik D, et al. Efficacy and safety of Rezūm system water vapor treatment for lower urinary tract symptoms secondary to benign prostatic hyperplasia. Urology 2015;86(5):1042–7.
27. Darson MF, Alexander EE, Schiffman ZJ, et al. Procedural techniques and multicenter postmarket experience using minimally invasive convective radiofrequency thermal therapy with Rezūm system for treatment of lower urinary tract symptoms due to benign prostatic hyperplasia. Res Rep Urol 2017;9:159–68.
28. Mollengarden D, Goldberg K, Wong D, et al. Convective radiofrequency water vapor thermal therapy for benign prostatic hyperplasia: a single office experience. Prostate Cancer Prostatic Dis 2018; 21:379–85.
29. Alegorides C, Fourmarier M, Eghazarian C, et al. Treatment of benign prostate hyperplasia using the Rezum® water vapor therapy system: Results at one year. Prog Urol 2020. https://doi.org/10.1016/j.purol.2020.05.004.
30. Johnston MJ, Noureldin M, Abdelmotagly Y, et al. Rezum water vapour therapy: promising early outcomes from the first UK series. BJU Int 2020; 126(5):557–8.
31. Siena G, Cindolo L, Ferrari G, et al. Water vapor therapy (Rezūm) for lower urinary tract symptoms related to benign prostatic hyperplasia: early results from the first Italian multicentric study. World J Urol. 2021 Mar 31;1–6. https://doi.org/10.1007/s00345-021-03642-4.
32. McVary KT, Rogers T, Mahon J, et al. Is sexual function better preserved after water vapor thermal therapy or medical therapy for lower urinary tract symptoms due to benign prostatic hyperplasia? J Sex Med 2018;15(12):1728–38.
33. Garcia C, Chin P, Rashid P, et al. Prostatic urethral lift: a minimally invasive treatment for benign prostatic hyperplasia. Prostate Int 2015;3(1):1–5.
34. Jones P, Rajkumar GN, Rai BP, et al. Medium-term outcomes of urolift (minimum 12 months follow-up): evidence from a systematic review. Urology 2016;97:20–4.
35. Roehrborn CG, Rukstalis DB, Barkin J, et al. Three year results of the prostatic urethral L.I.F.T. study. Can J Urol 2015;22(3):7772–82.
36. Roehrborn CG, Barkin J, Gange SN, et al. Five year results of the prospective randomized controlled prostatic urethral L.I.F.T. study. Can J Urol 2017; 24(3):8802–13.
37. Rukstalis D, Grier D, Stroup SP, et al. Prostatic Urethral Lift (PUL) for obstructive median lobes: 12 month results of the MedLift Study. Prostate Cancer Prostatic Dis 2019;22:411–9.
38. Miller LE, Chughtai B, Dornbier RA, et al. Surgical reintervention rate after prostatic urethral lift: systematic review and meta-analysis involving over 2,000 patients. J Urol 2020;204(5):1019–26.
39. Jones P, Rai BP, Aboumarzouk O, et al. UroLift: a new minimally-invasive treatment for benign prostatic hyperplasia. Ther Adv Urol 2016;8(6):372–6.
40. Page T, Veeratterapillay R, Keltie K, et al. Prostatic urethral lift (UroLift): a real-world analysis of outcomes using hospital episodes statistics. BMC Urol 2021;21:55.
41. Elterman DS, Zorn KC, Chughtai B, et al. Is it time to offer True Minimally Invasive Treatments (TMIST) for BPH? - A review of office-based therapies and introduction of a new technology category. Can J Urol 2021;28(2):10580–3.
42. Marcon J, Magistro G, Stief CG, et al. What's New in TIND? Eur Urol Focus 2018;4:40–2.
43. Porpiglia F, Fiori C, Amparore D, et al. Second-generation of temporary implantable nitinol device for the relief of lower urinary tract symptoms due to benign prostatic hyperplasia: results of a prospective, multicentre study at 1 year of follow-up. BJU Int 2019;123(6):1061–9.
44. Porpiglia F, Fiori C, Bertolo R, et al. 3-year follow-up of temporary implantable nitinol device implantation for the treatment of benign prostatic obstruction. BJU Int 2018;122:106–12.
45. Amparore D, Fiori C, Valerio M, et al. 3-Year results following treatment with the second generation of the temporary implantable nitinol device in men with LUTS secondary to benign prostatic obstruction. Prostate Cancer Prostatic Dis 2020. https://doi.org/10.1038/s41391-020-00281-5.
46. De Nunzio C, Cantiello F, Fiori C, et al. Urinary and sexual function after treatment with temporary implantable nitinol device (iTind) in men with LUTS: 6-month interim results of the MT-06-study. World J Urol 2020. https://doi.org/10.1007/s00345-020-03418-2.
47. Chughtai B, Elterman D, Shore N, et al. The iTind temporarily implanted nitinol device for the treatment of lower urinary tract symptoms secondary to benign prostatic hyperplasia: a multicenter, randomized, controlled trial. Urology 2020. https://doi.org/10.1016/j.urology.2020.12.022.
48. Kaplan SA, Pichardo M, Rijo E, et al. One-year outcomes after treatment with a drug-coated balloon catheter system for lower urinary tract symptoms related to benign prostatic hyperplasia. Prostate Cancer Prostatic Dis 2021. https://doi.org/10.1038/s41391-021-00362-z.
49. PRESS RELEASE. Medeon announces positive clinical results for XFLO minimally invasive BPH treatment device. In: madeonbio. 2021. Available at: https://www.medeonbio.com/wp-content/uploads/2021/01/Medeon-Press-20210127-Positive-Clinical-Results-for-XFLO-Minimally-Inv....pdf. Accessed May 11, 2021.

Future Platforms of Robotic Surgery

Sylvia L. Alip, MD[a,b], Jinu Kim, MD[a], Koon Ho Rha, MD[c], Woong Kyu Han, MD[c,*]

KEYWORDS

• Robotic urology • Robotic surgery • Telemanipulator systems • Robot-assisted laparoscopy • Single-incision surgery • Robotic endoscopy

KEY POINTS

- Robotic devices for surgery may be classified as semiactive, synergistic, and active, according to the degree of autonomy. Synergistic devices can be handheld, hands-on, or telemanipulator systems, according to the human body's movements.
- Several telemanipulator systems are licensed for commercial use and that are relevant to the urologic practice are the standard da Vinci, Avatera, Hinotori, Revo-i, Senhance, Versius, and Surgenius.
- Future trends include an exploration of more robust haptic systems that offer kinesthetic and tactile feedback; miniaturization and microrobotics; enhanced visual feedback with greater magnification and higher fidelity in detail; and autonomous robots.
- The role of the urologic surgeon in the operating room is ever expanding. The rise of robotics and the automation of devices do not serve to limit our role but rather allow for a richer realization of what it means to be a surgeon.

BRIEF HISTORY AND TERMINOLOGY OF ROBOTIC DEVICES FOR LAPAROSCOPY

The birth of robots in surgery and the idea of telepresence arose from necessity. One of the factors that drove these innovations was the need to provide surgical services to soldiers in remote areas. The U.S. military program Defense Advanced Research Projects (DARPA) developed the Bradley 557A, which first performed an ex vivo organ anastomosis telepresence surgery in 1994 using a microwave connection.[1] Moreover, as space exploration developed, the ability to perform long-distance operations was required for astronauts on years-long voyages. This need gave rise to the combination of a head-mounted display and data glove from NASA Ames Research Center with a telemanipulator from the Stanford Research Institute.[2] The second driving factor of these innovations is the infinite quest for better surgical quality as measured by certain outcomes, such as operation time and perioperative morbidity. This intuitively stems from the need for more predictable surgical interventions, with high degrees of accuracy in each action and minimal invasion.[3]

The first reported urologic robotic surgery was completed in the Imperial College London in 1988 by the Unimate Programmable Universal Manipulation Arm (PUMA; General Motors, MI, USA), a machine previously used for stereotactic brain biopsies. A transurethral resection of the prostate was simulated using a potato in an acrylic box attached to an artificial penis. The robot was fed a specially designed framework with a cutter assembly, and the area of the prostate was sectioned into a sequence of overlapping cuts. The PUMA made an axial cut on the forward stroke and a diathermic cauterization on the return stroke.[4]

[a] Department of Urology, Yonsei University College of Medicine, Urological Science Institute, 134 Shinchon-dong, Seodaemun-ku Seoul 120-752, South Korea; [b] Division of Urology, University of the Philippines – Philippine General Hospital, Manila, Philippines; [c] Department of Urology, Yonsei University College of Medicine, Urological Science Institute, 134 Shinchon-dong, Seodaemun-ku Seoul 120-752, South Korea
* Corresponding author.
E-mail address: hanwk@yuhs.ac

Urol Clin N Am 49 (2022) 23–38
https://doi.org/10.1016/j.ucl.2021.07.008

The Automated Endoscopic System for Optimal Positioning (AESOP; Computer Motion, CA, USA) designed by Sackier Wang[5] was the first robot to assist surgeons in the operating room in 1994.[6] The AESOP eliminated the need for a surgical assistant to hold the camera[7] by serving a foot pedal–controlled or hand remote–controlled camera holder and positioner. It afforded 14 inches of vertical movement with a 27-inch reach from its attachment at the surgical table rail, ushering in the concept of a surgeon's "third arm" that retains her faculties yet enhances the work[6] Subsequently, Wang[5] obtained DARPA funding to expand his vision of reproducing the movements of the arms of a surgeon. The Zeus robotic system (Computer Motion, CA, USA) was created and approved by the U.S. Food and Drug Administration in 2001 to assist blunt dissectors, retractors, graspers, and stabilizers during laparoscopic and thoracoscopic surgeries.[2] The Zeus had three robotic arms, one of which was the AESOP. Operation Lindbergh was performed with the Zeus: a robot-assisted laparoscopic cholecystectomy in a 68-year-old woman at a remote site in Strasbourg performed by Dr Jacques Marescaux from his surgeon console in New York. In 2003, Computer Motion was merged with Intuitive Surgical, and the development of Zeus was discontinued.

The Advanced Robotic Telemanipulator for Minimally Invasive Surgery (ARTEMIS; Karlsruhe Research Center, Germany) consisted of operating room table-mounted slave arms, each with six degrees of freedom. The surgeon console consisted of a joystick control for the endoscope and two master arms. Preclinical evaluation of a single-slave arm was conducted in porcine models for laparoscopic sigmoidectomy in 1996,[8] but the machine did not progress to further clinical studies.

Robotic surgery has advanced considerably since these pioneering machines. Especially in the past 10 years, robotic innovations have reached new heights. With the start of a new decade, surgeons are facing new dilemmas. As robotic devices become smaller and their capabilities for surgical use become broadly applicable, surgeons are faced with the challenge of redefining their role to incorporate these devices into clinical practice.

ROBOTIC CLASSIFICATION SYSTEMS

In 2008, due to wide dissemination of robotic surgical devices throughout the decade, members of the Society of American Gastrointestinal and Endoscopic Surgeons (SAGES) and Minimally Invasive Robotic Association convened to form a consensus on the various aspects of this new technological inclusion in health care. They defined robotic surgery as a surgical procedure or technology that adds a computer technology–enhanced device to the interaction between a surgeon and a patient during a surgical operation and assumes some degree of control previously completely reserved for the surgeon.[9] Since this consensus, many contemporary robotic classification systems have been proposed. However, not all have found utility from a surgeon's point of view. Most of these classification systems are broad and include all computer-aided devices that exist around the human body (some in other fields of study, such as engineering, industry, and so forth). The classification systems and model machines introduced in this section are those that are current and relevant to the medical perspective, with a focus on minimally invasive surgery and urology.

A 2019 classification from Schleer and colleagues[10] that draws from past classifications divides robotic systems for computer-aided surgery into three categories: active, semiactive, and synergistic. Active systems perform some subtasks autonomously under the supervision of the surgeon.[10] Semiactive systems physically constrain the actions of a surgeon to correspond to a predefined strategy. Synergistic systems provide a simultaneous shared control of an object by the robot and the surgeon. Synergistic systems are further subdivided into handheld, hands-on, and telemanipulated systems. Handheld surgical robots are manipulated by the surgeon without a stationary mechanical reference. Hands-on surgical robots are based on a stationary kinematic mechanism that is manually operated by a surgeon (the robot provides a mechanical constraint while the surgeon provides active motion). Telemanipulated systems exist in a master–slave configuration, whereby active motion provided by the surgeon is modified and transformed by a robotic system. The da Vinci and its forerunners ARTEMIS and AESOP-Zeus are telemanipulator systems.

This 2019 classification draws from past classifications. In 2003, Dario and colleagues3 defined handheld tools as enhanced tools endowed with a certain degree of embedded intelligence and autonomy. They are driven by the surgeon's hand but support it by correcting, amplifying, or attenuating her actions.[3] Some examples in this category are endoscopes, sensor-equipped laparoscopic graspers,[11] error-canceling microsurgical instruments, and scalpels with tremor compensation.[12] Because most pioneering applications of these handheld tools are in ophthalmology[13] and orthopedic surgery,[14] they are only mentioned briefly here, with their corresponding references.

An example of a hands-on device is the robot end effector that provides haptic feedback on planned boundaries using virtual fixtures and motion constraints; some types even provide tool positioning and immobilization for prolonged use. Specific systems include the ACROBOT[15] and MAKO[16] for orthopedics, Eye-robot[17] and MYNUTIA[18] for ophthalmology, PADyC for cardiac surgery,[19] and ROSA[20] and Neurobot[21] for neurosurgery.

More than 5000 devices have been developed in the field of computer-assisted surgery.[10] However, the focus of this review is on urologic robotic systems, most of which are telemanipulator systems. Historical devices are mentioned briefly, and robotic systems that have found greater utility, currently in development and use (have reached clinical studies on animals, cadaveric simulation, or human patients), are emphasized.

LICENSED TELEMANIPULATOR SYSTEMS

da Vinci

All landmark robotic studies that have paved the way for incorporating robotic surgery in most clinical pathways have been performed on the da Vinci system (Intuitive Surgical Inc, CA, USA). In clinical practice, robotic surgery has become synonymous with this platform. The company's latest development is a single-incision surgery system: the da Vinci SP platform.

The FDA granted initial clearance for the da Vinci SP surgical system in 2014. Final clearance was granted in early 2018, and customer shipments began in the third quarter of 2018. The single-port platform features a single rotatable arm inserted into a 25-mm cannula. The arm can hold three instruments, each with seven degrees of freedom. A full-articulated 3D endoscope can be controlled similarly in this arm. Several studies have already reported on favorable outcomes in renal surgery,[22] robotic perineal radical prostatectomy,[23] cystectomy,[24] partial prostatectomy,[25] and transperitoneal radical prostatectomy.[26,27] The latter studies retrospectively compared multi-port and single-port cohorts and found no significant differences in operative times. However, the single-port platform yielded a more favorable pain profile and a shorter hospital stay.

Despite the COVID-19 pandemic, 1,243,000 surgical procedures were performed in 2020 worldwide using the da Vinci surgical systems, besting its 2019 and 2018 numbers (1,229,000 and 1,038,000, respectively). Of these procedures, 876,000 were performed within the United States, and 134,000 of these US procedures were listed under the urology subspecialty.[28]

Avatera

The Avatera (avateramedical GmbH, Jena, Germany) is composed of a control unit (with a closed-system surgeon console with an integrated seat) and a surgical robot with four arms in a single boom (**Fig. 1**). Single-use surgical instruments are all 5 mm in diameter, with seven degrees of freedom. In addition, the system boasts of an ultralow noise level, with no external fans used. The company provides dry laboratory, wet laboratory, and on-site training. The Avatera obtained a CE mark in November 2019 for minimally invasive surgery. Each machine is estimated to cost approximately $1.1 M—half the cost of the more recent da Vinci models.[29,30]

Hinotori

The Hinotori robot (Medicaroid Corporation, Kobe, Japan) is composed of three components: the surgeon cockpit, operation unit, and vision unit.[31] The operation unit contains four arms in a single slender boom (**Fig. 2**). The uniqueness of the arms is in their "docking-free" design, which relies on the fulcrum or pivot-point, set by software.[32]

Hinotori received approval from the Japanese Ministry of Health, Labor and Welfare for commercial use in August 2020. The technology has been become accessible in its home country due to a dedicated training center in Kobe University Hospital International Clinical Cancer Research Center operating under the Japan Society for Endoscopic Surgery and the robot's inclusion into the national insurance the month following its regulatory approval. Distribution to various Japanese hospitals with an emphasis on urologic operations commenced in December 2020. The launch in international markets is slated for 2022.[31]

Revo-i

The Revo-i robotic surgical system (Meere Company Inc, Seongnam, Republic of Korea) is a telemanipulator that functions similarly to the da Vinci Si robot. The system (**Fig. 3**) consists of a closed-design surgeon console with precision grip finger controls and foot pedals for clutching and energy; a patient cart with four arms and seven degrees of freedom instruments; and a vision cart.[33]

In April 2010, Meere Company was selected as the major company for the development of a surgical robotic system for minimal invasion operations (Industrial Source Technology Development business of Ministry of Knowledge Economy). The robotic prototype was developed in 2007, and the MSR-1000 was introduced in 2009.[34] Since its introduction, the Revo-i has been examined in

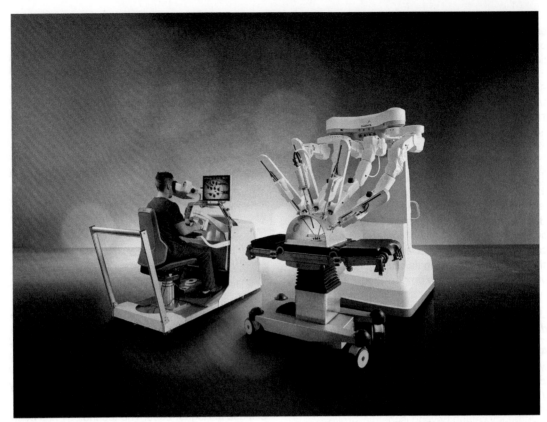

Fig. 1. The Avatera surgical robot and control unit. (*From* https://www.avatera.eu/en/home, with permission.)

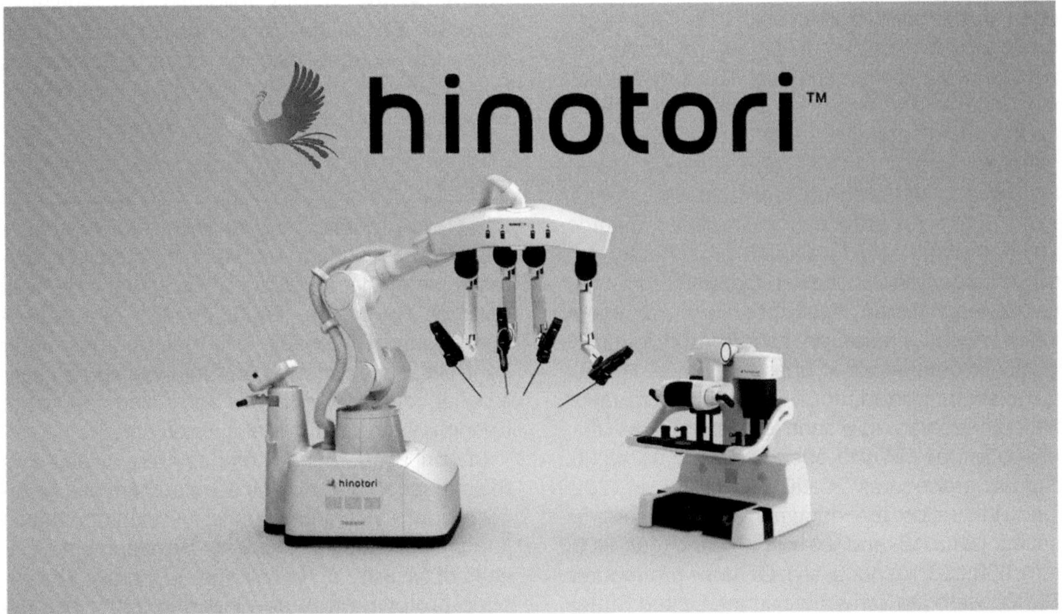

Fig. 2. The Hinotori operation unit and surgeon cockpit. (*From* © Medicaroid Corporation, https://www.medicaroid.com.)

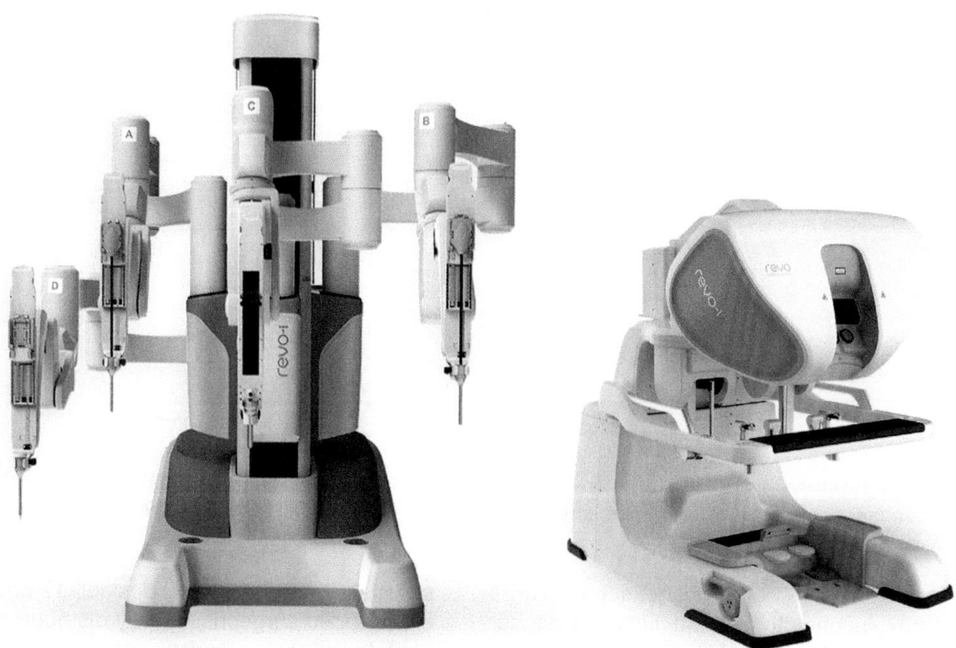

Fig. 3. Revo-i patient cart and surgeon console. (*From* © Revo Surgical, http://revosurgical.com.)

numerous studies,[34–37] especially those centered on urologic surgery.[38] The Korean Ministry of Food and Drug Safety granted commercial license to the company in 2018. Since then, the availability of the robotic system has expanded to various hospitals in South Korea, Russia, and Kazakhstan.[39]

Chang and colleagues conducted a prospective study in 17 patients with localized prostate cancer using the Revo-i through the Retzius-sparing approach.[38] This study described no perioperative major complications, no intraoperative complications, and no robotic malfunctions throughout the study. Of the 17 patients, one had biochemical recurrence and 15 were continent at 3 months after surgery.

Senhance

The Senhance telerobotic system (previously Telelap Alf-x; Asensus Surgical formerly Transenterix Surgical Inc; NC, USA) was first developed by SOFAR in Milan, Italy, and Tuebingen Scientific.[40] The system was approved for general surgical procedures in Europe in 2012 and obtained U.S. FDA approval in 2017.[41] The open system consists of a screen that allows for 2D-3D modes, a keyboard, and 2 to 4 laparoscopic-type handles that serve to control robotic working arms[42] (**Fig. 4**). Although the system has haptic sensation, an eye-tracking system (that requires preoperative calibration adapted to the surgeon's eyes), instrument reusability, and compatibility with most commercially available laparoscopic trocars, it lacks the additional "wristed" degrees of freedom found in competing systems[41] Testing on models for porcine nephrectomy[43] and vesicourethral anastomosis[44] was completed in 2014, and a short learning curve was ascertained. After several reports of feasibility in human patients, higher volume clinical studies in gynecology and colorectal surgery, as well as on-site credentialing and mentoring programs, and several studies examined using the Senhance system for robotic urologic operations.

Samalavicus and colleagues[45] performed 31 urologic operations (27 prostatectomies, 1 nephrectomy, 1 varicocelectomy, 1 pyeloplasty, 1 pyelolithotomy) in Lithuania. All patients had a body mass index less than 30, an American Society of Anesthesiologists score less than 3, and no previous operations. Two robot prostatectomies were converted to laparoscopy due to difficulties in pelvic anatomy, two required blood transfusions, and one required additional antibiotics postoperatively for epididymitis. There was one major complication (Clavien-Dindo Grade IIIA) for a urethral stricture, which needed urethral dilatation. However, the study noted no instrument malfunction in the cohort. In the study, at 30 days after surgery, 80.76% of Robot-assisted radical prostatectomy patients were continent (did not use pads).

In a larger study involving more than 100 patients in Croatia, Kastelan and colleagues performed extraperitoneal radical prostatectomy

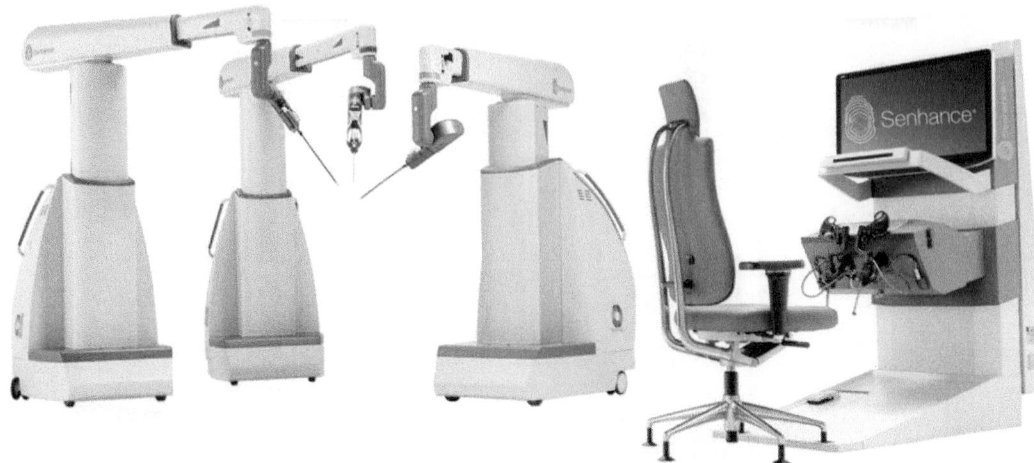

Fig. 4. Senhance robotic arms and open console. Senhance® Surgical System (*From* © Asensus Surgical US, Inc https://www.senhance.com/us/home.)

(with and without pelvic lymphadenectomy), adrenalectomy, nephrectomy, and kidney cyst surgeries with the Senhance system, and instructional videos are available as online supplements.[46,47] Some disadvantages of the system cited by this study are the longer setup, including docking time (which took an hour initially but improved in subsequent cases), and the large working space that the separate arms required. Advantages of the system included lower costs and the ability to easily convert to simple laparoscopy, should the need arise.

Early exploratory investigations into the Senhance system in the United States are limited to manual skills in simulation models (peg transfers and precision cutting). A study at Duke University showed that the system enables rapid learning regardless of the surgeon's experience level, with the haptic feedback function not having a significant effect on skills acquisition.[48]

Versius

The Versius surgical system (CMR Surgical, Cambridge, UK) (**Fig. 5**) provides wristed instruments with seven degrees of freedom. Each instrument and arm comes in a separately wheeled cart, comprising a mobile bedside unit.[49] Owing to its modular design, up to 3 bedside units may be used at a time. The handgrip is a game controller grip, which was reported as the most comfortable and easiest to use in preliminary modeling.[50] The entire control of the device is in the handheld unit, with no need for foot pedal controls.[51] The surgeon console is in an open design, allowing the surgeon to sit or stand. Instrument ports are 5 mm each.

In an IDEAL collaboration (Idea, Development, Exploration, Assessment, Long-term study) for surgical research (stage 0 design), 17 novice and experienced surgeons (equally distributed among obstetrician-gynecologists, upper gastrointestinal, colorectal, and urologic surgeons) and their teams were underwent a 3.5-day-long standardized Versius training program and were assessed in a cadaveric simulation on usability and task errors. Of more than 11,000 tasks performed, 98% were recorded as a pass or a pass with difficulty. The most common user errors were the failure to mention the possibility of trapping think cables on moving the bedside unit and the failure to maintain sterility. No failures in critical tasks occurred, and the study concluded usability, safety, and operational proficiency after undergoing training.

In a preclinical study published in 2020, Thomas and colleagues[51] performed 24 radical nephrectomies (transperitoneal and retroperitoneal) and radical prostatectomies (with or without lymphadenectomy; all transperitoneal, one Retzius-sparing) in porcine and cadaveric models. All procedures were completed, and no device-related or nondevice-related intraoperative complications occurred. All recovery pigs showed good recovery after surgery, and assessments at necropsy revealed the same.

The Versius system obtained its CE mark in March 2019. Since then, the Versius system has been studied in clinical practice. In the United Kingdom, it was used as a part of a COVID-19–protected robotic surgical center without perioperative complications.[52] Additionally, a novel two-console dual-field robotic approach was used for a transanal total mesorectal excision with two surgeons working synchronously on the robot.[53] This approach, compared with the existing laparoscopic-transanal approach, had the potential to reduce operative time. It was facilitated

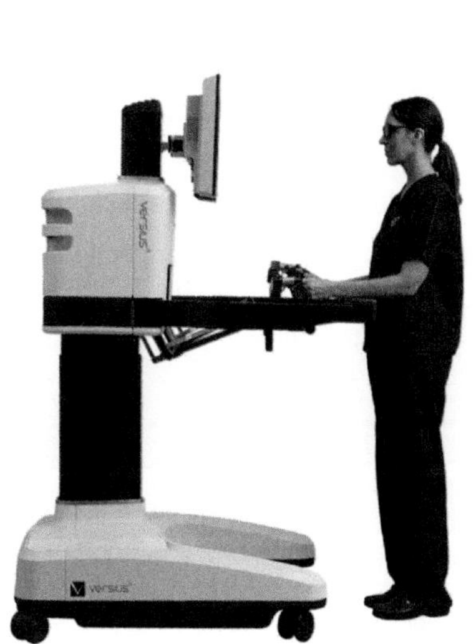

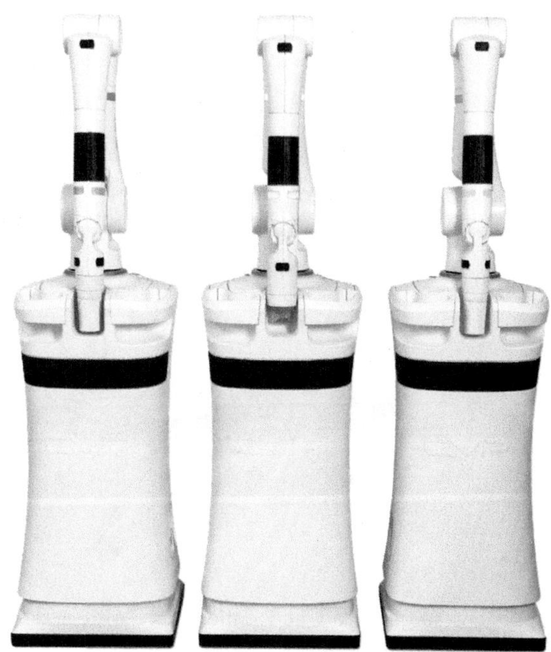

Fig. 5. Versius open surgeon console with surgeon standing and three modular bedside units. (*From* https://cmrsurgical.com/versius.)

by the modular flexibility of the Versius, with seven experimental bedside units coupled into two consoles.

Surgenius

The Surgenius system (Surgica Robotica Sp.A, Italy) obtained a CE Mark for Surgenius Beta in 2012 after *in vivo* trials and had plans for commercialization.[54] However, to date, no further data on the system have been published. The company's website states confidential development for their third model, the Surgenius Gamma.[55]

EXPERIMENTAL TELEMANIPULATOR SYSTEMS

The following systems are under investigation or in the initial stages of their developed. They are expected to gain traction in the coming years.

Enos

The Enos robotic single-access surgical system (Titan Medical Inc, Ontario, Canada) is a purpose-built telemanipulator for single-incision laparoscopic surgery. This system was previously known as Single Port Orifice Robotic Technology (SPORT) Surgical System but was rebranded in 2020. In a regulatory update,[56] the company announced that they would communicate with the U.S. FDA for their filing of a presubmission and additional investigational device studies in the first quarter of 2022. Commercial launch is slated for 2024.[57]

The system is composed of an open surgeon workstation and a patient cart. The patient cart uses a 25-mm insertion tube (**Fig. 6**), two articulating arms, and two lighted camera systems: a 2D high-definition camera and a 3D high-definition articulating camera.[57] Two 8-mm diameter multiarticulated instruments can be used through the insertion tube.[58] The SPORT is built on a previous model, the insertable robotic effector platform developed at the Advanced Robotics and Mechanism Applications Laboratory at Vanderbilt University.[59]

Under the name SPORT, the system was tested in 2019 in 12 minimally invasive general surgery procedures (cholecystectomy, Nissen fundoplication, splenectomy, and hepatic pedicle dissection) on porcine and cadaveric models.[58] Titanium clips were placed using a port separate from the insertion cannula inserted into a gel access platform in the same abdominal incision or through a separate port entirely. A lens wash feature provides lens cleaning intraabdominally, activated by the bedside assistant or the surgeon via his secondary screen. Insertion tube movement is not controlled by the surgeon, and repositioning was done by the bedside assistant.

Hugo Robotic-Assisted Surgery

In September 2019, Medtronic unveiled its Hugo RAS robotic telemanipulator system (**Fig. 7**)

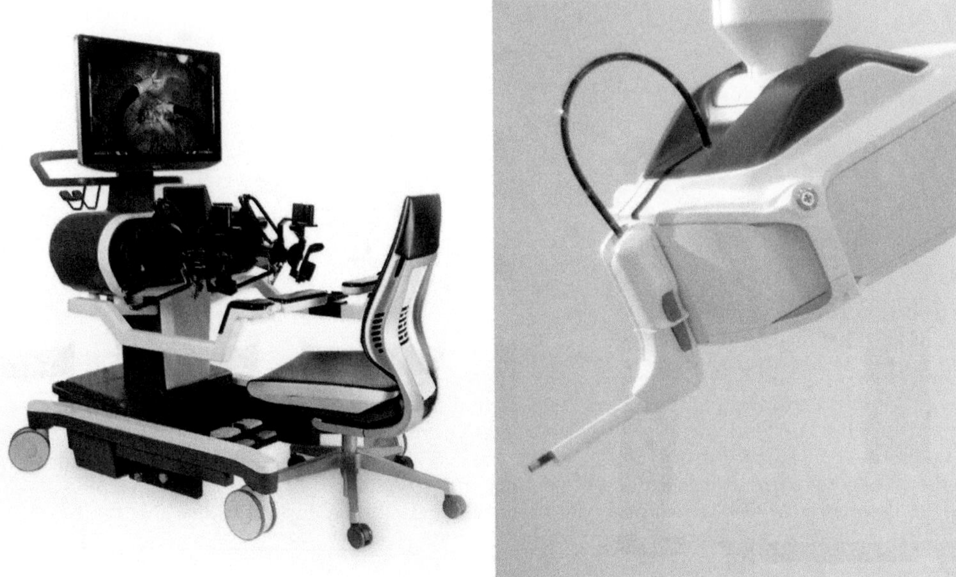

Fig. 6. Enos surgeon cart and patient cart with a camera protracted in the insertion tube. (*From* https://titanmedicalinc.com/enos/.)

(Medtronic PLC, Dublin, Ireland) by way of a cadaveric laparoscopic prostatectomy performed by Dr Joseph Wagner.[60,61] The promising feature of its design is versatility (utility in both laparoscopy and robotic surgery) and modularity (use of up to four arms). The endoscope is made in partnership with Karl Storz. End effectors are wristed and come with energy and stapling technology. Medtronic is pushing for a CE mark by the end of 2021.

MIRA

The MIRA system (Miniaturized *In Vivo* Robotic Assistant, Virtual Incision, University of Nebraska, Nebraska Innovation Campus, NE, USA), previously single-incision in vivo surgical robot is a purpose-built telemanipulator for single-incision laparoscopic surgery. The system is a bedside portable robot that weighs only two pounds (**Fig. 8**). The current model holds two 7 degrees of freedom instruments controlled by pistol-like handgrips, a bipolar fenestrated grasper, and monopolar shears. Its foot pedals control energy and the flex tip articulating endoscope, and its camera has motion tracking features. The device is mounted on the operating room table by a holding arm. The surgeon console has an open design, with a monitor and a smaller touchscreen. Critical features are the hand input devices that also provide haptic feedback to indicate workspace

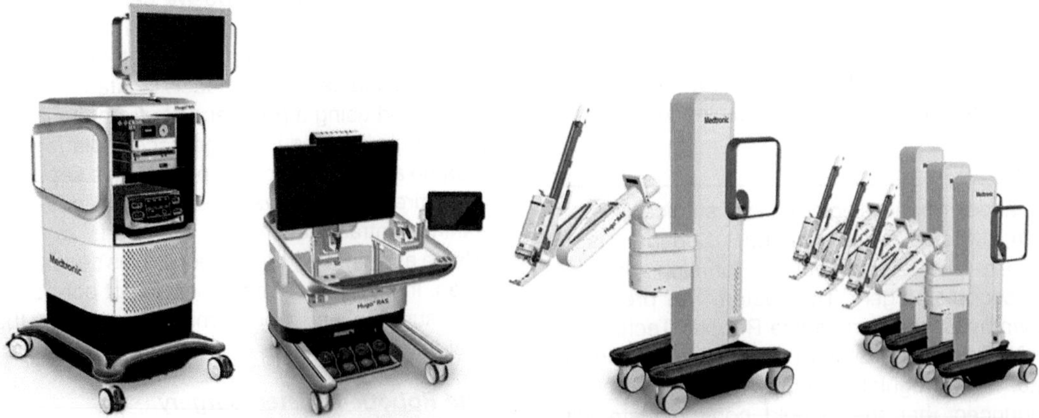

Fig. 7. Hugo robotic-assisted surgery (RAS) system vision cart, surgeon console, and mobile robotic arm units. (*From* Medtronic © https://www.medtronic.com/covidien/en-us/robotic-assisted-surgery/hugo-ras-system.html.)

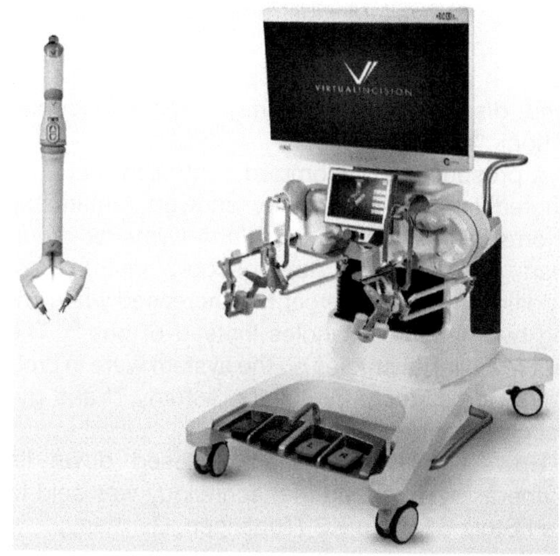

Fig. 8. The MIRA two-pound bedside portable robot and open surgeon console. (*From* MetraLabs GmbH | Neue Technologien und Systeme, https://www.mira-project.org/joomla-mira/.)

boundaries.[62] Because of its size, the strength of the MIRA lies in its modularity. Preliminary studies have discussed this option with multiple robots being used, each inserted into a single port[63]; this option will likely double robotic capability.

Cholecystectomy and colectomy were performed using the system in nonsurvival animal models.[63,64] In December 2020, the FDA granted the platform an investigational device exemption, which will allow clinical studies to be conducted in a limited number of U.S. hospitals.[62]

MiroSurge

The Miro robotic surgery platform (German Aerospace Center [DLR - Deutschen Zentrum für Luft-und Raumfahrt], Germany) was initially designed as a versatile robotic system that was built around four types of surgery: placement of pedicle screws, neurosurgical biopsies, laser osteotomies, and endoscopic telesurgery. Its versatility is hinged on a configurable or modular concept by a flexible tool interface, allowing the system to adapt to various surgical tasks. The MiroSurge is the dedicated configuration of the Miro platform for minimally invasive robotic abdominal and thoracic surgery. Each weighing a mere 10 kg, the robotic arm is made to resemble the human arm: there is a dedicated shoulder upper arm, elbow, forearm, and wrist. Unlike the da Vinci that uses a remote center of motion to address the fulcrum point constraint, the Mirosurge uses a moving fulcrum point, allowing for applications with a moving entry point such as the moving chest wall during respiration.[65] Its parent the Miro system allows for varying setups such as wall-, ceiling-, or table-mounted configurations. An additional option is available for haptic hand controllers (Omega, Sigma7, Force Dimension, Nyon, Switzerland), in combination with the German Aerospace Center's own Mica instruments that afford seven degrees of freedom. The MiroSurge did not progress into preclinical or clinical studies. Technical components of the MiroSurge have been licensed to Medtronic (Medtronic PLC, Dublin, Ireland).

Taurus II Robot

In 2015, Johnson & Johnson's Ethicon and Google Verily formed Verb Surgical with the intention of building on the work of SRI International (formerly Stanford Research Institute; CA, USA) and their Taurus line of robots.[66] In 2020, Johnson & Johnson announced the buyout of Google's shares as the latter exited the robotic venture.[67] Preclinical studies on the system have yet to be published.

Taurus II (Verb Surgical Inc, CA, USA) is one of the models studied by Gonzalez and colleagues[68] in robotic transfer learning for their dataset Dexterous Surgical Skill. The system has manipulators that exhibit seven degrees of freedom and force feedback. This study attempted to collect and analyze surgical gestures to enable transfer learning between different robots. Other robots studied were the YuMi and da Vinci Research Kit.

Other projects that entered the field but have yet to gain traction in preclinical studies are the Endobot (Rensselaer Polytechnic Institute, NY, USA),[69] the purpose-built single-site platform Single Port LapaRoscopy bImaNual roboT–Array of Robots Augmenting the Kinematics of Endoluminal Surgery Project (The BioRobotics Institute, Italy),[70] and the Surgeon's Operating Force-feedback Interface Eindhoven robot (Eindhoven University of Technology, Netherlands).[71]

HANDS-ON PLATFORMS

As previously defined, hands-on robots are based on a stationary kinematic mechanism (eg, mounted on an operating room table), with a surgeon providing dynamic motion. This section provides examples of hands-on platforms with clinical relevance to minimally invasive surgery and urology.

LODEM

The goal of the Locally Operated Detachable End-Effector Manipulator (LODEM; Osaka Institute of Technology, Osaka, Japan) and similar devices is to achieve robotically assisted surgery performed by a single surgeon working in a sterile area near the patient.[72] This requires a robot compact enough to be mounted in the sterile field of the abdomen, yet could achieve a wide range of movement within the patient's abdomen. To achieve this, the LODEM uses a spherical coordinate manipulator with a linear telescopic rail and two circular telescopic rails to achieve three degrees of freedom (pitch, yaw, insertion/extraction) and act as a third arm of the surgeon. The LODEM is controlled by a handheld interface with button switches attached to the surgeon's forceps.

Preclinical studies in swine showed the feasibility of the LODEM[73] with the surgeon controlling all three instruments. An assistant surgeon, however, is still needed to control the endoscope.

Raven II

Raven II is an open-source, low-cost research robotic platform consisting of both hardware and software. As a collaborative effort of American universities, it has been adopted by 18 research institutes worldwide.[74] The platform consists of a master console and slave robotic arms. An arm provides seven degrees of freedom, which is developed based on real-time Linux and is Robot Operating System compatible. The master control uses foot pedals to couple/decouple master/slave motion and work with various control devices. The Raven II is an improvement of the Raven I, with a more compact design and a better tool interface.[75]

The studies on the platform have focused on various novel control mechanisms and interfaces from a biomechanical engineering perspective.[76,77] One preclinical study simulated a semi-autonomous brain tumor ablation using a 3D printed surgical field.[78]

Other hands-on platforms such as the FDA-rejected SurgiBot (sold to Great Belief International China, from Asensus Surgical, NC, USA)[79] have yet to publish recent developments.

HANDHELD DEVICES

As previously defined, handheld surgical robots are manipulated by the surgeon without a stationary mechanical reference.

The handheld surgical robot Kymerax (Terumo Corporation, Tokyo, Japan) obtained its CE Mark in 2011.[80] It is an articulated reusable system that incorporates lateral and circular movements. The console can accommodate two instrument handles, which have buttons for pitch, yaw, and rotation. These handles are controlled in a pistol-like grip, with a release/engage trigger and rotation/deflection in its thumb controllers.[81] It has four available instruments that attach to the handle component, each of which is 8.8 mm in diameter: monopolar scissors, Maryland dissector, needle driver, and monopolar L-hook.[82]

A prospective randomized controlled trial conducted in a dry laboratory showed remarkably shorter learning curves with the Kymerax group than with standard laparoscopic instruments. Additionally, depth perception increased when using two handheld handles instead of one.[83] The first few clinical studies on the system were in urology: a prostatectomy,[84] nephrectomy,[80] and gynecology surgery.[85,86]

However, Terumo recently closed down its Kymerax system, and the technology was sold to Karl Storz SE & Co KG (Tuttlingen, Germany).

ROBOTIC SURGICAL DEVICES FOR ENDOSCOPIC AND PERCUTANEOUS UROLOGIC SURGERY

Aquabeam

The Aquabeam robotic system (PROCEPT Bio-Robotics, Inc, CA USA) achieved a CE mark in 2014 and FDA approval in 2017.[87] Its double-blinded randomized controlled trials WATER[88] and WATER II[89] showed equivalence with the current Transurethral Resection of the Prostate standard, and subsequent real-world data showed robust evidence of its efficacy and safety.[90] Additionally, it has been incorporated as an option in 30 to 80 mL prostates in clinical care guidelines.[91,92]

The system combines a transrectal ultrasound image map and a saline waterjet (heat-free) for hydroablation of excess tissue under general anesthesia. Its average resection time is less than 5 minutes. The system consists of three primary components: the console, the robotic handpiece, and a single-use probe.

Avicenna Roboflex

The Avicenna Roboflex system (ELMED, Ankara, Turkey) obtained a CE mark in 2013. It consists of a surgeon's console and a manipulator of a flexible ureterorenoscope. The console provides an adjustable seat with armrests and two manipulators of the endoscope: the right wheel enables deflection and the left horizontal joystick allows rotation, as well as advancing and retracting the instrument. As the robot drives the mechanics of the flexible ureterorenoscope, the handpiece of the latter is directly attached to the robot's master plate. Three exchangeable master plates are available for different flexible digital ureteroscopes (Karl Storz Flex X2; Olympus URF-V2; Wolf Cobra digital). The advantages in more fine-tuned control of the endoscope are readily apparent: the range of rotation (210° in each direction = 420°) is beyond human manual capabilities during classical flexible ureterorenoscopy (maximal 120°). In robotic retrograde intrarenal surgery (roboRIRS), 10° of movement with the wheel results in 3° deflection of the tip compared with 60° on manual control. The Roboflex has a memory function for easier advancement of the scope after straightening it for laser fiber insertion.[93]

A multicenter phase 2 trial[94] on 266 patients who underwent roboRIRS showed a 0.7% risk of technical failure and an average operative time of 96 minutes for an average stone load of 1.6 cm^3. The authors attributed the inclusion of relatively larger stones—an expansion of the RIRS indication—to the efficiency and ease of use of the manipulator. In a phase 3 randomized trial[95] of 132 patients, comparing standard flexible ureteroscopy to roboRIRS, the stone-free rate after 3 months was 89.4% and 92.4%, respectively; however, no *P*-values were computed for the study.

TURBot

The TURBot (Vanderbilt University, TN, USA) is a miniature multibackbone continuum robot that works as a telemanipulator in a master–slave fashion. It allows deployment of graspers, custom flexible cameras, and other imaging probes through its three 18-mm working channels. The TURBot is telemanipulated by a seven degree of freedom haptic device (Omega.7, Force Dimension). The foot pedal is used to switch control from the master device to the distal laser arm.

For its preclinical study in a porcine model, a custom-made resectoscope with an eternal 3/8″ sheath and 3-mm endoscope was used. The study found that the robot had the ability to reach all regions of the bladder using retroflexion and extension maneuvers, even the bladder neck. Some difficulties included that the distal laser arm had only two degrees of freedoms and that the grasper did not have robotic articulation.[96,97] In a 2020 study, a human bladder phantom model was used to conduct further improvements on the robot.

One discontinued robotic project for endoscopic urology surgery is the Sensei-Magellan (Hansen Medical, Mountain View, CA, USA).[93] The device was primarily designed for interventional radiology and cardiology procedures and is still in use in those indications. Another machine for which preclinical studies are forthcoming is an MRI-guided telemanipulator for percutaneous procedures (Harvard, MA, USA). This was presented in a study by Su and colleagues98 featuring a surgical master–slave device under continuous MRI guidance. The slave is a robot with six degrees of freedom for needle placement with a haptic sensor. It aims to reduce procedural time and ensure accuracy in percutaneous accesses.[98]

FUTURE DIRECTIONS

Haptic Feedback

Although it is intuitive that the widespread development of robotic and minimally invasive technologies should have brought about equal innovation in vision and tactile technology, the haptic sense has largely been trailing in advancement. For the surgeon, haptic information is created in a haptic feedback loop termed the perception–action cycle by first gleaning information from his environment (eg, by means of palpation) and acting on these characteristics (eg, by repositioning his tools). The challenge is to seamlessly integrate it into robotic surgical devices with kinematic precision (the instruments should move to the surgeon's commands accurately), kinetic fidelity (haptic information should be measured and rendered to minimize distortion when perceived by the user), and minimal temporal lags (specifically transport delays in the robotic system, which occur at mechanical interfaces and in electronic communications).[41]

In current systems, a better term is "haptic-enabled robotic systems", which is defined as systems that enable access to the information normally made available through haptics.[41] This is to say that haptic feedback is most often achieved through sensory substitution: examples are visual excessive force alerts, vibration alerts, color markings overlay, and warning sounds.[2] Several systems discussed earlier already incorporate these haptic substitutions in current models.

Enhanced Visual Feedback

Currently, the da Vinci Firefly technology (Intuitive Surgical, Sunnyvale, CA, USA) enables activation of an injected indocyanine green fluorescent dye from the surgeon console to visualize blood vessels. The widespread use of this technology has enabled more meticulous partial nephrectomy and pelvic lymph node dissection for prostate cancer.[99] Several other innovative uses are microdissection of testicular and vessels for chronic orchialgia[100]; inguinal lymphadenectomy with a partial penectomy[101]; prevention of digestive fistulas and ureteral strictures in ileal neobladders[102]; and exceptional detection of lymph nodes in combination with a gamma probe for prostate cancer.[103]

Tissue-specific fluorescent-tagged antibodies (fluorophobes) can target specific tumor cells and help surgeons visualize cancer in real time. Microscopic light-emitting diode sensors may provide information on tissue oxygen levels and whether an increased tissue force is causing tissue ischemia.[2]

Microrobotics

The interest in miniaturization has always been present in medicine and surgery. This is evident in the shift from open to endoscopic surgery, laparoscopic to natural orifice surgery, and multiport to single-port surgery. Several robots discussed earlier feature a light weight and portability. Moreover, research for smaller devices is driven by concerns about the costs of infrastructure, housing, sterility, and maintenance of numerous working parts of these devices. In a 2009 study, Joseph and colleagues[104] tested two joystick-controlled microrobotic cameras (1.5 × 7.5 cm) to assist in prostatectomy and nephrectomy in canine models. One prototype had cylindrical wheels to navigate to target locations in the abdominal cavity. The two procedures were completed successfully with a standard endoscope as a failsafe.[104]

At the forefront of microrobotic surgery are ophthalmology and vascular surgery. The OctoMag, developed by Kummer and colleagues,[105] uses an external electromagnetic field to operate an untethered microrobot with 5 degrees of freedom deployed into the vitreal space. Preclinical studies in porcine and lapine models have also been conducted on this microrobot.[106]

In vascular surgery, a magnetically actuated soft microrobotic system has been developed to increase the steerability of a conventional guidewire within the human body. The robot is attached to the tip of a guidewire and controlled by an external magnetic field. In vitro studies in a 3D coronary artery phantom have been completed using this system.[107] These models could pave the way for creating more precise ureteral- or calyceal-maneuvering systems for stone and tumor management.

Truly Autonomous Surgical Robotics

In 2008, the Robotic Consensus Group stated that a more accurate term for robotic technology was "remote telepresence manipulators" as available technology back then "[did] not generally function without the explicit and direct control of a human robot." As technology clearly has caught up with this definition, telemanipulators are relegated to one type of robot only, and developments on robotic autonomy and artificial intelligence have paved the way for a new outlook. Instead of the highest degree of automation, flexible automation is the aim.[108]

A more detailed discussion on artificial intelligence in urology can be found in the succeeding articles. Notably, real-life applications of artificial intelligence are far from the walking-and-talking robots depicted in popular culture. Most systems harness a large amount of data and integrate it into algorithms that are used for problem solving. Artificial intelligence can run the gamut of health care solutions, from diagnosis (cancer detection, genomic analysis) and staging (imaging interpretation) to histopathologic analysis and molecular-targeted treatment.

One example of a system that combines artificial intelligence and robotics is composed of a dual-arm collaborative robot (YuMi) and a wearable motion capture device that assists patients with dementia in movement and activities of daily living using motion tracking algorithms.[109]

Although various issues surround it, ethics is central to the discussion on autonomy. Many studies have explored autonomy in individual surgeon tasks such as suturing. These studies aim to increase accuracy or increase speed and efficiency. With the rapid growth in robotic autonomy and research that continues to push the envelope, the role of surgeons in the operating room is being reimagined. Although, at first glance, it may seem that the surgeon's role is relegated to machine operator, the surgeon's role may likely expand to include both the design and operation of these new novel systems.

CLINICS CARE POINTS

- Various robotic telemanipulator systems aid in enhancing surgical dexterity and efficiency. Each system has its own capability, peculiarity, and cost. Surgeons must especially be mindful of the risk-benefit ratio of a procedure when recommending robotic-assisted surgeries in their patients.
- Credentialing and certification of surgeons is integral to the standardization of surgical outcomes. As robotic surgery is in its infancy, more studies are needed to prove system equivalence, and to optimize the robot's integration into urologic training programs.

DISCLOSURE

The authors have nothing to disclose.

REFERENCES

1. Bowersox IC, Shah A, Jensen J, et al. Vascular applications of telepresence surgery: Initial feasibility studies in swine. J Vasc Surg 1996;23(2):281–7.

2. Ganapathi HP, Ogaya-pinies G, Rogers T, et al. Operative atlas of laparoscopic and robotic reconstructive urology. Oper Atlas Laparosc Robot Reconstr Urol 2017;3–11. https://doi.org/10.1007/978-3-319-33231-4.
3. Dario P, Hannaford B, Menciassi A. Smart surgical tools and augmenting devices. IEEE Trans Robot Autom 2003;19(5):782–92.
4. Davies BL, Hibberd RD, Coptcoat MJ, et al. A surgeon robot prostatectomy-a laboratory evaluation. J Med Eng Technol 1989;13(6):273–7.
5. Sackier JM, Wang Y. Surgical endoscopy from concept to development. Surg Endosc 1994;8(8):63–6.
6. Jacobs LK, Shayani V, Sackier JM. Determination of the learning curve of the AESOP robot. Surg Endosc 1997;11(1):54–5.
7. Unger S, Unger H, Bass R. Aesop robotic arm. Surg Endosc 1994;8:1131.
8. Schurr MO, Buess G, Neisius B, et al. Robotics and telemanipulation technologies for endoscopic surgery: A review of the ARTEMIS project. Surg Endosc 2000;14(4):375–81.
9. Herron DM, Marohn M, Advincula A, et al. A consensus document on robotic surgery. Surg Endosc Other Interv Tech 2008;22(2):313–25.
10. Schleer P, Drobinsky S, de la Fuente M, et al. Toward versatile cooperative surgical robotics: a review and future challenges. Int J Comput Assist Radiol Surg 2019;14(10):1673–86.
11. Rosen J, Brown JD, Chang L, et al. The blueDRAGON - A system for measuring the kinematics and the dynamics of minimally invasive surgical tools in-vivo. Proc IEEE Int Conf Robot Autom 2002;2:1876–81. https://doi.org/10.1109/robot.2002.1014814.
12. Yang S. Handheld micromanipulator for robot-assisted microsurgery [Dissertation]. Robotic Institute, Carnegie Mellon University. 2015.
13. Ang WT, Riviere CN, Khosla PK. Design and implementation of active error canceling in hand-held microsurgical instrument. IEEE Int Conf Intell Robot Syst 2001;2:1106–11.
14. Wagner A, Pott PP, Schwarz ML, et al. Control of a handheld robot for orthopedic surgery. IFAC Proc Vol 2004;37(14):477–82.
15. Jakopec M, Harris SJ, Rodriguez y Baena F, et al. The Acrobot® system for total knee replacement. Ind Robot An Int J 2003;30:61–6.
16. Hagag B, Abovitz R, Kang H, et al. RIO: robotic-arm interactive orthopedic system MAKOplasty: user interactive haptic orthopedic robotics. In: Rosen J, Hannaford B, Satava RM, editors. Surgical robotics. Boston: Springer; 2011. p. 219–46.
17. Taylor R, Jensen P, Whitcomb L, et al. A steady-hand robotic system for microsurgical augmentation. Int J Rob Res 1999;18:1201–10.
18. MYNUTIA. Available at: http://www.mynutia.com/. Accessed May 2, 2021.
19. Schneider O, Troccaz J. A six-degree-of-freedom passive arm with dynamic constraints (PADyC) for cardiac surgery appli- cation: preliminary experiments. Comput Aided Surg 2001;6:340–51.
20. Surgeons | medtech. Available at: http://www.medtech.fr/en/surgeons. Accessed May 2, 2021.
21. Davies B, Starkie S, Harris SJ, et al. Neurobot: a special-purpose robot for neurosurgery. In: Proceedings. ICRA'00. IEEE international conference on robotics and automation, 2000. New York: IEEE; 2000. p. 4103–8.
22. Maurice MJ, Ramirez D, Kaouk JH. Robotic laparoendoscopic single- site retroperitoneal renal surgery: initial investigation of a purpose- built single-port surgical system. Eur Urol 2017;71:643–7.
23. Ramirez D, Maurice MJ, Kaouk JH. Robotic perineal radical prostatectomyandpelvic lymphnodedissectionusingapurpose- built single-port robotic platform. BJU Int 2016;118:829–33.
24. Maurice MJ, Kaouk JH. Robotic radical perineal cystectomy and extended pelvic lymphadenectomy: initial investigation using a purpose-built single-port robotic system. BJU Int 2017;120:881–4.
25. Kaouk JH, Sagalovich D, Garisto J. Robot-assisted transvesical partial prostatectomy using a purpose-built single-port robotic system. BJU Int 2018;122:520–4.
26. Moschovas MC, Bhat S, Sandri M, et al. Comparing the approach to radical prostatectomy using the multiport da Vinci Xi and da Vinci SP robots: A propensity score analysis of perioperative outcomes. Eur Urol 2021;79(3):393–404.
27. Vigneswaran HT, Schwarzman LS, Francavilla S, et al. A comparison of perioperative outcomes between single-port and multiport robot-assisted laparoscopic prostatectomy. Eur Urol 2020;77(6):671–4.
28. Intutive surgical 2020 Annual Report. Available at: https://www.annualreports.com/HostedData/AnnualReports/PDF/NASDAQ_ISRG_2020.pdf. Accessed May 1, 2021.
29. Avatera. Available at: https://www.avatera.eu/avatera-system. Accessed May 5, 2021.
30. Evaluate news article. Available at: https://www.evaluate.com/vantage/articles/interviews/avatera-medical-becomes-newest-robotic-surgery-group-europe. Accessed May 5, 2021.
31. Sysmex website. Available at: http://sysmex.co.jp. Accessed May 2, 2021.
32. Medicaroid. Available at: https://www.medicaroid.com/en/product/hinotori/. Accessed May 2, 2021.
33. Revo Surgical website. Available at: http://revosurgical.com. Accessed June 22, 2021.

34. Abdel Raheem A, Troya IS, Kim DK, et al. Robot-assisted Fallopian tube transection and anastomosis using the new REVO-I robotic surgical system: feasibility in a chronic porcine model. BJU Int 2016; 118(4):604–9.
35. Kang CM, Chong JU, Lim JH, et al. Robotic cholecystectomy using the newly developed korean robotic surgical system, Revo-i: A preclinical experiment in a porcine model. Yonsei Med J 2017;58(5):1075–7.
36. Kang I, Hwang HK, Lee WJ, et al. First experience of pancreaticoduodenectomy using Revo-i in a patient with insulinoma. Ann Hepato-biliary-pancreatic Surg 2020;24(1):104.
37. Lim JH, Lee WJ, Park DW, et al. Robotic cholecystectomy using Revo-i Model MSR-5000, the newly developed Korean robotic surgical system: a preclinical study. Surg Endosc 2017;31(8):3391–7.
38. Chang KD, Abdel Raheem A, Choi YD, et al. Retzius-sparing robot-assisted radical prostatectomy using the Revo-i robotic surgical system: surgical technique and results of the first human trial. BJU Int 2018; 122(3):441–8. https://doi.org/10.1111/bju.14245.
39. Korea Accelerating Healthcare Cooperation with Central Asian Countries. Korea Ministry of Health and Welfare website. 2019. Available at: http://www.mohw.go.kr/eng/nw/nw0101vw.jsp?PAR_MENU_ID=1007&MENU_ID=100701&page=6&CONT_SEQ=349164. Accessed February 21, 2021.
40. Senhance. Available at: https://www.senhance.com/us/home. Accessed June 22, 2021.
41. Culmer P, Alazmani A, Mushtaq F, et al. Haptics in surgical robots. Amsterdam: Elsevier Inc; 2020. https://doi.org/10.1016/b978-0-12-814245-5.00015-3.
42. deBeche-Adams T, Eubanks WS, de la Fuente SG. Early experience with the Senhance®-laparoscopic/robotic platform in the US. J Robot Surg 2019;13(2):357–9.
43. Falavolti C, Gidaro S, Ruiz E, et al. Experimental nephrectomies using a novel telesurgical system: (The Telelap ALF-X)-A pilot study. Surg Technol Int 2014;25:37–41.
44. Gidaro S, Buscarini M, Ruiz E, et al. Telelap Alf-X: a novel telesurgical system for the 21st century. Surg Technol Int 2012;22(4):20–5.
45. Samalavicius NE, Janusonis V, Siaulys R, et al. Robotic surgery using Senhance® robotic platform: single center experience with first 100 cases. J Robot Surg 2020;14(2):371–6.
46. Kastelan Z, Knežević N, Hudolin T, et al. Extraperitoneal radical prostatectomy with the Senhance Surgical System robotic platform. Croat Med J 2019;60(6):556–7.
47. Kastelan Z, Hudolin T, Kulis T, et al. Upper urinary tract surgery and radical prostatectomy with Senhance ® robotic system: Single center experience—First 100 cases. Int J Med Robot 2021;17(4):e2269.
48. Hutchins AR, Manson RJ, Lerebours R, et al. Objective assessment of the early stages of the learning curve for the senhance surgical robotic system. J Surg Educ 2019;76(1):201–14.
49. CMR Surgical. Available at: https://cmrsurgical.com/versius. Accessed June 22, 2021.
50. Hares L, Roberts P, Marshall K, et al. Using end-user feedback to optimize the design of the Versius Surgical System, a new robot-assisted device for use in minimal access surgery. BMJ Surg Interv Heal Technol 2019;1(1):e000019.
51. Thomas BC, Slack M, Hussain M, et al. Preclinical evaluation of the Versius Surgical System, a new robot-assisted surgical device for use in minimal access renal and prostate surgery. Eur Urol Focus 2021;7(2):444–52.
52. Huddy JR, Crockett M, Nizar AS, et al. Experiences of a "COVID protected" robotic surgical centre for colorectal and urological cancer in the COVID-19 pandemic. J Robot Surg 2021;(0123456789). https://doi.org/10.1007/s11701-021-01199-3.
53. Atallah S, Parra-Davila E, Melani AGF. Assessment of the versius surgical robotic system for dual-field synchronous transanal total mesorectal excision (taTME) in a preclinical model: will tomorrow's surgical robots promise newfound options? Tech Coloproctol 2019;23(5):471–7.
54. Hoeckelmann M, Rudas IJ, Fiorini P, et al. Current capabilities and development potential in surgical robotics. Int J Adv Robot Syst 2015;12. https://doi.org/10.5772/60133.
55. Surgica Robotica—Medical Technology Solutions. Available at: http://www.surgicarobotica.com/. Accessed May 2, 2021.
56. Available at: https://www.businesswire.com/news/home/20201230005089/en/Titan-Medical-Provides-Regulatory-Update. Accessed May 8, 2021.
57. Titan Enos Website. Available at: https://titanmedicalinc.com/enos/. Accessed May 2, 2021.
58. Seeliger B, Diana M, Ruurda JP, et al. Enabling single-site laparoscopy: the SPORT platform. Surg Endosc 2019;33(11):3696–703.
59. Vanderbilt. Available at: https://engineering.vanderbilt.edu/news/2018/getting-robotic-surgical-tools-from-the-lab-to-the-operating-room/. Accessed May 8, 2021.
60. Medtronic Form8k (Public document). Available at: https://www.sec.gov/ix?doc=/Archives/edgar/data/1613103/000161310319000042/item701ras8k.htm. Accessed May 5, 2021.
61. Medtronic website. Available at: https://www.medtronic.com/covidien/en-us/robotic-assisted-surgery/hugo-ras-system.html. Accessed June 22, 2021.

62. Mira Website. Available at: https://www.mira-project.org/joomla-mira/. Accessed May 2, 2021.
63. Lehman AC, Wood NA, Farritor S, et al. Dexterous miniature robot for advanced minimally invasive surgery. Surg Endosc 2011;25(1):119–23.
64. Wortman TD, Mondry JM, Farritor SM, et al. Single-site colectomy with miniature in vivo robotic platform. IEEE Trans Biomed Eng 2013;60(4):926–9.
65. Hagn UA, Fröhlich FA, Le-tien L, et al. MiroSurge — Advanced user interaction modalities in minimally invasive robotic. Presence (Camb) 2021;19(5): 400–14.
66. Rassweiler JJ, Goezen AS, Klein J, et al. New robotic platforms. In: Robotic Urology, Third Edition. USA: Springer Publishing, 2018. p. 3–38. https://doi.org/10.1007/978-3-319-65864-3_1.
67. Johnson & Johnson. 2019. Available at: https://www.jnj.com/johnson-johnson-announces-agreement-to-acquire-remaining-stake-in-verb-surgical-inc. Accessed May 7, 2021.
68. Gonzalez GT, Kaur U, Rahman M, et al. From the dexterous surgical skill to the battlefield - A robotics exploratory study. Mil Med 2021;186: 288–94.
69. Kang H, Wen JT. EndoBot: A robotic assistant in minimally invasive surgeries. Proc IEEE Int Conf Robot Autom 2001;2:2031–6.
70. Sánchez A, Poignet P, Dombre E, et al. A design framework for surgical robots: Example of the Araknes robot controller. Rob Auton Syst 2014;62(9): 1342–52.
71. van den Bedem LJM. Realization of a demonstrator slave for robotic minimally invasive surgery. Doctoral degree 22-09- 2010; Department of Mechanical Engineering; Supervisors: M. Steinbuch and I.A.M.J. Broeders; Co-promotor: P.C.J.N. Ros- ielle. Eindhoven: Technische Universiteit Eindhoven; 2010. https://doi.org/10.6100/IR684 835.
72. Kawai T, Shin M, Nishizawa Y, et al. Mobile locally operated detachable end-effector manipulator for endoscopic surgery. Int J Comput Assist Radiol Surg 2015;10(2):161–9.
73. Kawai T, Hayashi H, Nishizawa Y, et al. Compact forceps manipulator with a spherical-coordinate linear and circular telescopic rail mechanism for endoscopic surgery. Int J Comput Assist Radiol Surg 2017;12(8):1345–53.
74. Li Y, Hannaford B, Rosen J. Raven: Open surgical robotic platforms. arXiv 2019;14(12):151–69.
75. Hannaford B, Rosen J, Friedman DW, et al. Raven-II: An open platform for surgical robotics research. IEEE Trans Biomed Eng 2013;60(4):954–9.
76. Despinoy F, Zemiti N, Forestier G, et al. Evaluation of contactless human–machine interface for robotic surgical training. Int J Comput Assist Radiol Surg 2018;13(1):13–24.
77. Forestier G, Petitjean F, Senin P, et al. Surgical motion analysis using discriminative interpretable patterns. Artif Intell Med 2018;91:3–11.
78. Hu D, Gong Y, Hannaford B, et al. Semi-autonomous simulated brain tumor ablation with ravenii surgical robot using behavior tree. IEEE Int Conf Robot Autom 2015;3868–75. https://doi.org/10.1109/ICRA.2015.7139738.Semi-autonomous.
79. Asensus Press Release. 2017. Available at: https://ir.asensus.com/news-releases/news-release-details/transenterix-announces-global-surgibot-system-agreement. Accessed May 8, 2021.
80. Terumo. 2011. Available at: https://www.prnewswire.co.uk/news-releases/terumo-announces-first-clinical-case-of-a-ce-certified-precision-drive-articulating-surgical-system-145276325.html. Accessed May 8, 2021.
81. Sieber MA, Fellmann-Fischer B, Mueller M. Performance of Kymerax© precision-drive articulating surgical system compared to conventional laparoscopic instruments in a pelvitrainer model. Surg Endosc 2017;31(10):4298–308.
82. Aykan S. Extraperitoneal laparoscopic radical prostatectomy with handheld articulating laparoscopic instruments driven by robotic technology. Haydarpasa Numune Train Res Hosp Med J 2018;60(3):314–6.
83. Hruby S, Pann R, Bernecker R, et al. A prospective randomized study of a new articulating laparoscopy device (Kymerax-Terumo) in the dry lab – part 1: Learning curve and objective skills assessment. Eur Urol Suppl 2013;12(1):e22–3.
84. Pérez-Lanzac de Lorca A, Rosety Rodriguez J, Okhunov Z, et al. Robot-assisted laparoendoscopic hybrid single-site radical prostatectomy: A novel technique using kymerax. Videourology 2013;27(5):10–3.
85. Hackethal A, Koppan M, Eskef K, et al. Handheld articulating laparoscopic instruments driven by robotic technology. First clinical experience in gynecological surgery. Gynecol Surg 2012;9(2): 203–6.
86. Iacoponi S, Terán M, De Santiago J, et al. Laparoscopic hysterectomy with a handheld robotic device in a case of uterine sarcoma. Taiwan J Obstet Gynecol 2015;54(1):84–5.
87. NIH Website. Available at: https://www.accessdata.fda.gov/cdrh_docs/reviews/DEN170024.pdf. Accessed May 2, 2021.
88. Gilling P, Barber N, Bidair M, et al. Three-year outcomes after Aquablation therapy compared to TURP: results from a blinded randomized trial. Can J Urol 2020;27(1):10072–9.
89. Desai M, Bidair M, Bhojani N, et al. Aquablation for benign prostatic hyperplasia in large prostates (80-150 cc): 2-year results. Can J Urol 2020;27(2): 10147–53.

90. Bach T, Gilling P, El Hajj A, et al. First multi-center all-comers study for the aquablation procedure. J Clin Med 2020;9(2):603.
91. Mottet N, Bellmunt J, Briers E, et al, members of the EAU – ESTRO – ESUR –SIOG Prostate Cancer Guidelines Panel. EAU – ESTRO – ESUR – SIOG Guidelines on Prostate Cancer. Edn. presented at the EAU Annual Congress Milan. Arnhem, The Netherlands: EAU Guidelines Office; 2021.
92. Parsons JK, Dahm P, Köhler TS, et al. Surgical management of lower urinary tract symptoms attributed to benign prostatic hyperplasia: AUA Guideline amendment 2020. J Urol 2020;204:799.
93. Rassweiler J, Fiedler M, Charalampogiannis N, et al. Robot-assisted flexible ureteroscopy: an update. Urolithiasis 2018;46(1):69–77.
94. Klein J-T, Fiedler M, Kabakci AS, et al. Pd18-08 multicenter phase ii study of the clinical use of the avicenna roboflex urs robot in robotic retrograde intrarenal stone surgery. J Urol 2016; 195(4S):e406–7.
95. Geavlete P, Saglam R, Georgescu D, et al. Robotic flexible ureteroscopy versus classic flexible ureteroscopy in renal stones: The initial Romanian experience. Chir 2016;111(4):326–9.
96. Sarli N, Del Giudice G, De S, et al. Preliminary porcine in vivo evaluation of a telerobotic system for transurethral bladder tumor resection and surveillance. J Endourol 2018;32(6):516–22.
97. Sarli N, Del Giudice G, De S, et al. TURBot: A system for robot-assisted transurethral bladder tumor resection. IEEE ASME Trans Mechatron 2020; 24(4):1452–63.
98. Su H, Shang W, Li G, et al. An MRI-guided telesurgery system using a fabry-perot interferometry force sensor and a pneumatic haptic device. Ann Biomed Eng 2017;45(8):1917–28.
99. Wu Y, Jing J, Wang J, et al. Robotic-assisted sentinel lymph node mapping with indocyanine green in pelvic malignancies: A systematic review and meta-analysis. Front Oncol 2019;9:1–8.
100. Goedde MA, Nguyen KD, Choi KB. Robotic microsurgical spermatic cord denervation for chronic orchialgia: A case series. J Am Osteopath Assoc 2021;121(1):29–34.
101. Sávio LF, Panizzutti Barboza M, Alameddine M, et al. Combined partial penectomy with bilateral robotic inguinal lymphadenectomy using near-infrared fluorescence guidance. Urology 2018; 113:251.
102. Petrut B, Bujoreanu CE, Porav-Hodade D, et al. Indocyanine green use in urology. J BUON 2021; 26(1):266–74.
103. Dell'Oglio P, Meershoek P, Maurer T, et al. A DROP-IN gamma probe for robot-assisted radioguided surgery of lymph nodes during radical prostatectomy. Eur Urol 2021;79(1):124–32.
104. Joseph JV, Oleynikov D, Rentschler M, et al. Microrobot assisted laparoscopic urological surgery in a canine model. J Urol 2008;180(5):2202–5.
105. Kummer MP, Abbott JJ, Kratochvil BE, et al. Octomag: An electromagnetic system for 5-DOF wireless micromanipulation. IEEE Trans Robot 2010; 26(6):1006–17.
106. Ullrich F, Bergeles C, Pokki J, et al. Mobility experiments with microrobots for minimally invasive intraocular surgery. Investig Ophthalmol Vis Sci 2013; 54(4):2853–63.
107. Jeon S, Hoshiar AK, Kim K, et al. A magnetically controlled soft microrobot steering a guidewire in a three-dimensional phantom vascular network. Soft Robot 2019;6(1):54–68.
108. Spath D, Braun M, Bauer W. Integrated human and automation systems. In: Nof SY, editor. Springer handbook of automation. Berlin, Heidelberg: Springer; 2009. p. 571–98.
109. Honghao LV, Yang G, Zhou H, et al. Teleoperation of collaborative robot for remote dementia care in home environments. IEEE J Transl Eng Heal Med 2020;8. https://doi.org/10.1109/JTEHM.2020.3002384.

A Call for Change. Can 3D Printing Replace Cadavers for Surgical Training?

Ahmed Ghazi, MD, FEBU, MHPE

KEYWORDS

• Simulation • Cadaver training • 3D printing • Physical reality • Hydrogel casting
• Minimal invasive surgery

KEY POINTS

- Cadavers have long been the gold standard of procedural surgical simulation.
- Advances in 3D printing technologies have led to the fabrication of high-fedility anatomical replicas but lack tissue consistency.
- By combining 3D printing and hydrogel casting we have successful fabricated a surgical rehearsal platform that enables the surgeon to experience all aspects of the procedure with tissue realism and anatomical accuracy.
- Objective and clinically relevant metrics incorporated into the model (e.g. Estimated blood loss and Positive tumor margins) have improved the educational impact of these models.
- Future directions include fabrication of patient specific surgical rehearsal platforms and applications for remote feedback and proctoring.

INTRODUCTION

According to the Oxford dictionary simulation has been defined as "A situation in which a particular set of conditions is created artificially to study or experience something that could exist in reality."[1] Health care simulations are centered around education, assessment, and research which can be achieved by some combination of low- and high-tech tools and a variety of settings from tabletop models to a realistic full-mission environment to provide a safe and supportive educational climate.[2] Skill acquisition solely from operating room experience is no longer sufficient for training given recent duty hour restrictions, amplified surgical training programs, increased surgical procedure complexity, limited operating room time, and increased medical litigation.[3] To compensate for this, regulatory bodies such as the Accreditation Council for Graduate Medical Education (ACGME) require surgical programs to provide simulation and skills laboratories to fulfill these needs.[4]

THE PAST OF PROCEDURAL SIMULATION IN UROLOGY

Since the birth of surgery, human cadavers have been used as models of anatomic training, experimentation, and to test new procedures. Cadavers have definitely stood up to the test of time even with increased regulation of their use and elevated costs.[5] In urology, the rapid advancement of laparoscopic and endoscopic technologies as well as increase in procedure complexity has led to the dissemination of virtual reality simulators as effective training tools.[6,7] However, these expensive tools remain limited to the initial phase of training, and significant progress is needed to address rapidly developing advanced skill acquisition required to enhance operating room (OR) performance.[8]

Advanced procedural simulation can be classified broadly into two categories: biological models (ex vivo and in vivo) and synthetic models. The greatest limitation of in vivo biological models (eg, porcine and canine models) is their relevant

Urology department, University of Rochester, 158 Sawgrass Drive, Rochester, NY 14642, USA
E-mail address: ahmed_ghazi@urmc.rochester.edu

Urol Clin N Am 49 (2022) 39–56
https://doi.org/10.1016/j.ucl.2021.08.001
0094-0143/22/

anatomic differences and difficulty in extrapolating the findings to humans. Generally, few proposed animal models have sufficient procedural similarity to a human model to be effective in achieving competency.[9] Furthermore, the ethical dilemma of animal studies and costs associated with extended veterinary care (before, during, and after the procedure) constitute major drawbacks.[10,11] Human cadavers (ex vivo biological models) remain undoubtedly the most reliable and realistic version in reducing the learning curve of procedures, improving patient safety, and experimenting with new surgical techniques.[12] However, to be relevant for surgical training, cadavers used should, as much as possible, maintain the natural color, texture, and flexibility of the living body which directly is dependent on their method of preservation. The three most common types of preservation are fresh frozen cadavers, Thiel's embalming method (TEM), and formalin-fixed cadavers.

While fresh frozen cadavers exhibit the most lifelike features, they require freezer storage facilities, have limited lifespan because of rapid putrefaction, exhibit infection hazards, and are in limited supply.[13] They are considered the most expensive with very high initial and running costs. Formalin-fixed cadavers can be kept at room temperature for years at very low cost, making it one of the preferred methods of embalming in research and anatomy training.[14] However, formaldehyde fixation leads to unnatural stiffness, coloring, and abnormal echogenicity limiting its usefulness for surgical practice.[15] Moreover, health hazards including irritation to skin and mucosa as well as carcinogenic properties from the vapors require additional precautions in the form of adequate covering and sophisticated ventilation systems.[16] TEM-prepared cadavers were specifically devised to include long-term structural preservation of organs in natural, fresh consistency, texture, color, and echogenicity of organs. TEM-prepared cadavers are sterile and do not release toxic or irritant vapors, thus minimizing the risk during handling of the specimens and the setup of the training activities,[14] making it more cost-effective than fresh frozen cadavers in the long run. Drawbacks include poor histologic quality, technically difficult, more time for embalming process, and inability to perfuse due to increased permeability of vessels.

Both expert and trainee surgeons agree that cadaveric simulation remains the "gold standard" for realistic procedural simulation despite their limited availability, high cost, and lack of specific pathology (eg, renal tumor), which is crucial to achieving advanced surgical proficiency.[17–19] However, the use of human cadavers has historically been and, in many ways, may remain controversial.[20] The right to a burial is a basic human right, and some may consider the use of cadavers for teaching purposes as a deprivation of that right. In fact, dissection of human cadavers has been characterized as an insult to the dead and the ultimate violation of a person's privacy.[21] Consequently, emerging technologies such as image reconstruction from medical images and 3D printing for the creation of customizable models, with the possibility to add increased functionality features (eg, color coding of vital structures, bleeding, and metrics for measuring performance), have been explored to revolutionize surgical training and help equate synthetic models to cadavers.[22]

THE PRESENT STATUS OF PROCEDURAL SIMULATION IN UROLOGY

3D Printing and Organ Modeling

Multiple centers have applied 3D printing to create physical models designed from patients' imaging to be used by the treating team for preoperative planning.[23–26] While the current practice is adequate for surgical planning, none of the available printed polymers have the ability to reproduce tissue properties permitting dissection, hemostasi,s and suturing. The Simulation Innovation Laboratory (SIL) at the Department of Urology, University of Rochester Medical Center, has developed a cost-effective technique using image segmentation, 3D printing technology, and polymer molding in creating an immersive, procedural simulation platform for the surgical rehearsal of a challenging urologic procedures. A molding technique allows different materials replicating the various mechanical properties of human tissue to be layered into a single model. For full immersion, the fabrication process also incorporated all steps of the procedure by the addition of surrounding organs and reproducing genuine operative metrics of performance (blood loss, tumor margins, ischemia time, urine leak, and the potential for complications) enabling practicing surgeons to obtain feedback and track performance. These features which we have collective referred to as "physical reality" set our approach apart from any other simulation platforms that create realistic models to be used in training of complex urologic procedures.

Fabrication of Hydrogel-Based Simulation Procedural Platforms

Construction of the organ phantoms

Polyvinyl alcohol (PVA) was used as it is a biocompatible and inexpensive hydrogel that can be adapted to mimic human tissue properties.[27] PVA can be altered to replicate the variable mechanical properties of different tissues such as tissue parenchyma, blood vessels, tumors, and fat by varying PVA concentration and number of processing (freeze/thaw) cycles that form polymeric bonds. The freezing/thawing cycle is completed at varying times depending on the object's size. PVA's phase change property is also critical for our fabrication process as the induction of cross-links through successive freeze/thaw cycles polymerizes it from an injectable gel into a progressively stiffer soild, with a texture that upholds its shape. To configure this PVA hydrogel into the geometry of a patient's specific anatomy, a combination of additive and subtractive methods is used.

If the model was obtained from exisiting patients' axial imaging, DICOM files are imported into Mimics 20.0 (Mimics, Materialise, Belgium) for segmentation. Segmentation is completed for each component of the patient's relevant anatomy and pathology (eg, in case of partial nephrectomy model, the kidney, including parenchyma, tumor, inferior vena cava and renal vein, abdominal aorta and renal artery, and urinary drainage system, is segmented) (**Fig. 1**A). Specific software tools such as thresholding, region growing tools, and multiple slide edit are used to increase the accuracy of the segmentation for noncontrasted structures. Each component was then converted to a 3D mesh and imported into 3-matic 12.0 (Mimics, Materialise, Belgium) to form a computer-aided design (CAD) model of the patient's anatomy (**Fig. 1**B). To recreate the functional aspects of the simulation model using PVA hydrogel, the CAD model is then converted into injection molds. An injection mold in its simplest form is designed by surrounding each CAD structure with a box, and using the Boolean difference operation, a cavity of the same shape is formed (**Fig. 1**C). PVA injected into these molds would retain the cavity geometry representative of the patient's anatomy. The number of molds 3D printed in a hard plastic depends on the model created for robot-assisted partial nephrectomy (RAPN); the three main injection molds are of the tumor, kidney, and renal hilum (**Fig. 1**D).

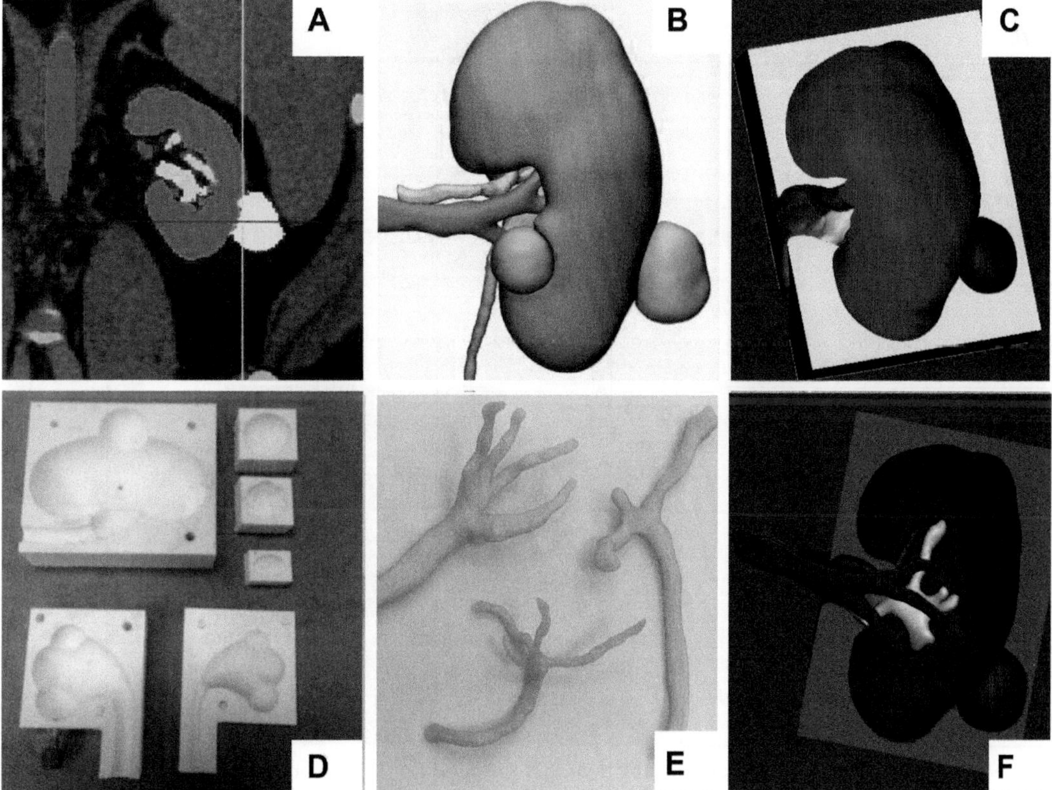

Fig. 1. Process for fabrication of robotic partial nephrectomy simulation using 3D printing and hydrogel molding. (*A*) Segmentation of patient's DICOM images; (*B*) smoothing of the mesh in 3-matic to generate a CAD; (*C*) Boolean subtraction of the CAD; (*D*) kidney, tumor, and hilum injection molds printed in PLA; (*E*) arterial, venous, and pelivcaliceal structures printed in dissolvable PVA; (*F*) registration of tumor, hollow vasculature and urine systems in the kidney mold.

To incorporate the functionalilty of the simulation platform, that is, bleeding and urine leakage in the kidney model, the hilar structures (arterial, venous, and calyx urinary systems) are printed using dissolvable PVA filaments using a Flashforge Creator Pro (Flashforge 3D technology Co; Zhejiang, China) and coated with processed PVA (**Fig. 1**E). Once the layers are solidified, the inner PVA filament is dissolved in water to create a hollow, watertight vascular and urinary system. All these structures are then registered into the primary mold and surrounded by fat. The kidney injection mold will form the kidney, encasing the preformed tumor and hilum to form a single entity (**Fig. 1**F). Each mold is injected with PVA previously tested to duplicate the mechanical properties of human kidneys as described in the following sections. The result is a simulated kidney that matches the patient anatomy.

Validation of models' mechanical properties

Our refined process of creating kidney phantoms in which each kidney component is fabricated separately within injection molds allows alterations in PVA formulations (varying PVA concentration, the number of freeze/thaw cycles [that form polymeric bonds], and fortification with other materials that can replicate the variable mechanical properties of different tissue densities) and can be individually injected into each layer.[27] Our mechanical validation was guided by studies demonstrating that porcine kidneys can be used as human surrogates.[28–30] For kidney testing, three tests were completed (**Fig. 2**A–C): (1) an unconfined uniaxial compression test that involves exerting a compressive force on a sample between two smooth platens and investigating the stress-strain behavior of the material, (2) indentation testing is a nondestructive method where an indentor is pressed into the sample and the resulting forces are measured, and (3) elastography that involves the use of ultrasound methods to measure the speed of shear waves through a sample. Functionally, the model is designed to recreate the effects of bleeding and suturing, and thus, customized testing methods were established to

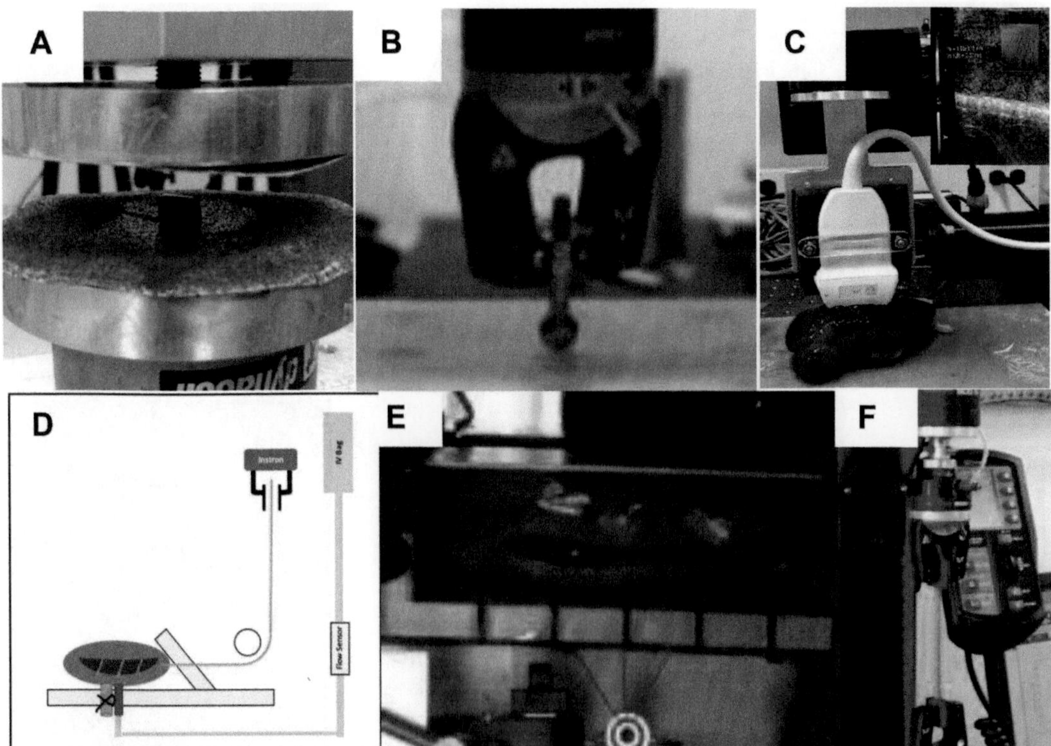

Fig. 2. Validation of mechanical properties of hydrogel formulation. (*A*) Unconfined compression testing, (*B*) indention testing, (*C*) ultrasound elastography testing, (*D*) graphic illustration of perfusion testing setup. Simulated blood is flowing though the catheter secured in the artery, and suture is secured to Instron testing instrument to apply the force to the suture (*red arrow*). (*E*) Renorrhaphy rip testing setup. A 3D-printed support tray with vertical slits to allow passage of the sutures, b visual cooptation of the renal capsule during testing of porcine kidney up to violation of clips through the edge of the renal capsule, (*F*) uniaxial stretch testing of the hydrogel and living renal vasculature.

study the flow of blood through both porcine and PVA kidneys with the aim to analyze their responses to the two types of suturing techniques used for closure of the parenchymal defect during an RAPN. These tests measured the tension applied to the first layer of running sutures required to achieve hemostasis and the tension applied to the second layer of parenchymal sutures for approximation of the parenchymal edges before tearing occurs in both an ex vivo porcine and the PVA kidney models during a simulated perfusion at 120 mm Hg (**Fig. 2**D, E). Our published results demonstrated that PVA kidneys, fabricated using 7% PVA at three freeze-thaw cycles, closely approximated the mechanical and functional properties of live kidney tissue.[31] Furthermore, artery and vein testing by uniaxial tension test (stretched up to a strain of 30% at a rate of 10 mm/min) was used to compare remnant iliac vessels from four liver transplantation operations to various PVA samples (**Fig. 2**F).

Development of procedural simulation platform (RAPN)

To recreate the entire operative experience, a full procedural rehearsal platform of the hydrogel kidney, surrounding musculature, peritoneum, fat, and any other pertinent organs defined by patient anatomy was fabricated (**Fig. 3**A). The rest of the relevant structures of the abdomen are constructed via the same process described to form the kidney. Correct anatomic layers were recreated starting with the posterior abdominal musculature, then the kidney, peritoneum, fat, mesentery, bowel, and liver or spleen were added one at a time within a custom pelvic trainer and exposed to a final processing cycle for organ adhesion (**Fig. 3**B). The trainer is covered in a simulated abdominal wall and rehearsal occurred using the Davinci surgical robot (Intuitive Surgical, Sunnyvale, CA) in a simulated OR environment (**Fig. 3**C). The emphasis was placed on a model incorporating all steps of the procedure including (1) exposure of the tumor-bearing kidney, (2) vascular control of the renal hilum, (3) identification and exposure of the renal mass, (4) excision of the tumor with negative margins, and (5) reconstruction by closure of medullary vascular and collecting system structures avoiding postoperative bleeding and urine leakage (**Fig. 3**D–F). The fabrication process also includes reproducing genuine operative metrics of performance (blood loss, tumor margins, ischemia time, and the potential for complications).

An Educational Design Framework (Simulation Innovation Laboratory Validation Process)

For simulation platforms that are fabricated to replicate the anatomy and pathology of target

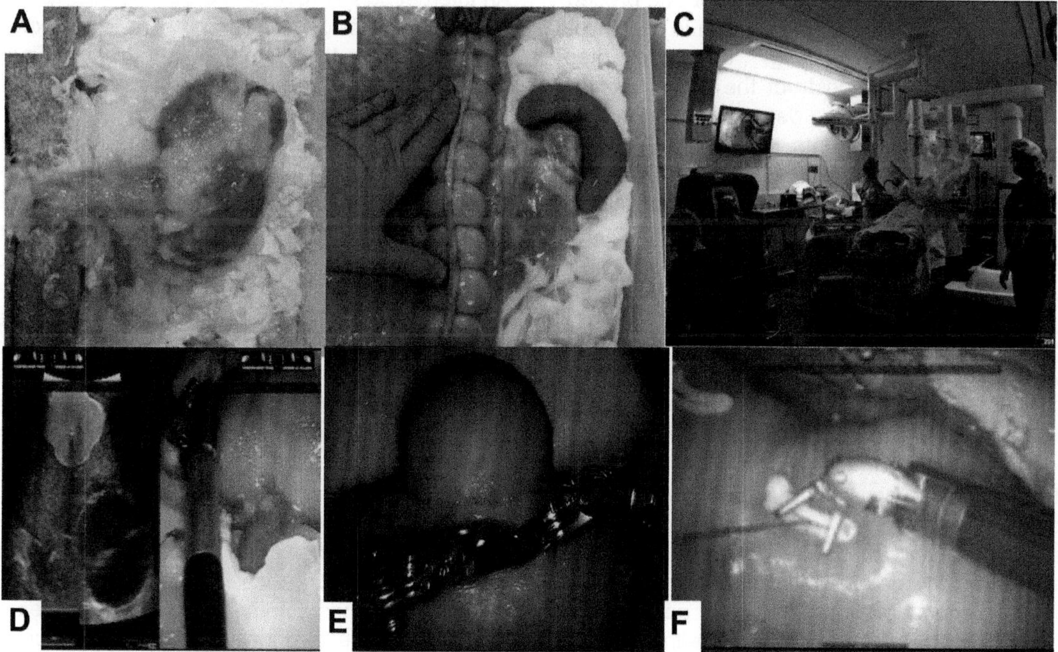

Fig. 3. (*A*) View of the kidney model surrounded by perinephric fat and anatomically placed on posterior abdominal wall muscles, (*B*) final partial nephrectomy trainer surrounded with peritoneum, abdominal fat, spleen, bowel, and mesentery. (*C*) Robot-assisted partial nephrectomy simulation. (*D*) Ultrasound examination of the model. (*E*) Resection of tumor mass with bleeding. (*F*) Renorrhaphy of the renal parenchyma.

organs as for in robot-assisted procedures, axial imaging from an idealized patient or specific patient provides the basis to guide the fabrication process. However, for advanced training models that have inherent complexities and focus on a particular skill set, an educational framework is required to define both relevant and irrelevant elements of the model with the most educational impact (eg, model for a HoLEP procedure would be inherently different from a UroLift model although both contain similar anatomic elements). To develop these, we used a backward design educational framework to identify and reach expert consensus on the essential elements, steps, and potential errors of a procedure for the development of high-fidelity procedural simulation platforms using a combination of 3-dimensional (3D) printing and hydrogel casting technology. This process was conducted in four phases.

Phase 1: delineating model requirements from the physicians' perspective

This first phase uses a hierarchical task analysis (HTA) to detail essential steps required to formulate necessary actions and decisions performed during the surgery.[32] HTA is an objective approach that deconstructs the surgical procedure into a hierarchy of tasks and subtasks, as well as offering the relationship among these tasks.[33] This approach has recently been implemented to outline the procedural steps for a robotic procedures and evaluate its representation in a physical model for simulation training.[34] During this step, expert surgeons deconstruct the procedure into discrete steps while also determining the necessary anatomic components, protocols, surgical instruments, and step-by-step surgical subtasks using a template. They also determine potential errors of commission (action carried out wrongly), omission (action not taken), and execution (action not completed as intended) for the procedure.

Phase 2: translating physicians' requirements to engineering tasks (deliverables)

Clinical perspectives obtained from the HTA are then translated into engineering and design deliverables using 4 criteria (anatomic fidelity, procedural relevance, physiologic fidelity, and methods for error identification) for each core component identified during the HTA. Anatomic fidelity is defined as the detailed anatomic representation of the component within the male genitourinary system. Procedural relevance is defined by the function of the core component in the simulator as it relates to the learning objective. In other words, these 2 criteria encompassed requirements for how the simulator would replicate anatomic structures within the context of procedural relevance: for a HoLEP model, a urethra (into which a scope can be introduced and is watertight), prostatic tissue (appropriate laser-tissue interaction), prostatic capsular plan (that can be bluntly dissected), and a verumontanum (landmark during enucleation). We sought to incorporate physiologic fidelity into the model, defined by the ability to detect potential procedural errors together with their corresponding methods for identification either intraoperatively or postoperatively (eg, perforation of prostatic capsule tested with appearance of yellow fat intraoperatively, residual adenoma, or injury to external sphincter that can be tested postoperatively).

Phase 3: establishing expert consensus

Individual templates from each expert surgeon are then compiled into a single document and put forth to achieve an expert consensus through a Delphi methodology. The Delphi methodology refers to a systematic process of collecting, evaluating, and tabulating expert opinion on a specific topic. The Delphi survey is a group facilitation technique, which is an iterative multistage process, designed to transform opinion into group consensus. A particular benefit of this approach is that it can sample the opinion of a group of experts which can be controlled by appropriate feedback and modification to drive findings toward a group consensus.[35] An internet survey (Google Forms; Google, Mountain View, CA) is generated and sent to an expert surgeon among the members of the panel. Each survey is divided into 4 sections (overall utility of the model, anatomic components of the model, tissue fidelity of various components within the model, and assessment of surgical performance). Panelists indicate their agreement with the proposed criteria in previous phases. Questions in which there was $\geq$80% agreement or disagreement were removed from the next round of the survey. Repeated iterations of anonymous voting continued over three rounds, where an individual's vote in the next round was informed by knowledge of the entire group's results in the previous round. Responders have the option of proposing new credentialing criteria during all rounds. New criteria are added to the following round and were voted upon along with the other questions. To be included in the final list of credentialing criteria, each survey item had to have reached group consensus by the end of the 3 survey rounds. Items that did not reach consensus were excluded from the final recommendations of this article.

During development of a HoLEP model, 250 overall questions addressed aspects to optimize a procedural simulation: overall utility, anatomic and procedural components, tissue fidelity, assessment of performance. A total of 85 out of 250 questions (34%) reached greater than 80% consensus, with 63.5% of these achieving 100% agreement. In summary, to address HoLEP training needs, a simulation-based physical model that was realistic, replicated all crucial procedural steps, and developed using a validated educational approach is required. Essential features of the model included realistic tissue texture, perfused to include a bleeding component, non-biohazardous nature of the model, with embedded objective metrics for performance evaluation, portable, easy to set up (reusable base with a hydrogel insert) (**Fig. 4**A–C). Anatomic components included a hollow bladder (with bladder neck and ureteric orifices), 100-gm prostate adenoma with a clear prostatic capsule, and a watertight urethra with verumontanum and external sphincter to replicate all steps of the procedure. Regarding tissue fidelity, fundamental tissue interactions included anatomic visual cues, laser-tissue interaction, instrument-tissue interaction, bleeding, and hemostasis. Performance metrics included a checklist with eight domains; flow of operation, plane identification, scope handling, blunt dissection, laser dissection and hemostasis, efficiency, autonomy, and morcellation.

Phase 4: development of a model prototype and testing

Prototype design: Based on the consensus reached for HTA requirements and engineering deliverables, a computer-aided design model consisting of all external and internal core structures are digitally rendered (**Fig. 4**D, E). After an iterative review and editing process using expert feedback, the computer-aided design model is transformed into a physical representation using a combination of 3D printing and hydrogel injection casting technologies. Different PVA hydrogel formulations are then injected into each respective cast and processed to achieve the desired properties (see **Fig. 4**C). After processing, each component is removed from its cast and molded in series to replicate the anatomic relationships between various organ components.

Prototype testing An iterative prototyping process was used to optimize the anatomic configuration, tissue fidelity, and procedural relevance of the prototype, while addressing any gaps in these qualities (adaptive testing). A postsimulation autopsy and analysis are conducted during a debriefing session between engineers and expert surgeons to ensure correct functioning of the model, detect any deviation from the established protocols, and establish

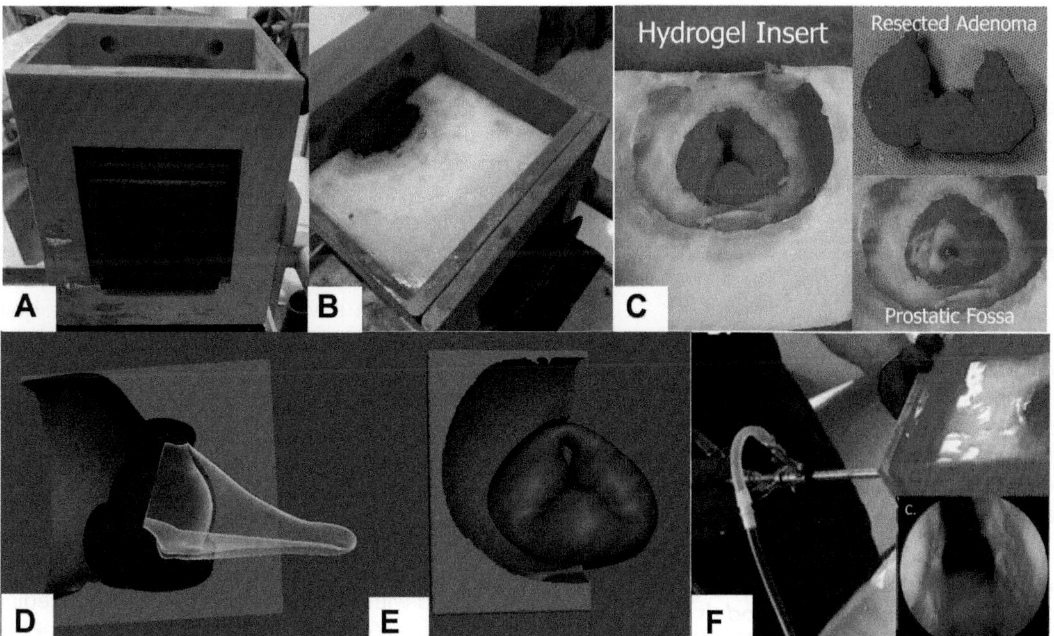

Fig. 4. HoLEP model. (*A*) 3D printed encasing unit for the HoLEP model, with a watertight flexible access. (*B*) Hydrogel insert containing the adenoma, capsule, urethra, and verumontanum. (*C*) Simulation autopsy with surgeons and engineers to debrief aspects of the model. CAD model based on the expert consensus: (*D*) lateral view, (*E*) anteroposterior view, (*F*) full immersion simulation in an operating room with all instruments (lower right insert of endoscopic view).

comparable textures used for realistic tactile element responses (see **Fig. 4**C, upper, lower right).

Over 5 iterations, changes included improved change in size and, in particular median lobe of the adenoma, alterations in the capsular plane to allow for realistic blunt and laser dissection, modification in PVA formulation to improve consistency of adenoma, improvement in the design of resectoscope access to prevent leakage, and integration of a fluid pump system to recycle fluid irrigation. A final full-immersion test was conducted under operating room conditions by a panel expert surgeon (**Fig. 4**F). All simulations used surgical instruments, completed surgical tasks, and protocols identified by the HTA. Questionnaires evaluating the simulation agreement with the HTA, realism, and value as a training tool was performed using a 5-point Likert scale, and all data are collected and stored in a deidentified manner using Research Electronic Data Capture (Nashville, TN). Descriptive statistics is used to analyze measures of central tendency (mean and median) and variability (SD and interquartile range) of data collected.

The HoLEP model fulfilled 78% (63/81) elements and lacked 17% (14/81). Categorically, 82%, 78%, 73%, and 82% were satisfied in overall utility, anatomic and procedural components, tissue fidelity, and assessment of performance, respectively (**Table 1**). The model contained all 9 anatomic components (except for bladder, ureteric orifices, lateral and median lobes, capsule, urethra), 7 objective evaluation metrics (except for injury of ureteric orifices or bladder neck, perforation of the bladder or prostate capsule), and 5 procedural steps except for hemostasis and morcellation. Laser and instrument tissue interactions achieved greater than 85% satisfaction. All experts agreed the model could provide a safe training alternative, be used to evaluate trainee performance, and trial new approaches in a risk-free environment.

This was the first consensus-based approach to design and fabricate a hydrogel HoLEP simulation with incorporated objective evaluation metrics capable of supplementing training. Continuing modifications will mainly include the addition of morcellation and bleeding to prepare for the next validation phase.

Embedded Clinically Relevant Objective Metrics in the Simulation Models

The primary focus for surgical skills simulators is to provide training for a specific tasks or procedure. Over the last decade, this concept of simulators has expanded to also include a means for evaluation of performance. It has been argued that training and assessment are simply two sides of the same coin.[36] Modern surgical simulators must also have the potential to evaluate surgical competence which has potential benefits of improved safety of surgical training processes, enhanced accreditation of specialists, and maintenance of skills.[37,38] Despite cadavers providing an ideal anatomic simulation platform for minimal invasive urologic procedures, the assessment of technical skill using cadavers remains more subjective than objective. Specifically, the Global Evaluative Assessment of Robotic Skills (GEARS)[39] is an assessment method that incorporates rating of multiple domains to calculate an overall score for surgical performance. Despite being considered objective performance metrics, they are in essence subjective measures that still require an expert to judge the performance on a worst to best scale. Owing to this lack of objective measures for assessing operating skills on a cadaver, researchers will have to rely on evaluation by expert surgeons. The use of objective scoring metrics that consider variances in technique between surgeons, rely on clinical relevance, and focus on the end result is preferable.[40]

From design to conception, we incorporated Clinically Relevant Objective Metrics (CROMS) pertinent to the procedure that is being modeled as a means of quantitative method for assessment of surgical performance. Furthermore, we explored the correlation between these proposed metrics and current gold standard metrics that have previously been linked to level of training. The techniques for incorporating these objective metrics into our models are divided into three main categorizes.

Registration of fluid filled structures, for example, blood vessels and urine laden cavities

To incorporate bleeding and urine leakage functionality within several procedural models, both positive and negative casting techniques are used. Vascular and urine-filled structures (hilum vasculature, prostate pedicle, bladder, pelvicalyceal system) are fabricated as previously described resulting in hollow arterial, venous, and urinary structures. Watertightness is checked before registering them in their anatomic configuration into the cast of the final organ or sequence for a procedural model. The organ model is perfused with artificial blood, resulting in bleeding when dissected (**Fig. 5**). To replicate urine leakage of the bladder within a robot-assisted radical prostatectomy (RARP) model, a multilayer, watertight bladder was fabricated that could be tested for any leaks (see **Fig. 5**). The tensile strength of the PVA bladder mucosa and muscle layer was tested

Table 1
The HoLEP model fulfilled 78% (63/81) elements and lacked 17% (14/81)

Elements	Grading for Each Point		
	Positive	Neutral	Negative
Section 1: Overall utility			
1a: Ultimate goals (5)	4	1	0
1b: essential features (6)	5	0	1
Total	9 82%	1 9%	1 9%
Section 2: Components			
2a: Anatomic components (9)	9	0	0
2b: 100-g prostate with median lobe no nodules	yes		
2c: Procedural steps (9)	5	1	3
Total	14 78%	1 6%	3 17%
Section 3: Tissue fidelity			
3a: Fundamental skills (6)	5	0	1
3b: fundamental tissue interactions (4)	3	0	1
3c: Anatomic visual cues (5)	3	0	2
3d: Laser-tissue interactions (7)	6	0	1
3e: Instrument-tissue interactions (6)	5	1	0
3f: Bleeding/Hemostasis (2)	0	0	2
Total	22 73%	1 3%	7 23%
Section 4: Assessment of surgical performance			
4a: Objective evaluation (7)	7	0	0
4b: Subjective evaluation (6)	4	1	1
4c: Objective measurement methods (1)	1	0	0
4d: Standard evaluation metrics (8)	6	0	2
Total	18 82%	1 5%	3 14%
Overall	63 78%	4 5%	14 17%

Categorically, 82%, 78%, 73%, and 82% were satisfied in overall utility, anatomic and procedural components, tissue fidelity, and assessment of performance, respectively.

in the development phase to ensure its adequacy for urethra-vesical anastomosis suture retention. After the anastomosis, a leak test consisting of the installation of 180 mL of saline into the urethra and the resulting binary measurement of positive (saline leak) or negative (no leak) was performed. Specimens with incomplete circumferential mucosal alignment and inadequate tissue approximation exhibited a positive leak, while those without did not demonstrate a leak, confirming our findings (**Fig. 6**A, B).

Sensors

Calibrated analog stretch sensors were aligned in the molds during the casting process within various hydrogel models specifically the neurovascular bundle (NVB) during RARP simulation (**Fig. 6**C, D). These could measure nerve tension applied during dissection of the NVB during the RARP model. A data-acquisition system involved a custom circuit and LabJack U6 DAQ using LJLogUD Software (LabJack, Lakewood, CO) is connected to the model to measure tension values during the nerve sparing component of the procedure. The stretch sensors were calibrated with the application of a controlled force to confirm appropriate corresponding voltage readings and were tested to ensure reliability. Tensile forces were applied across the sensor at 1-N increments until reaching 5 N as the corresponding voltages

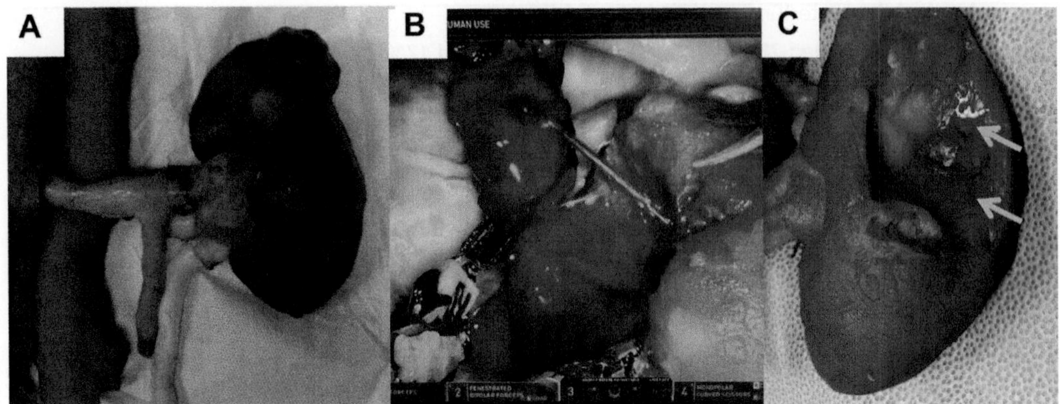

Fig. 5. Perfusion of the kidney model during robot-assisted partial nephrectomy. (*A*) Hydrogel kidney model with tumor, renal vasculature, and major vessels. (*B*) Arterial parenchymal bleeding occurring during resection of the tumor. (*C*) Examination of the resection base with *arrows* demonstrating bleeding channels.

were measured and an exponential curve was plotted. The sensors allowed the calculation of maximum force, average force, peak force frequency, and total energy applied to the NVB during the simulation.

Fluorescence

To enable the measurement of positive surgical margins, luminol, a chemical that exhibits chemiluminescence (Science Company Lakewood, CO), was added to the liquid PVA injected within the prostate mold in the RARP model and tumor in the RAPN model. The mixture remains inert throughout the entire freeze/thaw cycle and assembly process until hydrogen peroxide is added to the surgical bed after simulation to induce a chemiluminescent reaction illuminating any prostate PVA/luminol mixture left behind on

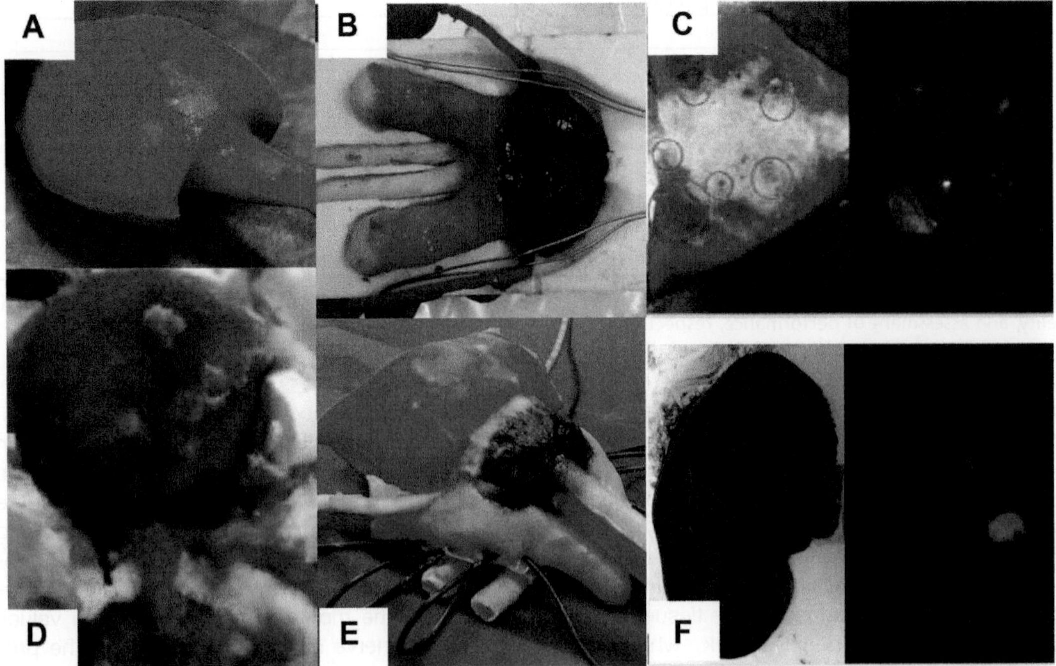

Fig. 6. Incorporated CROMS (Clinically Relevant Objective Metrics of Simulation). (*A*) Multilayered, watertight bladder in robot-assisted radical prostatectomy model. (*B*) Leak test of urethrovesical anastomosis after simulation by instillation of 180 cc of fluid. (*C*) Alignment of analog stretch sensors within the prostate mold. (*D*) Position of stretch sensors within the completed robot-assisted radical prostatectomy model. Fluorescence testing of positive margins. (*E*) Base of prostate resection in robot-assisted radical prostatectomy model. (*F*) Base of tumor resection in robot-assisted partial nephrectomy model (left, before; right, after activation of fluorescence).

the surgical bed (prostate/tumor remnant) (**Fig. 6**E, F).

Metric validation

Nerve-sparing robot-assisted radical prostatectomy On completion of each simulation, CROMS (forces applied to the NVB, surgical margins, and UVA leak rate) were collected. Nerve forces exported from the microcontroller using MATLAB (MathWorks Inc, Natick, MA) included maximum force, average force, peak force frequency, and total energy applied. Positive surgical margins were examined after each simulation by fluorescence lighting and qualitatively assessed (yes/no). Anastomosis leak was evaluated by instillation of 180 mL of saline for each subject in a binary fashion (yes/no), regardless of the degree of leakage. Video analysis of the NVB dissection was assessed by two blinded experts using the GEARS score, and anastomosis performance was also assessed using the task-specific scoring system of RACE (six metrics of performance assessed, for a final performance score out of 30). CROMS, clinical metrics, and task-specific expert objective performance ratings for the novice and the expert groups were compared to measure response process evidence (previously known as "construct validity"). GEARS scores were correlated with forces applied to the NVB. RACE scores were correlated with leak rates of the UVA. Statistical analysis was performed using SPSS version 24 by conducting Spearman's analysis between groups and evaluating the linear relationships between performance metrics and data output. Student's *t*-test was used to compare expert and novice continuous variables.

The maximum force (P = .011), average force (P = 160.011), and total energy (P = .003) applied to the NVB with incorporated sensors during the simulation were significantly lower for experts. Novices applied five times and 2.5 times greater maximal and average forces (N) than experts (**Fig. 7**A, B). Each UVA performed in the expert group was watertight on postsimulation leak test, whereas for six of the nine novices, the UVA procedures exhibited positive leakage of saline (P = .019). Furthermore, none of the experts' results showed positive surgical margins on postsimulation analysis compared to positive margin status in 7 of the novice group (P = .011). Video analysis of the nerve-sparing portion of the simulation using the validated GEARS assessment metric showed significantly higher total scores in the expert group (29.25 $\pm$ 0.96) than in the novice group (12.22 $\pm$ 3.24; P = .05), as well as significantly higher scores in every GEARS subcategory. Higher total GEARS score and force sensitivity (a subcategory of GEARS score that measures tissue handling, injury to adjacent structures, and fine control) correlated with lower total energy forces (Joules) applied during simulated NVB dissection (**Fig. 7**C). Using Spearman's Rank correlation, an inverse correlation coefficient (r value) of -0.66 (P = .019) and -0.87 (P = .000) was calculated

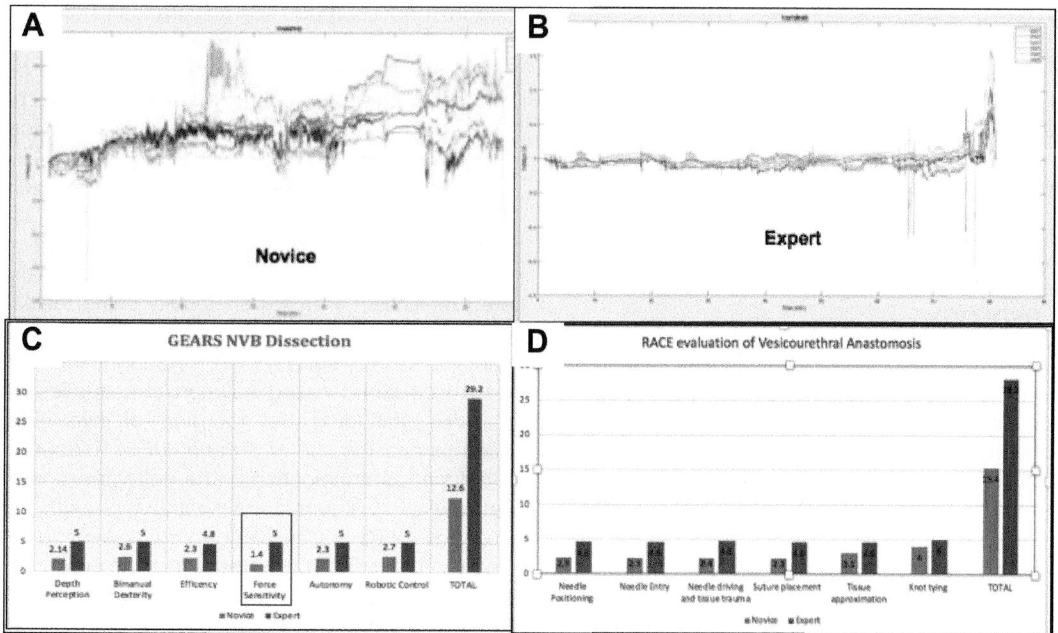

Fig. 7. Validity of CROMS. Print out of summative feedback of stretch data during NVB dissection (*A*) novice, (*B*) expert, (*C*) comparison of expert and novice GEARS rating, (*D*) comparison of expert and novice RACE rating.

between total energy/total GEARS score and total energy/force sensitivity score (GEARS subcategory), respectively. In video analysis of the UVA portion of the simulation using the validated RACE scores, the experts demonstrated a statistically significant superior performance in every category except knot-tying (**Fig. 7**D). Mean (±SD) RACE scores in the expert group were 28.2 (±1.64) out of 30, and the novice group obtained a mean (±SD) score of 15.44 (±5.36; $P = .003$). The UVA leak rate was highly correlated with total RACE score r value = −0.86 (0.000). Mean RACE scores were also significantly different between novices and experts ($P = .003$).

Robot-assisted partial nephrectomy Clinically relevant objective metrics of simulators (CROMS), including estimated blood loss (EBL), positive surgical margins, and persistent leakage of urine after violation of the pelivcaliceal system, were collected. Warm ischemia time (WIT) was defined as the period of renal artery clamping (min). EBL was defined by the volume in the suction after simulation (mL). A Positive Surgical Margin (PSM) was defined as the presence of fluorescence at the resected tumor base, after activation of the fluorescent dye. Experts demonstrated statistically significant differences over novices in all CROMS including WIT (11.94 ± 4.15 min vs 28.37 ± 11.7 min; $P < .001$) and EBL (232 ± 157 mL vs 996 ± 784 mL; $P < .001$), with the exception of PSM (one of 16 vs eight of 27; $P = .042$). A significant difference was seen in the GEARS scores between experts (22.13 ± 1.39) and novices (15.78 ± 2.82, $P < .001$). The correlation coefficient between each CROMS component and total GEARS score yielded an r (and P value) of −0.76 (<0.0001), −0.74 (<0.0001), 0.77 (<0.0001), and 0.21 (0.19) for console time, WIT, EBL, and PSMs, respectively. The strongest correlations were revealed by r scores closest to ±1.

THE FUTURE OF PROCEDURAL SIMULATION IN UROLOGY

Potential for Remote Learning

The pandemic COVID-19 outbreak is responsible for a major education crisis globally as almost the entire world is under lockdown, and all educational institutions including medical colleges are shut down. The key reason is to decrease the risk of exposure for medical students, residents, faculty, and laboratory technicians to contain the spread of Covid-19, which is an understandable concern. As the modern medical curriculum already allows restricted time for each subject, the potential for more remote learning opportunities necessitated modern surgical educators to discover novel methods using e-Learning.[41] In our own experience, e-learning was sufficient for teaching of basic surgical skills; however, instructor-led demonstrations was still essential for higher level knowledge acquisition and advanced skill refinement.[42] Mixed reality (MR) technologies compared to augmented and virtual reality are unique in their ability to interpose real-life view with real-time virtual information from a distant location over a cloud-based platform and would be ideal in providing remote feedback during complex procedures without the need for costly resources.[43,44] This technology combined with the portability, safety, and mitigation of any biohazardous risks would provide an ideal platform to enable both formative feedback (instructor-guided areas of improvement during the simulation) to guide progression of performance remotely. A hydrogel model for transrectal ultrasound (TRUS) biopsy procedure was fabricated to be compatible with a virtual (remote) learning environment. Relevant anatomy from DICOM files of a deidentified MRI scan with a 80-g prostate was segmented to create a CAD file that included the prostate, prostatic urethra, posterior prostate fascial layers, rectum, seminal vesicles, and vas deferens. The prostate was divided into 6 biopsy zones each denoted by a different color (left/right, base, mid, and apex) (**Fig. 8**). Six experts (median cases completed = 550) and six residents completed a TRUS biopsy with volumetric prostate evaluation, administration of local anesthetic, and 2 adequate biopsies of each zone in a standard outpatient procedure room equipped with an ultrasound using the model (**Fig. 9**). Experts took significantly less attempts and time per biopsy region, less time per attempt, with more accuracy (see **Fig. 3**), and reported significantly lower difficulty than novices (2.4 vs 3.7, $P = .001$; 59.8 vs 123.9, $P < .001$; 23.3 vs 31.3, $P = .001$; 3.0 vs 4.8, $P = .001$, respectively) (**Fig. 10**).

A TRUS biopsy simulation was piloted in an educational session where feedback was delivered remotely by an expert faculty using the MR Help Lightning software (Help Lightening, Birmingham AL, USA) (**Fig. 11**). MR Help Lightning software is a cloud-based solution that applies AR features, including the merging of two video streams and the use of 3D annotation to improve real-time communications. The software runs on virtually every smart device without requiring an app download via an electronic link sent to the trainee that will open on any Web browser. The software proved easy to set up, intuitive to use, and proved effective in delivering feedback to the trainee remotely which could offer the potential for virtual training sessions in urology.

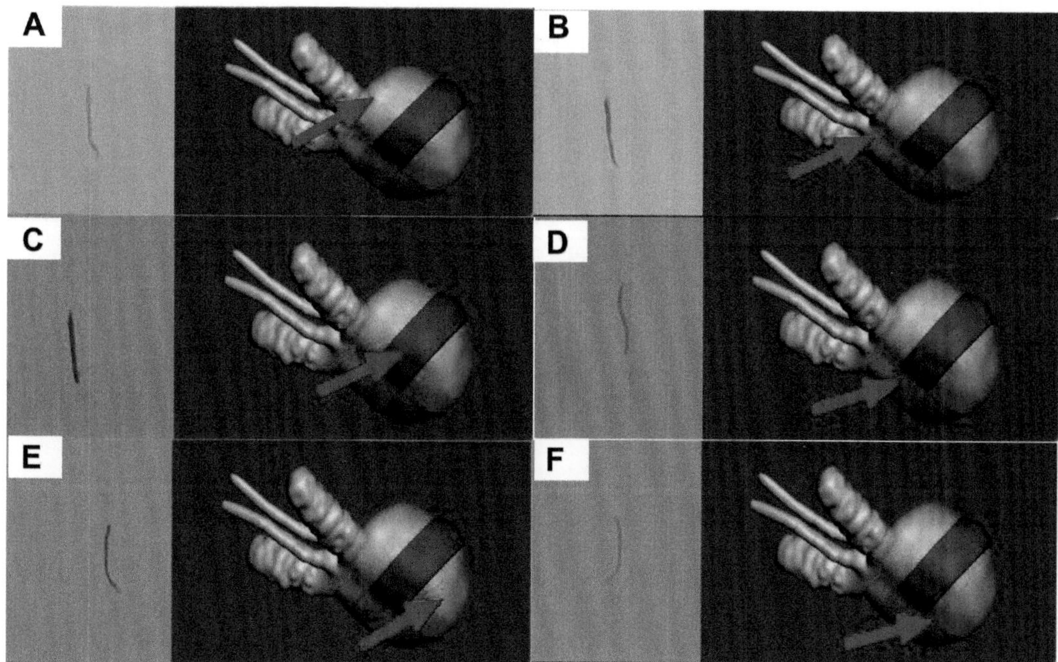

Fig. 8. Transrectal ultrasound (TRUS) biopsy model. CAD design of TRUS model containing seminal vesicle, rectum, and prostate divided into 6 color zones with corresponding cores from each zone (*A*) right base, (*B*) left base, (*C*) right mid-prostate, (*D*) left mid-prostate, (*E*) right apex, (*F*) left apex.

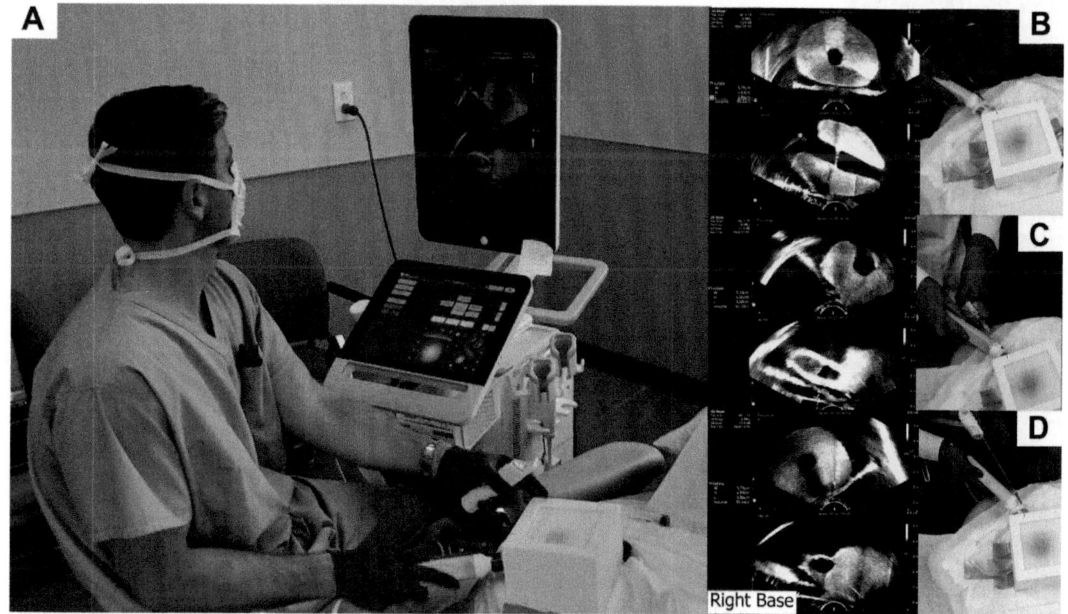

Fig. 9. Transrectal ultrasound (TRUS) biopsy full-immersion simulation. (*A*) Full-immersion simulation of TRUS model in clinic procedure room using ultrasound, (*B*) ultrasound examination of the prostate, (*C*) instillation of local anesthetic, (*D*) biopsy of right base region of the prostate.

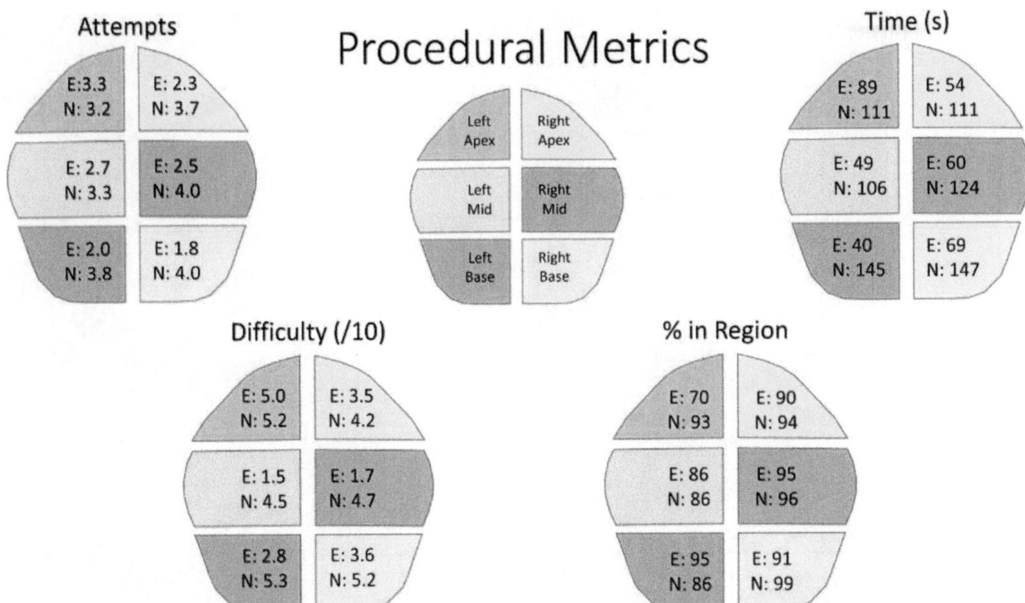

Fig. 10. Validation of the transrectal ultrasound (TRUS) biopsy model. Comparison of expert and novice performance regarding number of biopsy attempts, difficulty, percentage of core with correct color corresponding to the intended prostate zone, time to complete biopsy from prostate region.

Learning New Approaches

Cadaveric models remain the gold standard for realistic procedural simulation, despite the controversial use for routine surgical training.[17] However, in the initial phase of exploration, the focus is on determining their feasibility, safety profile, ideal approach, and potential complications in novel procedures.[12]The value of surgical rehearsal on cadavers before proceeding to actual live patient surgery for novel approaches is essential as they not only provide real human anatomic variability

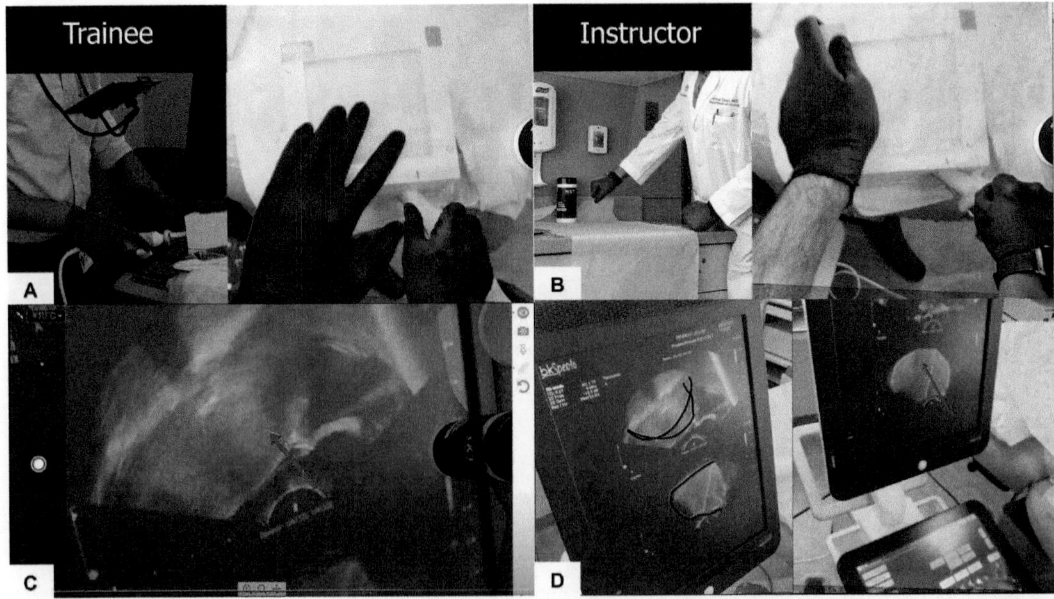

Fig. 11. Pilot for remote learning during TRUS simulation using Mixed reality software. (*A*) Trainee (*left*) completing simulation with view demonstrating overlay demonstrating direction of ultrasound probe (*right*), (*B*) instructor (*left*) in remote location using software to overlay his hand on the view from the trainee, (*C, D*) annotations that can be placed by instructor on trainee view.

but also are often relevant with common pathologic conditions of the vessels and viscera.[45] A procedure that has been gaining traction is a robot-assisted kidney transplant (RAKT) particularly using the robotic approach for recipient renal transplant vascular anatomists, retroperitonealization, and ureter reimplant requiring a minimum of 35 RAKT cases are necessary to reach reproducibility in terms of renal rewarming time (RWT), complications, and functional results.[46] Ultimately, this steep learning curve may lead to lower graft and patient survival rates, which can hinder the integration and success of RAKT for recipients. We sought to overcome these limitations by developing a high-fidelity perfused full-immersion nonbiohazardous RAKT training simulator consisting of both donor and recipient procedures by combining three-dimensional (3D) printing and hydrogel casting technologies. Using a similar technique described previously, a recipient pelvic cavity model was fabricated including bony pelvis, bladder, perfused right iliac arteries and veins, and watertight multilayered bladder (see **Fig. 11**). Each assembled simulation model is placed into a da Vinci abdominal trainer box and docked to the da Vinci surgical robot to complete all the necessary steps of the recipient transplantation operation, including peritoneal reflection and dissection, exposure of the bladder dome, regional hypothermia, positioning of the kidney, and finally, the arterial, venous, and ureterovesical anastomosis (with placement of J-stent) (**Fig. 12**).

The perfusion capacity and realistic tissue texture, confirmed by a series of mechanical tests, provided a full immersion environment, allowing a robotic naive transplant surgeon to achieve anastomosis times overlapping with published competency values. This provided evidence indicates that during the simulated procedure, the surgeon encountered levels of difficulty similar to that of live cases ensuring the transferability of the skills from simulation to patient.[47]

Patient-Specific Simulation

Patient-specific simulation refers to a training modality that directly emulates the task to be performed in vivo and requires simulations that focus on optimizing the preparation of practicing physicians immediately before the actual intervention for an individual patient.[48] This preoperative strategy marks a distinct shift in the use of simulation from a tool that allows practice of a specific skill (ie, training) to one that allows rehearsal of a specific event (ie, a patient's operation).[49] Patient-specific rehearsals would allow practicing surgeons to practice, plan, and address potential problems related to a specific patient's case, thus optimizing the real intervention.[50] However, the benefits of surgical rehearsals are limited in abdominal surgeries because of the absence of a realistic and immersive simulation platform that can adapt to the anatomic/pathologic variability of each patient, a task that would be almost impossible in cadavers. Our group at the Simulation Innovation Laboratory at the University of Rochester Medical has refined the process combining image segmentation, 3D printing, and

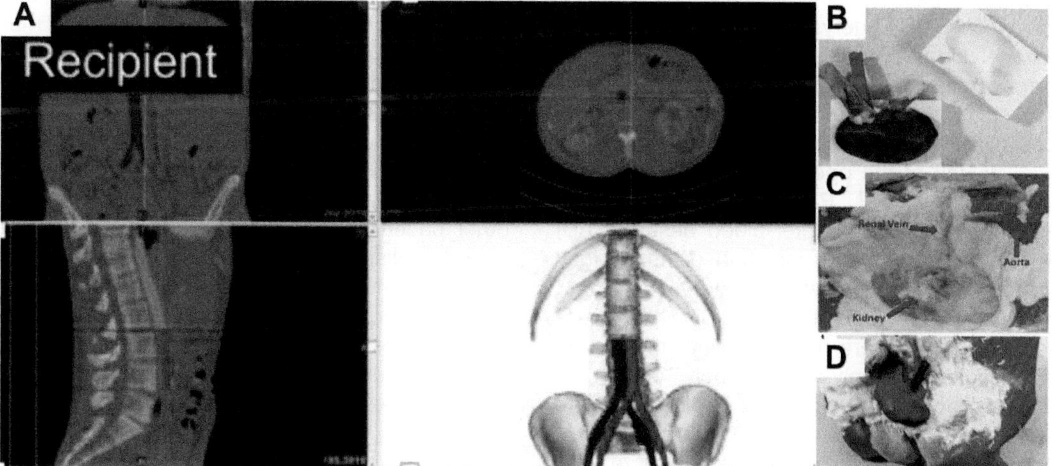

Fig. 12. Robot-assisted Kidney transplant simulation (recipient). (*A*) Segmentation of vasculature and bony pelvis of a patient receiving donor kidney, (*lower right*) CAD from recipient scan containing CAD from donor patient kidney, (*B*) donor kidney mold and kidney model with hollow vasculature, (*C*) pelvic model for kidney reimplant, revascularization, and positioning, (*D*) final view after robotic reimplant, revascularization, and positioning of donor kidney in recipient pelvis.

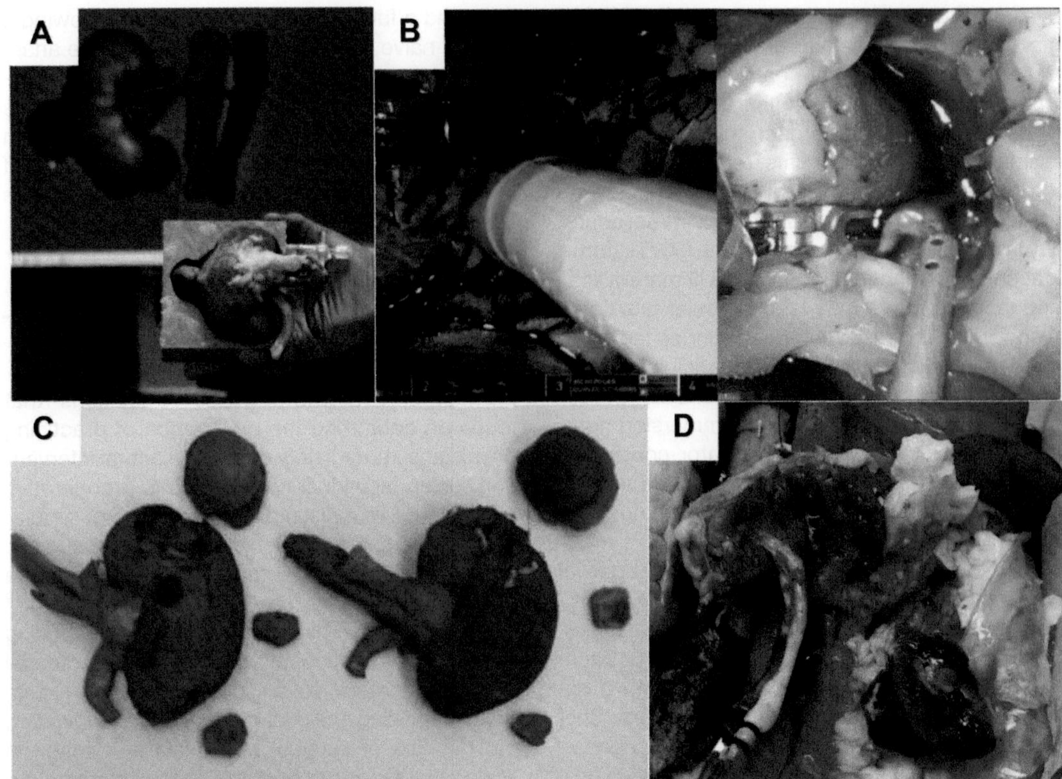

Fig. 13. Patient-specific simulation. (*A*) Computer design resulting from segmentation of the patients' CT scan in the background with personalized kidney model in its cast, (*B*) excision of a tumor with bleeding (left live surgery, right simulated rehearsal), (*C, D*) examination of the specimen after simulated rehearsals showing the excised lesions.

hydrogel molding, originally designed to fabricate realistic physical models for resident training to develop a patient-specific simulation platform for kidney cancer surgery. These patient-specific hydrogel kidney models represent an accurate portrayal of each patient's anatomic and pathologic characteristics with the capacity to reproduce tissue characteristics that replicate the entire gestalt of the operative experience for an RAPN procedure.[51] Patient CT scans were segmented into a computer-aided design (CAD) file and used to create injection casts. Kidney and tumor casts along with hollow vascular and urinary structures were 3D-printed. The hilar structures and tumor were registered into the kidney cast, injected with poly-vinyl alcohol (PVA) hydrogel, and processed to create the kidney phantom. Mechanical and functional testing protocols were completed to confirm that the properties of PVA matched the live tissue.[52] Anatomic accuracy was confirmed by CT scanning the phantom and creating another CAD, which was compared to the original patient CAD.[53] Full-procedural rehearsals were completed in eight patients with highly complex renal masses (average nephrometry score 9.9) 24 to 48 hours before their respective live surgeries. Clinically relevant metrics (WIT, estimated blood loss [EBL], and positive surgical margins) from each rehearsal and live case were 16.5 versus 15 minutes, 260 mL versus 265 mL, and negative margins consecutively. Wilcoxon-rank sum test showed a positive correlation for WIT ($P = .12$) and EBL ($P = .81$) between the rehearsal and the simulation[51] (**Fig. 13**). Expanding beyond other patient-specific platforms that rapidly produced realistic silicone models, this developed platform simulated kidney texture, anatomy, and perfusion, incorporating the surrounding perinephric fat, bowel, and musculature, including bleeding vessels simulating blood flow allowing for a full-immersion experience for the surgeon.

SUMMARY

The recent construction and validation of 3D-printed synthetic organ models has provided an opportunity to improve the safety, effectiveness, and efficiency of surgical education and training.

Innovations using a combination of 3D printing and polymer technologies to fabricate patient-specific, nonbiohazardous models based on imaging data and idealized models based on expert consensus with incorporated clinically relevant metrics for feedback and potential for patient-specific rehearsals is a game changer for surgical training. These models will provide equally effective pedagogic tools for surgeons to trial novel technologies and trainees safely meet mandated caseloads, potentially limiting the role of cadaveric simulation.

DISCLOSURE

No disclosures.

REFERENCES

1. Oxford University Press. Available at: http://www.oup.com.
2. Gordon J, Wilkerson W, Shaffer D, et al. 'Practicing' medicine without risk: students' and educators' responses to high-fidelity patient simulation. Acad Med 2001;76:469–72.
3. Pegden CD, Shannon RE, Sadowski RP. Introduction to simulation using SIMAN. 2nd edition. Hightstown (NJ): McGraw-Hill, Inc.; 1995.
4. Reznick RK. Teaching and testing technical skills. Am J Surg 1993;165:358–61.
5. Yiasemidou M, Gkaragkani E, Glassman D, et al. Cadaveric simulation: a review of reviews. Ir J Med Sci 2018;187(3):827–33.
6. Culligan P, Gurshumov E, Lewis C, et al. Predictive validity of a training protocol using a robotic surgery simulator. Female Pelvic Med Reconstr Surg 2014; 20:48–51.
7. Ahmed K, Jawad M, Abboudi M, et al. Effectiveness of procedural simulation in urology: a systematic review. J Urol 2011;186:26–34.
8. Ahmed K, Aydin A, Dasgupta P, et al. A novel cadaveric simulation program in urology. J Surg Educ 2015;72(4):556–65.
9. Mantica g, Pacchetti a, aimar r, et al. Developing a five-step training model for transperineal prostate biopsies in a naïve residents' group: a prospective observational randomised study of two different techniques. World J Urol 2019;37:1845–50.
10. Kobayashi E, Hishikawa S, Teratani T, et al. The pig as a model for translational research: overview of porcine animal models at Jichi Medical University. Transpl Res 2012;1(1):8.
11. Bestard Vallejo JE, Raventós Busquets CX, Celma Doménech A, et al. Pig model in experimental renal transplant surgery. Actas Urol Esp 2008;32(1):91–101.
12. Kaouk JH, Bertolo R. Single-site robotic platform in clinical practice: first cases in the USA. Minerva Urol Nefrol 2019;71(3):294–8.
13. Sharma M, Macafee D, Horgan AF. Basic laparoscopic skills training using fresh frozen cadaver: a randomized controlled trial. Am J Surg 2013; 206(1):23–31.
14. Hayashi S, Naito M, Kawata S, et al. History and future of human cadaver preservation for surgical training: from formalin to saturated salt solution method. Anat Sci Int 2016;91(1):1–7.
15. Okada R, Tsunoda A, Momiyama N, et al. Thiel's method of embalming and its usefulness in surgical assessments. Nihon Jibiinkoka Gakkai Kaiho 2012; 115(8):791–4.
16. Nielsen GD, Larsen ST, Wolkoff P. Re-evaluation of the WHO (2010) formaldehyde indoor air quality guideline for cancer risk assessment. Arch Toxicol 2017;91(1):35–61.
17. Gilbody J, Prasthofer AW, Ho K, et al. The use and effectiveness of cadaveric workshops in higher surgical training: a systematic review. Ann R Coll Surg Engl 2011;93(5):347–52.
18. Ross HM, Simmang CL, Fleshman JW, et al. Adoption of laparoscopic colectomy: results and implications of ASCRS hands-on course participation. Surg Innov 2008;15:179–83.
19. Villegas L, Schneider BE, Callery MP, et al. Laparoscopic skills training. Surg Endosc 2003;17:1879–88.
20. Hildebrandt S. Capital punishment and anatomy: history and ethics of an ongoing association. Clin Anat 2008;21(1):5–14.
21. Hasan TI. Dissection humane? J Med Ethics Hist Med 2011;4:4.
22. Thomas MP. The role of simulation in the development of technical competence during surgical training: a literature review. Int J Med Educ 2013;4:48–55.
23. Schmauss D, Gerber N, Sodian R. Three-dimensional printing of models for surgical planning in patients with primary cardiac tumors. J Thorac Cardiovasc Surg 2013;145(5):1407–8.
24. Schmauss D, Juchem G, Weber S, et al. Three-dimensional printing for perioperative planning of complex aortic arch surgery. Ann Thorac Surg 2014;97(6):2160–3.
25. Komai Y, Sakai Y, Gotohda N, et al. A novel 3-dimensional image analysis system for case-specific kidney anatomy and surgical simulation to facilitate clampless partial nephrectomy. Urology 2014;83: 500–7.
26. Silberstein JL, Maddox MM, Dorsey P, et al. Physical models of renal malignancies using standard cross-sectional imaging and 3-dimensional printers: a pilot study. Urology 2014;84:268–73.
27. Li P, Jiang S, Yu Y, et al. Biomaterial characteristics and application of silicone rubber and PVA hydrogels mimicked in organ groups for prostate brachytherapy. J Mech Behav Biomed Mater 2015;49:220–34.
28. Umale S, Deck C, Bourdet N, et al. Experimental mechanical characterization of abdominal organs: liver,

kidney & spleen. J Mech Behav Biomed Mater 2013; 17:22–33.

29. Farshad M, Barbezat M, Flueler P, et al. Material characterization of the pig kidney in relation with the biomechanical analysis of renal trauma. J Biomech 1999;32(4):417–25.
30. Snedeker JG, Barbezat M, Niederer P, et al. Strain energy density as a rupture criterion for the kidney: impact tests on porcine organs, finite element simulation, and a baseline comparison between human and porcine tissues. J Biomech 2005;38(5):993–1001.
31. Melnyk R, Ezzat B, Belfast E, et al. Mechanical and functional validation of a perfused, robot-assisted partial nephrectomy simulation platform using a combination of 3D printing and hydrogel casting. World J Urol 2020;38:1631–41.
32. Demirel D, Butler KL, Halic T, et al. A hierarchical task analysis of cricothyroidotomy procedure for a virtual airway skills trainer simulator. Am J Surg 2016;212:475–84.
33. Sarker SK, Chang A, Albrani T, et al. Constructing hierarchical task analysis in surgery. Surg Endosc 2008;22:107–11.
34. Myers EN, Anderson-Montoya BL, Fanaso HT, et al. Robotic sacrocolpopexy simulation model and associated hierarchical task analysis. Obstet Gynecol 2019;133:905–9.
35. Collins JW, Marcus HJ, Ghazi A, et al. Ethical implications of AI in robotic surgical training: a Delphi consensus statement. Eur Urol Focus 2021. https://doi.org/10.1016/j.euf.2021.04.006.
36. Satava RM. Assessing surgery skills through simulation. Clin Teach 2006;3:107–11.
37. Holmboe ES, Sherbino J, Long DM, et al. The role of assessment in competency-based medical education. Med Teach 2010;32(8):676–82.
38. McGaghie W, Issenberg B, Cohen E, et al. Does simulation-based medical education with deliberate practice yield better results than traditional clinical education? a meta-analytic comparative review of the evidence. Acad Med 2011;86(6): 706–71.
39. Sánchez R, Rodríguez O, Rosciano J, et al. Robotic surgery training: construct validity of Global Evaluative Assessment of Robotic Skills (GEARS). J Robot Surg 2016;10(3):227–31.
40. van Hove PD, Tuijthof GJ, Verdaasdonk EG, et al. Objective assessment of technical surgical skills. Br J Surg 2010;97(7):972–87.
41. Okland TS, Pepper JP, Valdez TA. How do we teach surgical residents in the COVID-19 era? J Surg Educ 2020;77:1005–7.
42. McGann KC, Melnyk R, Saba P, et al. Implementation of an E-Learning Academic Elective for Hands-On Basic Surgical Skills to Supplement Medical School Surgical Education. J Surg Educ 2020 Jul-Aug;78(4):1164–74.
43. Gerup J, Soerensen CB, Dieckmann P. Augmented reality and mixed reality for healthcare education beyond surgery: an integrative review. Int J Med Educ 2020;11:1–18.
44. Hu HZ, Feng XB, Shao ZW, et al. Application and prospect of mixed reality technology in medical field. Curr Med Sci 2019;39(1):1–6. Epub 2019 Mar 13. Erratum in: Curr Med Sci. 2021 Feb;41(1):188.
45. Holland JP, Waugh L, Horgan A, et al. Cadaveric hands-on training for surgical specialties: is this back to the future for surgical skills development? J Surg Educ 2011;68(2):110–6.
46. Gallioli A, Territo A, Boissier R, et al. Learning curve in robot-assisted kidney transplantation: results from the european robotic urological society working group. Eur Urol 2020;78(2):239–47.
47. Saba P, Belfast E, Melnyk R, et al. Development of a high-fidelity robot-assisted kidney transplant simulation platform using three-dimensional printing and hydrogel casting technologies. J Endourol 2020;34(10): 1088–94.
48. Rogers DA, Elstein AS, Bordage G. Improving continuing medical education for surgical techniques: applying the lessons learned in the first decade of minimal access surgery. Ann Surg 2001;233:159–66.
49. Hislop SJ, Hedrick JH, Singh MJ, et al. Simulation case rehearsals for carotid artery stenting. Eur J Vasc Endovasc Surg 2009;38:750–4.
50. Willaert W, Aggarwal R, Daruwalla F, et al. Simulated procedure rehearsal is more effective than a preoperative generic warm-up for endovascular procedures. Ann Surg 2012;255:1184–9.
51. Ghazi A, Saba P, Melnyk R, et al. Utilizing 3D printing and hydrogel casting for the development of patient-specific rehearsal platforms for robotic assisted partial nephrectomies. Urology 2020. https://doi.org/10.1016/j.urology.2020.10.023.
52. Melnyk R, Ezzat B, Belfast E, et al. Mechanical and functional validation of a perfused, robot-assisted partial nephrectomy simulation platform using a combination of 3D printing and hydrogel casting. World J Urol 2020;38:1631–4.
53. Melnyk R, Oppenhimer D, Ghazi A. How specific are patient-specific simulations? Analyzing the accuracy of 3D-printing and modeling to create patient-specific rehearsals for complex urological procedures. WJU 2021.

Emerging Intraoperative Imaging Technologies in Urologic Oncology

Parwiz Abrahimi, MD, PhD[a,b], Timothy McClure, MD[a,b,c,*]

KEYWORDS

• Intraoperative imaging • Surgical margins • Ultrasound • Narrow-band imaging
• Photodynamic imaging • Cerenkov luminescence imaging • Light reflectance spectroscopy

KEY POINTS

- New imaging technologies can help to identify hard-to-see tumors and improve surgical margins in urologic oncology.
- 5-aminolevulinic acid, 68-Ga-PSMA Cerenkov Luminescence Imaging and Light reflectance spectroscopy are promising intraoperative imaging modalities in prostate cancer but require larger studies for validation.
- Nephron-sparing surgery can be aided with ultrasonography and fluorescence imaging techniques including indocyanine green, 5-ALA and antibody-fluorochrome conjugates can to identify tumor margins but may be limited to exophytic tumors.
- Bladder cancer diagnosis and treatment can be improved with enhanced cystoscopy with narrow-band imaging and photodynamic imaging.

Urologic care has advanced considerably over the last several decades as new innovations in endoscopic and robotic surgery have come to the forefront. As surgical cases become more complex and challenging, intraoperative imaging technologies are increasingly being used. Safe and complete resection of tumor is the key objective in cancer surgery and advanced imaging techniques have been shown to improve surgical outcomes for kidney, prostate, and bladder surgery. This article discusses emerging intraoperative imaging technologies, their uses in urologic surgery, and the limits to their implementation.

PROSTATE

Radical prostatectomy (RP) has been the standard treatment for men with localized prostate cancer (CaP) with the ideal treatment trifecta being oncologic control and preservation of potency and urinary continence.[1] Despite advancements in surgical technique, including robotic assistance, complete tumor resection has been a major factor in treatment failure.[2] Positive surgical margins (PSMs) can occur in 10% to 35% of RP cases and are associated with an increased risk of biochemical recurrence as well as use of adjuvant radiation and androgen-deprivation therapies.[3,4] The standard workflow for diagnosis in the United States includes transrectal ultrasound, PET/computed tomography (CT), and MRI, which can help identify locally advanced tumors, stratify PSM risk and help to guide surgical planning. Intraoperative sampling of frozen sections for histopathological review is the current workhorse in assessing margin status. Advanced intraoperative fresh-frozen section analysis such as NeuroSAFE are attempts to improve this workflow; however, it can be time consuming, subject to sampling bias, and requires additional pathology

[a] Department of Urology, New York Presbyterian Hospital; [b] Weill Cornell Medical College, 525 East 68th Street Starr 946, New York, NY 10065, USA; [c] Department of Radiology, New York-Presbyterian Hospital
* Corresponding author. Weill Cornell Medical College, 525 East 68th Street Starr 946, New York, NY 10065, USA
E-mail address: tim047@med.cornell.edu

Urol Clin N Am 49 (2022) 57–63
https://doi.org/10.1016/j.ucl.2021.08.002
0094-0143/22/

personnel.[5] Three novel intraoperative imaging technologies have shown early promise in overcoming the limitations of frozen sections 5-aminolevulinic acid (5-ALA), ^{68}Ga-PSMA Cerenkov luminescence imaging (CLI), and light reflectance spectroscopy (LRS).

5-Aminolevulinic Acid

5-ALA is a nonproteinogenic amino acid that is converted to protoporphyrin IX (PPIX) within the mitochondria of cells.[6] PPIX emits red light after excitation with blue-violet (405 nm) light. Cancerous cells will accumulate higher doses of PPIX than noncancerous cells.[6] 5-ALA can be administered orally several hours before surgery or delivered by orogastric tube intraoperatively for adequate uptake by the CaP cells, with weak fluorescence detected in benign epithelial cells and none in the adjacent stroma.[7] Several small cohort studies have used specialized endoscopic cameras to demonstrate photodynamic detection in RP is feasible, safe, and integrates seamlessly into laparoscopic and robotic approaches.[8–10] In the largest of these studies, Fukuhara and colleagues[9] evaluated 52 patients with 5-ALA based photodynamic diagnosis (PDD) and demonstrated sensitivity of 75% and specificity of 87%. Like other applications of PDD (eg, blue light cystoscopy), there is a significant learning curve for interpretation. This can be complicated because the depth of penetration of blue light is limited to the surface and the intensity of detected red fluorescence is a function of the accumulation of PPIX, which can lead to false negatives in samples with shorter margin lengths, cases of extraprostatic extension where the tumor cells were covered with prostatic capsule or fat, or when PPIX is released, such as occurs with heat degeneration from electrocautery.[9] For that same reason, nonmalignant prostate cells undergoing physiologic hyperplasia can also result in false-positive signals. Additional studies are needed, ideally optimizing 5-ALA dosages, timing, and route of administration, to validate these findings.

^{68}Ga-PSMA Cerenkov Luminescence Imaging

Prostate-specific membrane antigen (PSMA) is highly expressed in the prostate and is expressed in much greater concentrations in CaP cells and this has been exploited in PET/CT staging using radiolabeled antibodies and ligands targeting PSMA.[11,12] Unlike PET imaging, which relies on γ-annihilation photons, CLI measures photons produced by charged particles emitted by radiolabeled molecules like ^{68}Ga-PSMA that travel faster than the speed of light through a medium, such as prostate tissue.[13] Cerenkov photons are highly attenuated in biological tissues and thus limited to their detection to superficial surfaces, a feature that is exploited in assessing margins. A recent single-center prospective study evaluated the feasibility and accuracy of ^{68}Ga-PSMA CLI and demonstrated the feasibility of intraoperative identification of margin status.[14] The resected tumor specimen was evaluated in an imaging chamber under both white light and CLI, and allowed identification of PSMs. However, because the radiotracer is excreted renally into the bladder and ^{68}Ga has a higher mean positron range, there was a false-positive rate of 28%, mostly around the prostate base. This study, although promising, highlights the limitations of ^{68}Ga-PSMA CLI, particularly with respect to renal excretion. Nonrenally excreted tracers such as ^{18}F-PSMA-1007 may be beneficial but has different tracer kinetics and would require additional nuclear medicine expertise.[15]

Light Reflectance Spectroscopy

LRS exploits the differential interaction between cancerous and noncancerous matter with electromagnetic radiation and it has been shown that benign prostate tissue has a lower light scattering coefficient than CaP.[16] The first study using LRS to analyze ex vivo prostate specimens to assess surgical margin status reported sensitivity of 86% and specificity of 85% in a study of 17 high-grade prostates.[17] A follow-up study from the same group demonstrated 91.3% sensitivity in identifying Gleason grade $\geq$7 after technique refinement, which decreases to 80.4% with inclusion of Gleason score 6.[18] The drop off in sensitivity likely reflects the morphologic and cellular differences between Gleason grades and benign tissue and may not be as clinically relevant given the indolent nature of Gleason 6 CaP. Major limitations of this imaging modality include lack of real-time data processing, small field-of-view of the detection probe making scanning the entirety of the prostatic surface impractical, and contaminating sources of light absorption and scattering by blood and inflammatory infiltrates in the prostatic specimen would limit the in vivo application.

KIDNEY

The management of renal cell carcinoma (RCC) has evolved significantly with the adoption of nephron-sparing surgery (NSS).[19] Partial nephrectomy has similar oncologic outcomes to radical nephrectomy and has been shown to lower morbidity, improve renal recovery, and has favorable patient survival rates compared to radical nephrectomy in the long-term.[20–24] A key objective in NSS is obtaining negative surgical margins balanced against the need to minimize the amount of normal parenchymal tissue that is excised and the size of that margin appears less important than complete tumor excision.[25] PSMs are reported to occur in 0% to 7% of reported cases performed for RCC, are associated with higher risk pathologies, and, although controversial, can increase the risk for recurrence as well as the need for total nephrectomy.[26] The complex anatomy of the kidney and tumor margin can be elucidated using ultrasound and fluorescence-based imaging technologies during NSS.

Ultrasonography

Ultrasonography (US) has been the mainstay imaging technique to assist in partial nephrectomy and is commonly applied in the open, laparoscopic, and robotic-assisted laparoscopic approaches. The placement of an ultrasonographic transducer directly on the capsular surface of the kidney improves the spatial resolution compared to transabdominal approach and physical examination alone.[27] This can help aid the surgeon in real-time to identify critical anatomic relationships of the primary lesion including the location and size of the tumor, its relationship to renal sinus fat, renal pelvis, peritumoral vascularity, as well as satellite lesions that may not have been apparent on preoperative imaging.[28–30] Endoscopic US probes can be integrated into the workflow of pure laparoscopic or robotic-assisted surgery with the image cast parallel on the console screen.[31,32] Although commonly used to identify renal masses preoperatively and intraoperatively, most studies evaluating margin status on partial nephrectomy specimens use ex vivo US. These reports have demonstrated promising sensitivities (100%) and specificities (97%) with mean durations of US imaging of 1 ± 1 minute.[33,34] However, because this approach involves imaging the specimen after they have been excised, the major disadvantages of this approach are the consequent reclamping and reresection if a positive PSM is found and, in the laparoscopic setting, the loss of pneumoperitoneum with specimen extraction. One study by Alharbi and colleagues[35] evaluated a technique where excised renal masses were examined with ultrasound in a saline-filled specimen bag in vivo. They reported a sensitivity of 99% and specificity of 75% with only a minor increase (41 sec) in total warm ischemia time, including a case where PSM was detected on US and allowed the surgeon to resect a deeper rim of tissue. Additional studies are needed to determine the accuracy of this intracorporeal approach in assessing margin status in a larger cohort and whether this approach is equivalent to macroscopic evaluation by the surgeon.

Fluorescence

Because US is operator dependent, cannot be used concurrently during tumor excision and if there is a PSM, this has to be remapped to the resection cavity, complementary technologies have been evaluated to identify the tumor in a more continuous fashion. Near-infrared fluorescence (NIRF) imaging is seeing increasing usage with the increased adoption of robotic systems. This technology is based on fluorescent dyes and can provide an enhanced anatomic view of the field that can aid tumor resection as well as help identify vessels for selective arterial clamping to minimize vascular compromise of the remaining kidney. Indocyanine green (ICG) is a nontoxic cyanine-based dye that can be injected intravenously to identify critical structures during surgical dissection. One favorable feature of ICG is that it binds to plasma proteins, including bilitranslocase. Many renal tumors have reduced bilitranslocase expression and therefore have reduced ICG signals compared with normal parenchyma.[36] The consequent hypofluorescence can be used to discriminate the renal mass and mass-parenchymal interface during dissection.[37]

There have been several studies using ICG to assess the adequacy of tumor resection. Mitsui and colleagues[38] were the first to report the use of NIRF/ICG for assessing surgical margin status in NSS. They reported ex vivo examination of the margins revealed negative surgical margins and also that fluorescence in the kidney persisted up to 60 minutes after ICG infusion, allowing for examination of the cavity after tumor excision and positing this could lead to improved margin status. However, another group reported no difference in the positive margin rate in a single institution which included a negative control (6% ICG vs 8.5% control).[39] In addition, while they did report a decrease in total clamp time, there were no significant differences in functional outcomes. Lastly, because of overlying normal parenchymal tissue on their surfaces, the application of NIRF/ICG to endophytic tumors is limited.

5-ALA administered orally before NSS could be observed on RCCs at the time of surgery and allowed for in vivo inspection of the resection site and comparison to resected specimen.[40] This approach had a reported sensitivity of 95% and specificity of 94% for identifying renal masses, predict the type of lesion with an accuracy of

94%, and was able to identify both cases of PSM in the study. Some limitations of systemic 5-ALA include considering of case complexity to timing with the peak fluorescent signal (in hours), phototoxic skin reaction, and possible hypotension.[41]

Antibodies that are conjugated to fluorescent tags can also be used to delineate tumors. Carbonic anhydrase IX (CAIX), recognized by the monoclonal antibody girentuximab, is a cell surface protein that is upregulated on clear cell RCC tumors. In 2018, a phase I dose-escalation study of girentuximab dually conjugated to an NIR dye and radioprobe was used to successfully localize and contrast tumor from normal parenchyma intraoperatively including identifying when the perinephric fact overlies the tumor and in endophytic tumors, 2 limitations of NIRF/ICG.[42] An additional benefit of this approach is that the same tracer could be used preoperatively for PET/CT to identify the location of the primary tumor and/or metastases.

BLADDER

Bladder cancer is the most expensive cancer to treat on a per-patient basis in the United States.[43] The cost is in part driven by the need for surveillance, including frequent cystoscopies, due to high rates of recurrence. Regular cystoscopy, also known as white light cystoscopy (WLC), is the standard of care in the evaluation and monitoring of bladder cancer, and is coupled with transurethral resection of bladder tumor (TURBT) as a diagnostic and therapeutic procedure. WLC and TURBT have an underappreciated, but significant, learning curve because of the need to visually inspect for bladder abnormalities and ensure completeness of TURBT.[44] Bladder cancers can display various morphologic features and flat lesions, such as carcinoma in situ, can be difficult to discern from normal urothelium and thus high rates of recurrence seen in bladder cancer can also result from missed lesions or residual tumor burden.[45,46] In the setting of nonpapillary tumors and persistently positive urine cytologies, random biopsies of normal appearing mucosa have been the recommendation.[47] To improve diagnosis and staging of bladder tumors by enhanced visualization, narrow-band imaging (NBI) and photodynamic imaging (PDI) have emerged as the most promising technologies, and both are represented in the latest American Urological Association guidelines for bladder cancer management.[48]

Enhanced cystoscopy with PDI is an optical imaging technology that requires preprocedural administration of the photodynamic compound hexaminolevulinate (HAL), which is FDA approved for intravesical use, and like 5-ALA accumulates more within cancerous tissues and is metabolized to PPIX, which fluoresces red after excitation with blue-violate (405 nm) light.[49] PDI, therefore, requires specialized cystoscope and camera head capable of emitting blue light. In several meta-analyses of randomized controlled trials, PDI was superior to WLC alone in 20.7% of patients with additional Ta or T1 tumors,[50] additional detection of 39% with respect to CIS,[51] more complete tumor resection.[51,52] However, because fluorescence may be affected by changes associated with intravesical therapy or inflammation, and interpretation of the fluorescence may also be subject to a learning curve, false-positive diagnoses can lead to unnecessary biopsies, although this rate does not appear to be more than WLC alone and has to be balanced against the consequences of missed diagnoses with WLC.[53]

In contrast to PDI, NBI relies on narrowing the bandwidth of white light emitted into specific wavelengths that penetrate the bladder mucosa and are absorbed by hemoglobin, thereby increasing the visibility of blood vessels including tumor-associated vasculature. This technology requires specialized cystoscopes capable of NBI but can be incorporated for office cystoscopy use because it does not require instillation of special contrast agents. Several studies examining the efficacy of NBI have demonstrated its utility in enhancing tumor detection in comparison to WLC, including improved sensitivity of CIS detection,[54] reduced recurrence rates, and fewer numbers of recurrent tumors,[55] additional detection rates of non-muscle invasive bladder cancer (NMIBC) and carcinoma *in situ* (CIS) of upwards of 25%,[56,57] as well as improve urologists WLC skills.[58] In 2016, a large prospective randomized single-blind multicenter study demonstrated NBI and WLC achieved similar overall recurrence rates 12 months after TURBT (27.1% vs 25.4%, respectively) but that NBI-enhanced TURBT reduced the likelihood of disease recurrence in low-risk patients (27.3% vs 5.6%).[59] False-positive diagnoses are also common during the initial learning curve, post-BCG, and inflammatory states.

SUMMARY

As urologic care advances, the use of intraoperative imaging tools developed to help aid the surgeon is becoming more common. For prostate, kidney, and bladder cancer, identification and complete resection are critical for optimal oncological control. This article focused on the latest intraoperative applications of several emerging and innovative imaging modalities and each has its strengths and weaknesses. There is no one-size-fits-all approach to imaging, and there may never be. Urologists will have to choose between competing technologies and familiarize themselves with their applications to provide the best care for patients. Learning curves, assessment times, access to proprietary technology, and additional nonsurgical personnel are just some factors that will determine which technologies are adopted. Despite perceived benefits of implementing these various intraoperative imaging tools, more long-term data are needed to determine whether those in this article actually improve patient outcomes.

CLINICS CARE POINTS

- Identification of the extent of prostate, kidney and bladder tumors during surgery can be challenging, and new intraoperative imaging modalities can help reduce.
- 5-ALA, ^{68}Ga-PSMA CLI, LRS have been used to improve completion of prostate tumor resection but are limited by false positive signal rates.
- Nephron-sparing surgery can be aided by both ultrasound and fluorescence imaging, however additional studies are needed to prove this improves positive surgical margin rates.
- Narrow-band and photodynamic imaging can improve sensitivity of detecting bladder tumors and reduce recurrence rates.

DISCLOSURE

The authors have nothing to disclose.

REFERENCES

1. Bianco FJ, Scardino PT, Eastham JA. Radical prostatectomy: Long-term cancer control and recovery of sexual and urinary function ("trifecta"). Urology 2005;66(5 SUPPL):83–94.
2. Ploussard G, Agamy MA, Alenda O, et al. Impact of positive surgical margins on prostate-specific antigen failure after radical prostatectomy in adjuvant treatment-naïve patients. BJU Int 2011;107(11): 1748–54.
3. Bolla M, van Poppel H, Tombal B, et al. Postoperative radiotherapy after radical prostatectomy for high-risk prostate cancer: Long-term results of a randomised controlled trial (EORTC trial 22911). Lancet 2012;380(9858):2018–27.
4. Ohori M, Wheeler TM, Katt'an MW, et al. Prognostic significance of positive surgical margins in radical prostatectomy specimens. J Urol 1995;154(5): 1818–24.
5. Schlomm T, Tennstedt P, Huxhold C, et al. Neurovascular structure-adjacent frozen-section examination (NeuroSAFE) increases nerve-sparing frequency and reduces positive surgical margins in open and robot-assisted laparoscopic radical prostatectomy: Experience after 11 069 consecutive patients. Eur Urol 2012;62(2):333–40.
6. Batlle C. Porphyrins, Porphyrias, cancer and model for carcinogenesis photodynamic therapy-A. J Photochem Photobiol B 1993;20:5–22.
7. Zaak D, Sroka R, Khoder W, et al. Photodynamic Diagnosis of Prostate Cancer Using 5-Aminolevulinic Acid-First Clinical Experiences. Urology 2008; 72(2):345–8.
8. Inoue K, Ashida S, Fukuhara H, et al. Application of 5-aminolevulinic acid-mediated photodynamic diagnosis to robot-assisted laparoscopic radical prostatectomy. Urology 2013;82(5):1175–8.
9. Fukuhara H, Inoue K, Kurabayashi A, et al. Performance of 5-aminolevulinic-acid-based photodynamic diagnosis for radical prostatectomy. BMC Urol 2015;15(1):78.
10. Ganzer R, Blana A, Denzinger S, et al. Intraoperative photodynamic evaluation of surgical margins during endoscopic extraperitoneal radical prostatectomy with the use of 5-aminolevulinic acid. J Endourol 2009;23(9):1387–94.
11. Maurer T, Eiber M, Schwaiger M, et al. Current use of PSMA–PET in prostate cancer management. Nat Rev Urol 2016;13(4):226–35.
12. Perera M, Papa N, Roberts M, et al. Gallium-68 prostate-specific membrane antigen positron emission tomography in advanced prostate cancer—updated diagnostic utility, sensitivity, specificity, and distribution of prostate-specific membrane antigen-avid lesions: a systematic review and meta-analysis. Eur Urol 2020;77(4):403–17.
13. Robertson R, Germanos MS, Li C, et al. Optical imaging of Cerenkov light generation from positron-emitting radiotracers. Phys Med Biol 2009;54(16): N355–65.
14. Darr C, Harke NN, Radtke JP, et al. Intraoperative 68Ga-PSMA cerenkov luminescence imaging for surgical margins in radical prostatectomy: a feasibility study. J Nucl Med 2020;61(10):1500–6.
15. Giesel FL, Hadaschik B, Cardinale J, et al. F-18 labelled PSMA-1007: biodistribution, radiation dosimetry and histopathological validation of tumor lesions in prostate cancer patients. Eur J Nucl Med Mol Imaging 2017;44(4):678–88.
16. Sharma V, Olweny EO, Kapur P, et al. Prostate cancer detection using combined auto-fluorescence and light reflectance spectroscopy: ex vivo study

of human prostates. Biomed Opt Express 2014;5(5): 1512–29.

17. Morgan MSC, Lay AH, Wang X, et al. Light reflectance spectroscopy to detect positive surgical margins on prostate cancer specimens. J Urol 2016; 195(2):479–84.
18. Lay AH, Wang X, Morgan MSC, et al. Detecting positive surgical margins: utilisation of light-reflectance spectroscopy on ex vivo prostate specimens. BJU Int 2016;118(6):885–9.
19. Novick AC. Nephron-sparing surgery for renal cell carcinoma. Annu Rev Med 2002;53:393.
20. Leibovich BC, Blute ML, Cheville JC, et al. Nephron sparing surgery for appropriately selected renal cell carcinoma between 4 and 7 cm results in outcome similar to radical nephrectomy. J Urol 2004;171: 1066.
21. Becker F, Siemer S, Hack M, et al. Excellent long-term cancer control with elective nephron-sparing surgery for selected renal cell carcinomas measuring more than 4 cm. Eur Urol 2006;49:1058.
22. Kim JM, Song PH, Kim HT, et al. Comparison of partial and radical nephrectomy for pT1b renal cell carcinoma. Korean J Urol 2010;51:596.
23. Crispen PL, Boorjian SA, Lohse CM. Outcomes following partial nephrectomy by tumor size. J Urol 2008;180:1912.
24. Margulis V, Tamboli P, Jacobsohn KM, et al. Oncological efficacy and safety of nephron-sparing surgery for selected patients with locally advanced renal cell carcinoma. BJU Int 2007;100:1235.
25. Lam JS, Bergman J, Breda A, et al. Importance of surgical margins in the management of renal cell carcinoma. Nat Clin Pract Urol 2008;5:308.
26. Marszalek M, Carini M, Chlosta P, et al. Positive surgical margins after nephron-sparing surgery. Eur Urol 2012;61(4):757–63.
27. Gilbert BR, Russo P, Zirinsky K, et al. Intraoperative sonography: application in renal cell carcinoma. J Urol 1988;139(3):582–4.
28. Bhosale PR, Wei W, Ernst RD, et al. Intraoperative sonography during open partial nephrectomy for renal cell cancer: does it alter surgical management? Am J Roentgenol 2014;203(4):822–7.
29. Polascik TJ, Meng M v, Epstein JI, et al. Intraoperative sonography for the evaluation and management of renal tumors: experience with 100 patients. J Urol 1995;154:1676.
30. Assimos DG, Boyce H, Woodruff RD, et al. Intraoperative renal ultrasonography: a useful adjunct to partial nephrectomy. J Urol 1991;146:1218.
31. Kaczmarek BF, Sukumar S, Petros F, et al. Robotic ultrasound probe for tumor identification in robotic partial nephrectomy: Initial series and outcomes. Int J Urol 2013;20(2):172–6.
32. Kaczmarek BF, Sukumar S, Kumar RK, et al. Comparison of robotic and laparoscopic ultrasound probes for robotic partial nephrectomy. J Endourol 2013;27(9):1137–40.
33. Desmonts A, Tillou X, le Gal S, et al. A new technique for ensuring negative surgical margins during partial nephrectomy: the ex vivo ultrasound control. Prog Urol 2013;23(12):966–70.
34. Doerfler A, Cerantola Y, Meuwly J-Y, et al. Ex vivo ultrasound control of resection margins during partial nephrectomy. J Urol 2011;186(6):2188–93.
35. Alharbi FM, Chahwan CK, le Gal SG, et al. Intraoperative ultrasound control of surgical margins during partial nephrectomy. Urol Ann 2016;8(4):430.
36. Golijanin DJ, Marshall J, Cardin A, et al. Bilitranslocase (BTL) is immunolocalised in proximal and distal renal tubules and absent in renal cortical tumors accurately corresponding to intraoperative near infrared fluorescence (NIRF) expression of renal cortical tumors using intravenous indocyanine green (ICG). J Urol 2008;179(4S):137.
37. Tobis S, Knopf JK, Silvers CR, et al. Near infrared fluorescence imaging after intravenous indocyanine green: initial clinical experience with open partial nephrectomy for renal cortical tumors. Urology 2012; 79(4):958–64.
38. Mitsui Y, Shiina H, Arichi N, et al. Indocyanine green (ICG)-based fluorescence navigation system for discrimination of kidney cancer from normal parenchyma: application during partial nephrectomy. Int Urol Nephrol 2012;44(3):753–9.
39. Krane LS, Manny TB, Hemal AK. Is near infrared fluorescence imaging using indocyanine green dye useful in robotic partial nephrectomy: a prospective comparative study of 94 patients. Urology 2012; 80(1):110–8.
40. Hoda MR, Popken G. Surgical outcomes of fluorescence-guided laparoscopic partial nephrectomy using 5-aminolevulinic acid-induced protoporphyrin IX. J Surg Res 2009;154(2):220–5.
41. Waidelich R, Stepp H, Baumgartner R, et al. Clinical experience with 5-aminolevulinic acid and photodynamic therapy for refractory superficial bladder cancer. J Urol 2001;165(6 Part 1):1904–7.
42. Hekman MC, Rijpkema M, Muselaers CH, et al. Tumor-targeted dual-modality imaging to improve intraoperative visualization of clear cell renal cell carcinoma: a first in man study. Theranostics 2018; 8(8):2161–70.
43. Mossanen M, Gore JL. The burden of bladder cancer care: direct and indirect costs. Curr Opin Urol 2014;24(5):487–91.
44. Poletajew S, Krajewski W, Kaczmarek K, et al. The learning curve for transurethral resection of bladder tumour: how many is enough to be independent, safe and effective surgeon? J Surg Educ 2020; 77(4):978–85.
45. Brausi M, Collette L, Kurth K, et al. Variability in the recurrence rate at first follow-up cystoscopy after

TUR in stage Ta T1 transitional cell carcinoma of the bladder: a combined analysis of seven EORTC studies. Eur Urol 2002;41(5):523–31.

46. Sfakianos JP, Kim PH, Hakimi AA, et al. The effect of restaging transurethral resection on recurrence and progression rates in patients with nonmuscle invasive bladder cancer treated with intravesical bacillus Calmette-Guérin. J Urol 2014;191(2):341–5.
47. Babjuk M, Burger M, Compérat EM, et al. European association of urology guidelines on non-muscle-invasive bladder cancer (TaT1 and carcinoma in situ)-2019 update. Eur Urol 2019;76(5):639–57.
48. Chang SS, Boorjian SA, Chou R, et al. Diagnosis and treatment of non-muscle invasive bladder cancer: AUA/SUO guideline. J Urol 2016;196(4):1021–9.
49. Daneshmand S, Schuckman AK, Bochner BH, et al. Hexaminolevulinate blue-light cystoscopy in non-muscle-invasive bladder cancer: review of the clinical evidence and consensus statement on appropriate use in the USA. Nat Rev Urol 2014;11(10):589–96.
50. Burger M, Grossman HB, Droller M, et al. Photodynamic diagnosis of non–muscle-invasive bladder cancer with hexaminolevulinate cystoscopy: a meta-analysis of detection and recurrence based on raw data. Eur Urol 2013;64(5):846–54.
51. Kausch I, Sommerauer M, Montorsi F, et al. Photodynamic diagnosis in non–muscle-invasive bladder cancer: a systematic review and cumulative analysis of prospective studies. Eur Urol 2010;57(4):595–606.
52. Daniltchenko DI, Riedl CR, Sachs MD, et al. Long-term benefit of 5-aminolevulinic acid fluorescence assisted transurethral resection of superficial bladder cancer: 5-year results of a prospective randomized study. J Urol 2005;174(6):2129–33.
53. Stenzl A, Burger M, Fradet Y, et al. Hexaminolevulinate guided fluorescence cystoscopy reduces recurrence in patients with nonmuscle invasive bladder cancer. J Urol 2010;184(5):1907–14.
54. Herr HW, Donat SM. A comparison of white-light cystoscopy and narrow-band imaging cystoscopy to detect bladder tumour recurrences. BJU Int 2008;102(9):1111–4.
55. Herr HW, Donat SM. Reduced bladder tumour recurrence rate associated with narrow-band imaging surveillance cystoscopy. BJU Int 2011;107(3):396–8.
56. Xiong Y, Li J, Ma S, et al. A meta-analysis of narrow band imaging for the diagnosis and therapeutic outcome of non-muscle invasive bladder cancer. PLoS One 2017;12(2):e0170819.
57. Li K, Lin T, Fan X, et al. Diagnosis of narrow-band imaging in non-muscle-invasive bladder cancer: a systematic review and meta-analysis. Int J Urol 2013;20(6):602–9.
58. Bryan RT, Shah ZH, Collins SI, et al. Narrow-band imaging flexible cystoscopy: a new user's experience. J endourology 2010;24(8):1339–43.
59. Naito S, Algaba F, Babjuk M, et al. The clinical research office of the endourological society (CROES) multicentre randomised trial of narrow band imaging–assisted transurethral resection of bladder tumour (TURBT) versus conventional white light imaging–assisted TURBT in primary non–muscle-invasive bladder cancer patients: trial protocol and 1-year results. Eur Urol 2016;70(3):506–15.

Artificial Intelligence Applications in Urology

Reporting Standards to Achieve Fluency for Urologists

Andrew B. Chen, MD[a], Taseen Haque, BA[b], Sidney Roberts, BA[b], Sirisha Rambhatla, PhD[c], Giovanni Cacciamani, MD[a], Prokar Dasgupta, MD[d], Andrew J. Hung, MD[a,*]

KEYWORDS

• Machine learning • Artificial intelligence • Urology • Deep learning • Review

KEY POINTS

- Applications of artificial intelligence are increasing in multiple disciplines, including medicine and urology.
- Artificial intelligence literacy is critical for clinicians participating in research.
- Although the reporting of methodologies and outcomes varies in the literature, reporting standards can serve as a foundation for future evaluation of medical research in artificial intelligence.

INTRODUCTION

The past few years have seen enormous growth in artificial intelligence (AI) applications in a multitude of disciplines, including medicine.[1,2] This rising interest in AI, and machine learning (ML) more specifically, is reflected in the increased research output (ie, registered clinical trials and published articles), devices obtaining regulatory approval in the United States, and entrepreneurial funding of health care startups.[3]

Similarly, there is increasing literature supporting its use in urology.[4] Although there have been impressive results in the field, there is an evident gap in medical education in preparing future clinicians for discussions regarding AI.[3] Understanding the differences between AI, ML, deep learning, and subsets such as neural networks is merely the first step in achieving fluency in this growing field. The complexity of the topic is such that some authors have even proposed curricula that would require further in-depth exploration of the hard sciences (physics and computational sciences such as coding, algorithms, and mechatronic engineering) to adequately train the next generation of AI-competent physicians.[5]

Given the importance of AI and its impact on the practice of medicine, an AI-literate workforce is critical. Misconceptions can limit people's ability to use, collaborate with, and act as critical consumers of AI.[6] Despite the growing popularity of AI in urology, education of urologists remains limited. This finding is no surprise, because even newly trained physicians graduate with little to no exposure to AI and ML within the medical curriculum.[3] In addition, the variability in reported information within the subfields of oncology, infertility, endourology, and general urology increases the heterogeneity of documented outcomes and methodologies reported in publications. With the broad spectrum of applications of AI in urology, it is critical to develop a method to standardize

[a] USC Institute of Urology, 1441 Eastlake Avenue Suite 7416, Los Angeles, CA 90089, USA; [b] Keck School of Medicine of USC, 1441 Eastlake Avenue Suite 7416, Los Angeles, CA 90089, USA; [c] Viterbi School of Engineering at USC, 1441 Eastlake Avenue Suite 7416, Los Angeles, CA 90089, USA; [d] King's College London, King's Health Partners, 145 Harley Street, London W1G 6BG, UK
* Corresponding author.
E-mail address: Andrew.hung@med.usc.edu

Urol Clin N Am 49 (2022) 65–117
https://doi.org/10.1016/j.ucl.2021.07.009
0094-0143/22/

reporting to assist in readability and distribution of information to clinicians.

Although the ultimate goal would be to establish a foundation where all physicians would be able to understand the construction of algorithms, critically evaluate the datasets powering the outputs, and understand any limitations in the approach, a more attainable first step would be to establish baseline AI literacy without the need for supplemental degrees or education. Herein, we perform a narrative review of the literature of AI and ML in urology and propose a checklist of reporting standards for articles reporting outcomes of AI and ML to improve readability for clinicians and evaluate the current state of the literature.

METHODS

A literature search was performed. Articles between 2012 and 2020 using the search terms "urology", "artificial intelligence," "machine learning" were vetted and categorized by the application of AI in urology. Review articles, editorial comments, articles with no full-text access, and nonurologic studies were excluded.

A checklist of reporting standards was created in a multi-disciplinary fashion. Three investigators independently evaluated (AC, TH, SR) all articles under the proposed checklist of competencies. **Box 1** lists our proposed reporting standards.

RESULTS

Our initial search yielded 400 articles, but after excluding duplicates and after full-text review and examination of article references, the 112 most relevant articles were included in the final analysis. Similar to our previous work, we classified articles into 3 categories of AI applications: diagnosis, outcome prediction, and surgical skill analysis.[4]

Box 1
Lists of proposed reporting standards

Reporting standards

Algorithm/model

Neural network architecture

Preprocessing methodology disclose

Size of dataset

Number of features

Train/test explanation

Train/test split

Cross-validation or Monte Carlo runs

Lay term explanation of AI methodology

Performance metrics

Implications/significance and discussion of how AI/ML advances the field

Comparison with traditional methods

Feature ranking

Diagnosis

Disease diagnosis was found to be the most common application of AI/ML in urology. There were 73 of the 112 articles in the final analysis reporting AI and ML algorithms automating and improving the detection of pathologies.

Prostate cancer

As the most common malignancy seen by urologists, 44 of the 73 (60.2%) articles used algorithms to find new ways of detecting prostate cancer. Applications include the analysis of serum studies, urine studies, novel biomarkers, radiomics, clinical variables, pathology slides, and electronic health records (**Table 1**). Connell and colleagues[7] examined the clinical, urine-derived cell-free messenger RNA and urine cell DNA methylation data to diagnose clinically significant prostate cancer with an area under the curve (AUC) of 0.89. The growth of natural language processing can also help to streamline research and analysis. Leyh-Bannurah and associates[8] analyzed 3679 electronic health records to accurately report primary and secondary Gleason patterns, tumor stage, nodal stage, tumor volume, and surgical margin, all with greater than 90% agreement. Radiomics involves the high-throughput extraction of radiologic features from clinical imaging.[9] Varghese and colleagues[10] identified the best ML classifier for prostate cancer risk stratification and compared it with the Prostate Imaging Reporting and Data System Version 2 (PI-RADS v2). They found better performance in the high-risk class (F-score, 0.69 vs 0.52; precision, 0.57 vs 0.45; recall, 0.86 vs 0.61), albeit with a similar AUC in the total dataset (0.71 vs 0.73).[10]

Bladder cancer

A total of 7 studies were identified involving detection of bladder cancer with AI. Shkolyar and colleagues[11] used a convolutional neural network, CystoNet, to automate tumor detection on cystoscopy with a sensitivity and specificity of 90.9% and 98.6%, respectively. Additional modalities include atomic force microscopy, urine biomarkers, MRI, and computed tomography (CT) urogram as input data in the detection of bladder cancer (**Table 2**).

Kidney cancer

The diagnosis of renal cell carcinoma (RCC) remains challenging in certain subsets of cases. In

Table 1
Prostate Cancer Diagnosis

Study	Application	Category	Subcategory	Algorithms/ Models (List)	Neural Network: Architecture (Descriptor) (Y, N, N/A)	Preprocessing Methodology Disclose (Y/N)	Reporting Size of Dataset (n)	No. of Features	Train/Test Explanation (Y/N)	Train-Test Split	Cross-Validation or Monte Carlo Runs (Y/N)	Lay Term Explanation of AI Methodology	Performance Metrics_ x000 B_	Implications/ Significance Discussion of How AI/ML Advances the Field (Y/N)	Comparison to Traditional Method (Y/N)	Feature Ranking (Y/N)
Sapre 2014	Prostate cancer risk Stratification with plasma microRNA	Diagnosis	Prostate cancer	Hierarchical clustering	N/A	Y	70	12	Y	N/A	N	N	N/A	N	N	Y
	Prostate cancer risk stratification with urine microRNA	Diagnosis	Prostate cancer	Hierarchical clustering	N/A	Y	34	13	Y	34:36	N	N	AUC	N	N	Y
Mortensen 2019	Prostate weight from PET/CT scan	Diagnosis	Prostate cancer	Convolutional neural network	Y	Y	145	Not explained	Y	145:45	N	N	N/A	Y	N	N
	PET scan SUV_{max} from PET/ CT scan	Diagnosis	Prostate cancer	Convolutional neural network	Y	Y	145	Not explained	Y	145:46	N	N	N/A	Y	N	N
	PET scan SUV_{mean} from PET/ CT scan	Diagnosis	Prostate cancer	Convolutional neural network	Y	Y	145	Not explained	Y	145:47	N	N	N/A	Y	N	N
	PET Vol from PET/CT scan	Diagnosis	Prostate cancer	Convolutional neural network	Y	Y	145	Not explained	Y	145:48	N	N	N/A	Y	N	N
	TLU from PET/CT scan	Diagnosis	Prostate cancer	Convolutional neural network	Y	Y	145	Not explained	Y	145:49	N	N	N/A	Y	N	N
Nitta 2019	Predict prostate cancer based off temporal PSA	Diagnosis	Prostate cancer	Artificial neural network	N	N	512	4	Y	N/A	Y	Y	AUC	Y	N	Y
	Predict prostate cancer based off temporal PSA	Diagnosis	Prostate cancer	Support vector machine	N/A	N	512	4	Y	N/A	Y	Y	AUC	Y	N	Y
	Predict prostate cancer based off temporal PSA	Diagnosis	Prostate cancer	Random forest	N/A	N	512	4	Y	N/A	Y	Y	AUC	Y	N	Y

(continued on next page)

Table 1
(*continued*)

Study	Application	Category	Subcategory	Algorithms/ Models (List)	Neural Network: Architecture (Descriptor) (Y, N, N/A)	Preprocessing Methodology Disclose (Y/N)	Reporting Size of Dataset (n)	No. of Features	Train/Test Explanation (Y/N)	Train-Test Split	Cross-Validation or Monte Carlo Runs (Y/N)	Lay Term Explanation of AI Methodology	Performance Metrics_ x000 B_	Implications/ Significance Discussion of How AI/ML Advances the Field (Y/N)	Comparison to Traditional Method (Y/N)	Feature Ranking (Y/N)
Osman 2019	Diagnose Gleason score from radiomics	Diagnosis	Prostate cancer	Least absolute shrinkage and selection operator	N/A	Y	342	522	Y	80%:20%	Y	N	AUC	Y	N	N
	Diagnose risk group from radiomics	Diagnosis	Prostate cancer	ElasticNet	N/A	Y	342	522	Y	80%:20%	Y	N	AUC	Y	N	N
Johnson 2020	Prostate cancer detection from 25 gene panel urine test	Diagnosis	Prostate cancer	Random forest	N/A	Y	1010	25	N	N/A	Y	N	AUC Sensitivity Specificity	N	N	N
Connell 2020	Detection of clinically significant prostate cancer from urine cell-free RNA and cell DNA methylation	Diagnosis	Prostate cancer	Random forest	N/A	Y	197	12	Y	N/A	N	N	AUC	Y	N	Y
Bernatz 2020	Detect clinically significant prostate cancer in the peripheral zone with multiparametric MRI radiomics	Diagnosis	Prostate cancer	Support vector machine	N/A	Y	73	105	Y	N/A	Y	N	AUC	Y	N	Y
	Detect clinically significant prostate cancer in the peripheral zone with multiparametric MRI radiomics	Diagnosis	Prostate cancer	Random forest	N/A	Y	73	105	Y	N/A	Y	N	AUC	Y	N	Y
	Detect clinically significant	Diagnosis	Prostate cancer	Neural network	N	Y	73	105	Y	N/A	Y	N	AUC	Y	N	Y

	prostate cancer in the peripheral zone with multiparametric MRI radiomics														
Kan 2020	Detecting benign PIRADS3 lesions on multiparametric MRI	Diagnosis	Prostate cancer	Logistic regression	N/A	Y	287	Not explained	Y	200:59	Y	Y	AUC Accuracy Sensitivity Specificity	Y	N	Y
	Detecting benign PIRADS3 lesions on multiparametric MRI	Diagnosis	Prostate cancer	Support vector machine	N/A	Y	287	Not explained	Y	200:59	Y	Y	AUC Accuracy Sensitivity Specificity	Y	N	Y
	Detecting benign PIRADS3 lesions on multiparametric MRI	Diagnosis	Prostate cancer	Extreme gradient boosting	N/A	Y	287	Not explained	Y	200:59	Y	Y	AUC Accuracy Sensitivity Specificity	Y	N	Y
	Detecting benign PIRADS3 lesions on multiparametric MRI	Diagnosis	Prostate cancer	Random forest	N/A	Y	287	Not explained	Y	200:59	Y	Y	AUC Accuracy Sensitivity Specificity	Y	N	Y
Algohary 2018	Identify clinically significant prostate cancer in active surveillance patients with MRI	Diagnosis	Prostate cancer	Quadratic discriminant analysis	N/A	Y	56	5	Y	60%:40%	Y	Y	Accuracy, sensitivity, specificity	Y	Y	Y
	Identify clinically significant prostate cancer in active surveillance patients with MRI	Diagnosis	Prostate cancer	Random forest	N/A	Y	56	5	Y	60%:40%	Y	Y	Accuracy, sensitivity, specificity	Y	Y	Y
	Identify clinically significant prostate cancer in active surveillance patients with MRI	Diagnosis	Prostate cancer	Support vector machine	N/A	Y	56	5	Y	60%:40%	Y	Y	Accuracy, sensitivity, specificity	Y	Y	Y

(continued on next page)

Table 1
(continued)

Study	Application	Category	Subcategory	Algorithms/ Models (List)	Neural Network: Architecture (Descriptor) (Y, N, N/A)	Preprocessing Methodology Disclose (Y/N)	Reporting Size of Dataset (n)	No. of Features	Train/Test Explanation (Y/N)	Train-Test Split	Cross-Validation or Monte Carlo Runs (Y/N)	Lay Term Explanation of AI Methodology	Performance Metrics_ x000 B_	Implications/ Significance Discussion of How AI/ML Advances the Field (Y/N)	Comparison to Traditional Method (Y/N)	Feature Ranking (Y/N)
Fehr et al. 2015	Diagnose Gleason score on multiparametric MRI	Diagnosis	Prostate cancer	AdaBoost	N/A	Y	147	18	Y	N/A	Y	Y	Accuracy, sensitivity, s pecificity	Y	N	Y
	Diagnose Gleason score on multiparametric MRI	Diagnosis	Prostate cancer	AdaBoost	N/A	Y	147	18	Y	N/A	Y	Y	Accuracy, sensitivity, specificity	Y	N	Y
	Diagnose Gleason score on multiparametric MRI	Diagnosis	Prostate cancer	Support vector machine	N/A	Y	147	18	Y	N/A	Y	Y	Accuracy, sensitivity, specificity	Y	N	Y
	Diagnose Gleason score on multiparametric MRI	Diagnosis	Prostate cancer	Support vector machine	N/A	Y	147	18	Y	N/A	Y	Y	Accuracy, sensitivity, specificity	Y	N	Y
	Diagnose Gleason score on multiparametric MRI	Diagnosis	Prostate cancer	Support vector machine	N/A	Y	147	18	Y	N/A	Y	Y	Accuracy, sensitivity, specificity	Y	N	Y
	Diagnose Gleason score on multiparametric MRI	Diagnosis	Prostate cancer	Support vector machine	N/A	Y	147	18	Y	N/A	Y	Y	Accuracy, sensitivity, specificity	Y	N	Y
Ginzburg et al. 2017	Detect prostate cancer on MRI	Diagnosis	Prostate cancer	Logistic regression	N/A	N	80	10	Y	N/A	Y	N	AUC	N	Y	N
Iordanescu et al. 2015	Identify prostate cancer and cancer aggressiveness on MRI and proton MR spectroscopy	Diagnosis	prostate cancer	Support vector machine	N/A	Y	31	7	Y	Y	Y	N	AUC, accuracy, sensitivity, specificity	Y	Y	Y
Qian et al. 2014	Detect prostate cancer on MRI	Diagnosis	Prostate cancer	Random forest	N/A	Y	26	10,000	Y	25:1	Y	Y	Accuracy	N	N	Y

Sun et al 2017	Detect prostate cancer on MRI	Diagnosis	Prostate cancer	Support vector machine	N/A	Y	5	2	Y	10:1	Y	N	AUC, accuracy	N	Y	N
Imani et al. 2015	Identify prostate cancer on transrectal ultrasound examination	Diagnosis	Prostate cancer	jICA	Y	Y	12	64	Y	12:1	Y	Y	AUC, accuracy, sensitivity, specificity	N	Y	N
Del Grossi et al. 2014	Diagnosis of prostate cancer from clinical variables and PSA	Diagnosis	Prostate cancer	Logistic regression	N/A	Y	500	6	Y	1:1	Y	N	Accuracy	N	N	Y
	Diagnosis of prostate cancer from clinical variables and PSA	Diagnosis	Prostate cancer	Artificial neural network	N	Y	500	6	Y	1:1	Y	N	Accuracy	N	N	Y
	Diagnosis of prostate cancer from clinical variables and PSA	Diagnosis	Prostate cancer	Artificial neural network	N	Y	500	6	Y	1:1	Y	N	Accuracy	N	N	Y
	Diagnosis of prostate cancer from clinical variables and PSA	Diagnosis	Prostate cancer	Decision tree (alternating)	N/A	Y	500	6	Y	1:1	Y	N	Accuracy	N	N	Y
	Diagnosis of prostate cancer from clinical variables and PSA	Diagnosis	Prostate cancer	Decision tree (PART)	N/A	Y	500	6	Y	1:1	Y	N	Accuracy	N	N	Y
Regnier-Coudert et al. 2012	Diagnose organ confined prostate cancer based on patient clinical and pathologic data from biopsy	Diagnosis	Prostate cancer	k-Nearest neighbor	N/A	Y	>7500	10	Y	N/A	Y	Y	AUC	Y	N	N
	Diagnose extraprostatic extension based on patient clinical and pathologic data	Diagnosis	Prostate cancer	k-Nearest neighbor	N/A	Y	>7500	10	Y	N/A	Y	Y	AUC	Y	N	N
	Diagnose SVI invasion of prostate cancer based on	Diagnosis	Prostate cancer	k-Nearest neighbor	N/A	Y	>7500	10	Y	N/A	Y	Y	AUC	Y	N	N

(continued on next page)

Table 1
(continued)

Study	Application	Category	Subcategory	Algorithms/ Models (List)	Neural Network: Architecture (Descriptor) (Y, N, N/A)	Prepro-cessing Method-ology Disclose (Y/N)	Reporting Size of Dataset (n)	No. of Features	Train/Test Explanation (Y/N)	Train-Test Split	Cross-Validation or Monte Carlo Runs (Y/N)	Lay Term Explanation of AI Method-ology	Performance Metrics_ x000 B_	Implications/ Significance Discussion of How AI/ML Advances the Field (Y/N)	Comparison to Traditional Method (Y/N)	Feature Ranking (Y/N)
	patient clinical and pathologic data															
	Diagnose lymph node involvement of prostate cancer based on patient clinical and pathologic data	Diagnosis	Prostate cancer	k-Nearest neighbor	N/A	Y	>7500	10	Y	N/A	Y	Y	AUC	Y	N	N
	Diagnose organ confined prostate cancer based on patient clinical and pathologic data from biopsy	Diagnosis	Prostate cancer	Random forest	N/A	Y	>7500	10	Y	N/A	Y	Y	AUC	Y	N	N
	Diagnose extraprostatic extension based on patient clinical and pathologic data	Diagnosis	Prostate cancer	Random forest	N/A	Y	>7500	10	Y	N/A	Y	Y	AUC	Y	N	N
	Diagnose SVI invasion of prostate cancer based on patient clinical and pathologic data	Diagnosis	Prostate cancer	Random forest	N/A	Y	>7500	10	Y	N/A	Y	Y	AUC	Y	N	N
	Diagnose lymph node involvement of prostate cancer based on patient clinical and pathologic data	Diagnosis	Prostate cancer	Random forest	N/A	Y	>7500	10	Y	N/A	Y	Y	AUC	Y	N	N
	Diagnose organ confined prostate cancer based on patient clinical and pathologic data from biopsy	Diagnosis	Prostate cancer	Logistic regression	N/A	Y	>7500	10	Y	N/A	Y	Y	AUC	Y	N	N
	Diagnose extraprostatic extension based	Diagnosis	Prostate cancer	Logistic regression	N/A	Y	>7500	10	Y	N/A	Y	Y	AUC	Y	N	N

on patient clinical and pathologic data														
Diagnose SVI invasion of prostate cancer based on patient clinical and pathologic data	Diagnosis	Prostate c ancer	Logistic regression	N/A	Y	>7500	10	Y	N/A	Y	Y	AUC	Y	N	N
Diagnose lymph node involvement of prostate cancer based on patient clinical and pathologic data	Diagnosis	Prostate cancer	Logistic regression	N/A	Y	>7500	10	Y	N/A	Y	Y	AUC	Y	N	N
Diagnose organ confined prostate cancer based on patient clinical and pathologic data from biopsy	Diagnosis	Prostate cancer	Artificial neural network	Y	Y	>7500	10	Y	N/A	Y	Y	AUC	Y	N	N
Diagnose extraprostatic extension based on patient clinical and pathologic data	Diagnosis	Prostate cancer	Artificial neural network	Y	Y	>7500	10	Y	N/A	Y	Y	AUC	Y	N	N
Diagnose SVI invasion of prostate cancer based on patient clinical and pathologic data	Diagnosis	Prostate cancer	Artificial neural network	Y	Y	>7500	10	Y	N/A	Y	Y	AUC	Y	N	N
Diagnose lymph node involvement of prostate cancer based on patient clinical and pathologic data	Diagnosis	Prostate cancer	Artificial neural network	Y	Y	>7500	10	Y	N/A	Y	Y	AUC	Y	N	N
Diagnose organ confined prostate cancer based on patient clinical and pathologic data from biopsy	Diagnosis	Prostate cancer	Radial basis function network	N/A	Y	>7500	10	Y	N/A	Y	Y	AUC	Y	N	N
Diagnose extraprostatic extension based on patient clinical and pathologic data	Diagnosis	Prostate cancer	Radial basis function network	N/A	Y	>7500	10	Y	N/A	Y	Y	AUC	Y	N	N
Diagnose SVI invasion of prostate cancer based on patient	Diagnosis	Prostate cancer	Radial basis function network	N/A	Y	>7500	10	Y	N/A	Y	Y	AUC	Y	N	N

(continued on next page)

Table 1
(*continued*)

Study	Application	Category	Subcategory	Algorithms/ Models (List)	Neural Network: Architecture (Descriptor) (Y, N, N/A)	Prepro-cessing Method-ology Disclose (Y/N)	Reporting Size of Dataset (n)	No. of Features	Train/Test Explanation (Y/N)	Train-Test Split	Cross-Validation or Monte Carlo Runs (Y/N)	Lay Term Explanation of AI Method-ology	Performance Metrics_ x000 B_	Implications/ Significance Discussion of How AI/ML Advances the Field (Y/N)	Comparison to Traditional Method (Y/N)	Feature Ranking (Y/N)
	clinical and pathologic data															
	Diagnose lymph node involvement of prostate cancer based on patient clinical and pathologic data	Diagnosis	Prostate cancer	Radial basis function network	N/A	Y	>7500	10	Y	N/A	Y	Y	AUC	Y	N	N
	Diagnose organ confined prostate cancer based on patient clinical and pathologic data from biopsy	Diagnosis	Prostate cancer	Support vector machine	N/A	Y	>7500	10	Y	N/A	Y	Y	AUC	Y	N	N
	Diagnose extraprostatic extension based on patient clinical and pathologic data	Diagnosis	Prostate cancer	Support vector machine	N/A	Y	>7500	10	Y	N/A	Y	Y	AUC	Y	N	N
	Diagnose SVI invasion of prostate cancer based on patient clinical and pathologic data	Diagnosis	Prostate cancer	Support vector machine	N/A	Y	>7500	10	Y	N/A	Y	Y	AUC	Y	N	N
	Diagnose lymph node involvement of prostate cancer based on patient clinical and pathologic data	Diagnosis	Prostate cancer	Support vector machine	N/A	Y	>7500	10	Y	N/A	Y	Y	AUC	Y	N	N
	Diagnose organ confined prostate cancer based on patient clinical and pathologic	Diagnosis	Prostate cancer	Naïve Bayes classifier	N/A	Y	>7500	10	Y	N/A	Y	Y	AUC	Y	N	N

	data from biopsy														
	Diagnose extraprostatic extension based on patient clinical and pathologic data	Diagnosis	Prostate cancer	Naïve Bayes classifier	N/A	Y	>7500	10	Y	N/A	Y	Y	AUC	Y	N	N
	Diagnose SVI invasion of prostate cancer based on patient clinical and pathologic data	Diagnosis	Prostate cancer	Naïve Bayes classifier	N/A	Y	>7500	10	Y	N/A	Y	Y	AUC	Y	N	N
	Diagnose lymph node involvement of prostate cancer based on patient clinical and pathologic data	Diagnosis	Prostate cancer	Naïve Bayes classifier	N/A	Y	>7500	10	Y	N/A	Y	Y	AUC	Y	N	N
Neuhaus et al. 2013	Detect prostate cancer using peptide biomarker in seminal plasma	Diagnosis	Prostate cancer	Random forest	N/A	Y	125	26	Y	50:75	Y	N	AUC, accuracy, sensitivity, specificity	N	Y	N
	Detect prostate cancer using peptide biomarker in seminal plasma	Diagnosis	Prostate cancer	Random forest	N/A	Y	125	26	Y	50:75	Y	N	AUC, accuracy, sensitivity, specificity	N	Y	N
Wang et al. 2013	Diagnose and predict castration-resistant prostate cancer	Diagnosis	Prostate cancer	Support vector machine	N/A	Y	50	20	Y	N/A	Y	Y	AUC, accuracy, sensitivity, specificity	Y	Y	N
	Diagnose and predict castration-resistant prostate cancer	Diagnosis	Prostate cancer	Support vector machine	N/A	Y	50	20	Y	N/A	Y	Y	AUC, accuracy, sensitivity, specificity	Y	Y	N
Kwak et al 2017	Automated detection of prostate cancer on prostate	Diagnosis	Prostate cancer	k-Nearest neighbor	Y	Y	653 (samples)	Not explained	Y	172:481	Y	N	AUC	No	Y	N

(continued on next page)

Table 1
(continued)

Study	Application	Category	Subcategory	Algorithms/ Models (List)	Neural Network: Architecture (Descriptor) (Y, N, N/A)	Preprocessing Methodology Disclose (Y/N)	Reporting Size of Dataset (n)	No. of Features	Train/Test Explanation (Y/N)	Train-Test Split	Cross-Validation or Monte Carlo Runs (Y/N)	Lay Term Explanation of AI Methodology	Performance Metrics_ x000 B_	Implications/ Significance Discussion of How AI/ML Advances the Field (Y/N)	Comparison to Traditional Method (Y/N)	Feature Ranking (Y/N)
	tissue specimen slide															
Nguyen et al. 2017	Automated Gleason scoring on prostate tissue specimen slide	Diagnosis	Prostate cancer	Random forest	N/A	Y	141 (samples)	11	Y	Not Disclosed	Y	Y	AUC	Y	Y	N
	Automated Gleason scoring on prostate tissue specimen slide	Diagnosis	Prostate cancer	Logistic regression	N/A	Y	141 (samples)	11	Y	Not Disclosed	Y	Y	AUC	Y	Y	N
Gertych et al. 2015	Identify prostate cancer on pathology slides images	Diagnosis	Prostate cancer	Support vector machine	N/A	Y	230 (specimens and images)	Not explained	Y	19:191	Y	N	Other	Y	Y	N
	Identify prostate cancer on pathology slides images	Diagnosis	Prostate cancer	Random forest	N/A	Y	230 (specimens and images)	Not explained	Y	19:191	Y	N	Other	Y	Y	N
Habes et al. 2014	Estimate prostate volume on MRI	Diagnosis	Prostate cancer	Support vector machine	N/A	Y	53	Not explained	Y	Not Disclosed	Y	N	Accuracy	Y	Y	N
Bonekamp et al 2018	Characterization of prostate lesions detected during prospective MRI interpretation	Diagnosis	Prostate cancer	Random forest	N/A	Y	316	282	Y	183:133	Y	N	AUC, Accuracy, sensitivity, specificity	Y	Y	Y
Kwon et al 2018	Classify clinically significant prostate cancer in multiparametric MRI	Diagnosis	Prostate cancer	Classification and regression trees	N/A	Y	344	216	Y	204:140	Y	Y	AUC	N	Y	Y
	Classify clinically significant prostate cancer in multiparametric MRI	Diagnosis	Prostate cancer	Random forest	N/A	Y	344	216	Y	204:140	Y	Y	AUC	N	Y	Y
	Classify clinically significant prostate cancer in multiparametric MRI	Diagnosis	Prostate cancer	Least absolute shrinkage and selection operator	N/A	Y	344	216	Y	204:140	Y	Y	AUC	N	Y	Y

Lindgren Belal et al 2018	Development of a deep learning-based method for segmentation of bones in CT scans and test its accuracy compared with manual delineation	Diagnosis	Prostate cancer	Convolutional neural network	Y	Y	46	Not explained	Y	100:50	Y	Y	Other	Y	Y	N
Citak-Er et al. 2014	Predict Gleason score on multiparametric MRI	Diagnosis	Prostate cancer	Linear discriminant analysis	N/A	N	33	7	Y	N/A	Y	Y	Accuracy, sensitivity, specificity	N	N	N
	Predict Gleason score on multiparametric MRI	Diagnosis	Prostate cancer	Support vector machine	N/A	N	33	7	Y	N/A	Y	Y	Accuracy, sensitivity, specificity	N	N	N
	Predict Gleason score on multiparametric MRI	Diagnosis	Prostate cancer	Linear discriminant analysis	N/A	N	33	7	Y	N/A	Y	Y	Accuracy, sensitivity, specificity	N	N	N
	Predict Gleason score on multiparametric MRI	Diagnosis	Prostate cancer	Support vector machine	N/A	N	33	7	Y	N/A	Y	Y	Accuracy, sensitivity, specificity	N	N	N
Gatidis et al. 2015	Detect prostate cancer on PET scan/MRI	Diagnosis	Prostate cancer	Fuzzy C-means	N/A	Y	16	5	Y	15:1	Y	Y	Accuracy	Y	Y	Y
	Detect prostate cancer on PET scan/MRI	Diagnosis	Prostate cancer	Fuzzy C-means	N/A	Y	16	5	Y	15:1	Y	Y	Accuracy	Y	Y	Y
	Detect prostate cancer on PET/MRI	Diagnosis	Prostate cancer	Fuzzy C-means	N/A	Y	16	5	Y	15:1	Y	Y	Accuracy	Y	Y	Y
	Detect prostate cancer on PET/MRI	Diagnosis	Prostate cancer	Fuzzy C-means	N/A	Y	16	5	Y	15:1	Y	Y	Accuracy	Y	Y	Y
Haq et al. 2015	Identify prostate cancer on MRI	Diagnosis	Prostate cancer	Support vector machine	N/A	N	16	25	Y	15:1	Y	Y	AUC	Y	Y	Y
Merisaari et al. 2017	Predict Gleason score on multiparametric MRI	Diagnosis	Prostate cancer	Logistic regression	N/A	N	81	4	Y	N/A	Y	No	AUC	N	N	N

(continued on next page)

Table 1
(continued)

Study	Application	Category	Subcategory	Algorithms/ Models (List)	Neural Network: Architecture (Descriptor) (Y, N, N/A)	Preprocessing Methodology Disclose (Y/N)	Reporting Size of Dataset (n)	No. of Features	Train/Test Explanation (Y/N)	Train-Test Split	Cross-Validation or Monte Carlo Runs (Y/N)	Lay Term Explanation of AI Methodology	Performance Metrics_ x000 B_	Implications/ Significance Discussion of How AI/ML Advances the Field (Y/N)	Comparison to Traditional Method (Y/N)	Feature Ranking (Y/N)
Rampun et al. 2016	Detect prostate cancer on MRI	Diagnosis	Prostate cancer	Best node search	N/A	Y	45	215	Y	N/A	Y	N	AUC, accuracy, Sensitivity	Y	N	Y
	Detect prostate cancer on MRI	Diagnosis	Prostate cancer	ADTree	N/A	Y	45	215	Y	N/A	Y	N	AUC, accuracy, Sensitivity	Y	N	Y
	Detect prostate cancer on MRI	Diagnosis	Prostate cancer	Random forest	N/A	Y	45	215	Y	N/A	Y	N	AUC, accuracy, Sensitivity	Y	N	Y
	Detect prostate cancer on MRI	Diagnosis	Prostate cancer	Artificial neural network	N	Y	45	215	Y	N/A	Y	N	AUC, accuracy, Sensitivity	Y	N	Y
	Detect prostate cancer on MRI	Diagnosis	Prostate cancer	Naïve Bayes classifier	N/A	Y	45	215	Y	N/A	Y	N	AUC, accuracy, Sensitivity	Y	N	Y
	Detect prostate cancer on MRI	Diagnosis	Prostate cancer	Support vector machine	N/A	Y	45	215	Y	N/A	Y	N	AUC, accuracy, Sensitivity	Y	N	Y
	Detect prostate cancer on MRI	Diagnosis	Prostate cancer	k-Nearest neighbor	N/A	Y	45	215	Y	N/A	Y	N	AUC, accuracy, Sensitivity	Y	N	Y
	Detect prostate cancer on MRI	Diagnosis	Prostate cancer	Meta-vote (best 2)	N/A	Y	45	215	Y	N/A	Y	N	AUC, accuracy, Sensitivity	Y	N	Y
	Detect prostate cancer on MRI	Diagnosis	Prostate cancer	Meta-vote (best 3)	N/A	Y	45	215	Y	N/A	Y	N	AUC, accuracy, Sensitivity	Y	N	Y
Tiwari et al. 2013	Predict Gleason score on multiparametric MRI	Diagnosis	Prostate cancer	Random forest + SeSMiK-GE (benign vs malignant tissue)	N/A	N	29	34	Y	20:9; 28:1	Y	Y	AUC	Y	N	N
	Predict Gleason score on multiparametric MRI	Diagnosis	Prostate cancer	SeSMik (low vs high grade cancer)	N/A	N	29	34	Y	20:9; 28:1	Y	Y	AUC	Y	N	N
Kim et al. 2017	Predict prostate cancer extracapsular extension using clinical data	Diagnosis	Prostate cancer	Backpropagation network	N/A	N	944	4	Y	850:94	Y	N	Accuracy	Y	Y	N
	Predict prostate cancer extracapsular extension using clinical data	Diagnosis	Prostate cancer	Support vector machine	N/A	N	944	4	Y	850:94	Y	N	Accuracy	Y	Y	N
	Predict prostate cancer extracapsular extension using clinical data	Diagnosis	Prostate cancer	Naïve Bayes classifier	N/A	N	944	4	Y	850:94	Y	N	Accuracy	Y	Y	N

	Predict prostate cancer extracapsular extension using clinical data	Diagnosis	Prostate cancer	Best node search	N/A	N	944	4	Y	850:94	Y	N	Accuracy	Y	Y	N
	Predict prostate cancer extracapsular extension using clinical data	Diagnosis	Prostate cancer	Classification and regression trees	N/A	N	944	4	Y	850:94	Y	N	Accuracy	Y	Y	N
	Predict prostate cancer extracapsular extension using clinical data	Diagnosis	Prostate cancer	Random forest	N/A	N	944	4	Y	850:94	Y	N	Accuracy	Y	Y	N
Kim et al. 2016	Predict prostate cancer extracapsular extension using clinical data	Diagnosis	Prostate cancer	Generalized linear model (pT2 vs pT3)	N/A	N	108	34	Y	74:34	Y	Y	AUC	Y	N	Y
Aubertin et al. 2018	Predict presence and/or staging of prostate cancer from Raman spectroscopy	Diagnosis	Prostate cancer	Artificial neural network	Y	N	32	4	Y	31:1	Y	N	AUC, accuracy, sensitivity, specificity	Y	N	N
	Predict presence and/or staging of prostate cancer from Raman spectroscopy	Diagnosis	Prostate cancer	Artificial neural network	Y	N	32	4	Y	31:1	Y	N	AUC, accuracy, sensitivity, specificity	Y	N	N
	Predict presence and/or staging of prostate cancer from Raman spectroscopy	Diagnosis	Prostate cancer	Artificial neural network	Y	N	32	4	Y	31:1	Y	N	AUC, accuracy, sensitivity, specificity	Y	N	N
	Predict presence and/or staging of prostate cancer from Raman spectroscopy	Diagnosis	Prostate cancer	Artificial neural network	Y	N	32	4	Y	31:1	Y	N	AUC, accuracy, sensitivity, specificity	Y	N	N
	Predict presence and/or staging of prostate cancer from Raman spectroscopy	Diagnosis	Prostate cancer	Artificial neural network	Y	N	32	4	Y	31:1	Y	N	AUC, accuracy, sensitivity, specificity	Y	N	N
	Predict presence and/or staging of prostate cancer from Raman spectroscopy	Diagnosis	Prostate cancer	Artificial neural network	Y	N	32	4	Y	31:1	Y	N	AUC, accuracy, sensitivity, specificity	Y	N	N
		Diagnosis			Y	N	32	4	Y	31:1	Y	N		Y	N	N

(continued on next page)

Table 1
(*continued*)

Study	Application	Category	Subcategory	Algorithms/ Models (List)	Neural Network: Architecture (Descriptor) (Y, N, N/A)	Preprocessing Methodology Disclose (Y/N)	Reporting Size of Dataset (n)	No. of Features	Train/Test Explanation (Y/N)	Train-Test Split	Cross-Validation or Monte Carlo Runs (Y/N)	Lay Term Explanation of AI Methodology	Performance Metrics_ x000 B_	Implications/ Significance Discussion of How AI/ML Advances the Field (Y/N)	Comparison to Traditional Method (Y/N)	Feature Ranking (Y/N)
	Predict presence and/or staging of prostate cancer from Raman spectroscopy		Prostate cancer	Artificial neural network									AUC, accuracy, sensitivity, specificity			
Kwak et al. 2017 (2)	Tissue segmentation model for prostate cancer	Diagnosis	Prostate cancer	Multiview boosting classifier	N/A	N	205 (tissue samples)	845	Y	101:104	Y	Y	AUC	Y	Y	N
	Detecting prostate cancer on tissue preparation	Diagnosis	Prostate cancer	Multiview boosting classifier	N/A	N	667 (tissue samples)	845	Y	163:504	Y	Y	AUC	Y	Y	N
Salman et al. 2014	Detect prostate cancer in histologic imaging	Diagnosis	Prostate cancer	k-Nearest neighbor	N/A	N	75 (tissue sample images)	54	Y	15:60	N	No	Other	Y	Y	N
Gorelick et al. 2013	Identify prostate cancer on pathology slide images	Diagnosis	Prostate cancer	AdaBoost	N/A	N	15	134	Y	80%:20%	Y	Y	Accuracy	Y	N	N
Bleker 2020	Quantify the phenotype of clinically significant the peripheral zone prostate cancer from multiparametric MRI	Diagnosis	Prostate cancer	Random forest	N/A	N	206	92	Y	130:76	N	Y	AUC, sensitivity	Y	Y	N
	Quantify the phenotype of clinically significant the peripheral zone Prostate cancer from multiparametric MRI	Diagnosis	Prostate cancer	Random forest	N/A	N	206	92	Y	130:76	N	Y	AUC, sensitivity	Y	Y	N
	Quantify the phenotype of clinically significant peripheral zone prostate cancer from	Diagnosis	Prostate cancer	Extreme gradient boosting	N/A	N	206	92	Y	130:76	N	Y	AUC, sensitivity	Y	Y	N

	multiparametric MRI													
	Quantify the phenotype of clinically significant the peripheral zone prostate cancer from multiparametric MRI	Diagnosis	Prostate cancer	Random forest	N/A	N	206	92	Y	130:76	N	Y	AUC, sensitivity	Y	Y	N
Leyh-Bannurah 2018	Automated extraction of detailed pathologic prostate cancer data from narratively written electronic health records	Diagnosis	Prostate cancer	Natural Language Processing	N/A	Y	3679 (EHRs)	9	Y	70%:30%	N	Y	Other	Y	N	N
Wildboer 2019	Assess potential of ML based on B-mode, shear wave elastography and dynamic contrast enhanced ultrasound radiomics for localizing prostate cancer lesions	Diagnosis	Prostate cancer	Random forest	N/A	N	48	15	Y	N/A	Y	Y	AUC	N	N	N
Varghese 2019	Identify the best performing classifier for prostate cancer risk stratification based on multiparametric MRI-derived radiomic features derived from a sizable cohort.	Diagnosis	Prostate cancer	Logistic regression	N/A	Y	121	110	Y	68:53	Y	Y	AUC, F-measure, other	Y	Y	N
	Identify the best performing classifier for prostate cancer risk stratification based on multiparametric MRI-derived	Diagnosis	Prostate cancer	Linear support vector machine	N/A	Y	121	110	Y	68:53	Y	Y	AUC, F-measure, other	Y	Y	N

(continued on next page)

Table 1
(continued)

Study	Application	Category	Subcategory	Algorithms/ Models (List)	Neural Network: Architecture (Descriptor) (Y, N, N/A)	Prepro-cessing Method-ology Disclose (Y/N)	Reporting Size of Dataset (n)	No. of Features	Train/Test Explanation (Y/N)	Train-Test Split	Cross-Validation or Monte Carlo Runs (Y/N)	Lay Term Explanation of AI Method-ology	Performance Metrics_ x000 B_	Implications/ Significance Discussion of How AI/ML Advances the Field (Y/N)	Comparison to Traditional Method (Y/N)	Feature Ranking (Y/N)
	radiomic features derived from a sizable cohort.															
	Identify the best performing classifier for prostate cancer risk stratification based on multiparametric MRI-derived radiomic features derived from a sizable cohort.	Diagnosis	Prostate cancer	Quadratic support vector machine	N/A	Y	121	110	Y	68:53	Y	Y	AUC, F-measure, other	Y	Y	N
	Identify the best performing classifier for prostate cancer risk stratification based on multiparametric MRI-derived radiomic features derived from a sizable cohort.	Diagnosis	Prostate cancer	Cubic support vector machine	N/A	Y	121	110	Y	68:53	Y	Y	AUC, F-measure, other	Y	Y	N
	Identify the best performing classifier for prostate cancer risk stratification based on multiparametric MRI-derived radiomic features derived from a sizable cohort.	Diagnosis	Prostate cancer	Gaussian support vector machine	N/A	Y	121	110	Y	68:53	Y	Y	AUC, F-measure, other	Y	Y	N
	Identify the best performing classifier for	Diagnosis	Prostate cancer	Kernel-based support	N/A	Y	121	110	Y	68:53	Y	Y	AUC, F-measure, other	Y	Y	N

	prostate cancer risk stratification based on multiparametric MRI-derived radiomic features derived from a sizable cohort.			vector machine												
	Identify the best performing classifier for prostate cancer risk stratification based on multiparametric MRI-derived radiomic features derived from a sizable cohort.	Diagnosis	Prostate cancer	Linear discriminant analysis	N/A	Y	121	110	Y	68:53	Y	Y	AUC, F-measure, other	Y	Y	N
	Identify the best performing classifier for prostate cancer risk stratification based on multiparametric MRI-derived radiomic features derived from a sizable cohort.	Diagnosis	Prostate cancer	Random forest	N/A	Y	121	110	Y	68:53	Y	Y	AUC, F-measure, other	Y	Y	N
van Sloun 2019	To exploit deep learning to perform automatic, real-time prostate (zone) segmentation on TRUS images from different scanners	Diagnosis	Prostate cancer	Convolutional neural network	Y	Y	78	10,00,000	Y	54:24	Y	Y	Accuracy	Y	Y	N
Truong 2019	predicting high-risk lesions on 3 T multiparametric prostate MRI	Diagnosis	Prostate cancer	Support vector machine	N/A	N	1483	4	Y	1269:214	Y	Y	AUC	Y	Y	N

Abbreviations: jiCA, joint independent component analysis; PSA, prostate-specific antigen; SesMiK-GE, semi supervised multi kernel (SeSMiK) graph embedding; SUV_{max}, maximum standardized uptake value; SUV_{mean}, mean standardized uptake value; SVI, seminal vesicle invasion; TRUS, transrectal ultrasound,

Table 2
Bladder Cancer Diagnosis

Study	Application	Category	Subcategory	Algorithms/ Models (List)	Neural Network: Architecture	Preprocessing Methodology Disclose (Y/N)	Reporting Size of Dataset (n)	No. of Features	Train/Test Explanation (Y/N)	Train-Test Split?	Cross-Validation or Monte Carlo Runs (Y/N)	Lay Term Explanation of AI Methodology	Performance Metrics	Implications/ Significance Discussion of How AI/ML Advances the Field (Y/N)	Comparison to Traditional Method (Y/N)	Feature Ranking (Y/N)
Shkolyar 2019	Bladder tumor detection from cystoscopy	Diagnosis	Bladder cancer	Convolutional neural network	N	T	100	Not explained	Y	100:54	N	N	Sensitivity Specificity	Y	N	N
Sokolov 2018	Bladder cancer detection from atomic force microscopy	Diagnosis	Bladder cancer Bladder cancer Bladder cancer	Random forest Extremely randomized forest Gradient boosting trees	N/A	Y	68	Not explained	Y	N/A	Y	Y	AUC Accuracy Sensitivity Specificity	Y	Y	Y
Alanee 2020	Detect bladder cancer in urine and assess programmed death ligand 1 status	Diagnosis	Bladder cancer	Random forest	N/A	N	65	16	Y	90:10	Y	N	Accuracy	Y	N	Y
Alanee 2019	Detect bladder cancer from adaptive genetic algorithms with flow cytometry technology	Diagnosis	Bladder cancer	AGA (Adaptive Genetic Algorithms) Random forest	N/A	Y	50	16	Y	N/A	Y	Y	Accuracy Sensitivity Specificity	Y	Y	N
Xu 2017	Diagnose bladder cancer from MRI	Diagnosis	Bladder cancer Bladder cancer Bladder cancer bladder Cancer Bladder cancer	Support vector machine Support vector machine Random forest Random forest Support vector machine	N/A	N	62	22 29	Y	N/A	Y	N	Accuracy AUC	Y	N	Y

Garapati 2017	Diagnose bladder cancer stage from CT urogram	Diagnosis	Bladder cancer	Linear discriminant analysis	Y	Y	76	27	Y	N/A	Y	N	AUC	N	Y	Y
			Bladder cancer	Artificial neural network												
			Bladder cancer	Support vector machine												
			Bladder cancer	Random forest				91								
Shao 2017	Detect bladder cancer with urine metabolomic profile	Diagnosis	bladder Cancer	Decision tree	N/A	N	152	6	Y	100:47	Y	Y	Accuracy Sensitivity Specificity	N	N	Y

particular, differentiation of oncocytoma and RCC remains difficult owing to overlap in radiologic features. Pedersen and colleagues trained a convolutional neural network on CT images with a known RCC or oncocytoma diagnosis with an ability to classify with an AUC of 0.946 on an external validation set.[12] Although 5 of the articles also investigated the diagnosis of RCC via various imaging modalities, Zheng and colleagues[13] identified a biomarker cluster of metabolites to diagnose RCC with an accuracy of 94.74% (**Table 3**).

Testicular cancer

The histology of lymph nodes in patients with nonseminomatous germ cell tumors remains indeterminate based solely on classic radiologic interpretation of CT scans. Baessler and colleagues[14] trained a gradient boosted tree with radiomic features to differentiate between benign and malignant lymph nodes with an accuracy of 81% (**Table 4**).

Pediatric urology

Hydronephrosis remains a key subject of investigation in pediatric urology. Smail and colleagues classified hydronephrosis via the Society for Fetal Urology scale via a convolutional neural network within 1 grade of the provided label with 94% accuracy, an exact accuracy of 51%, and 78% when differentiating low versus high grades.[15] The remaining 3 articles also examined hydronephrosis through classifying obstruction and determining voiding cystourethrogram findings from renal ultrasound examination (**Table 5**).

General urology

AI and ML algorithms applied to general urology explored a broad range of diagnostics including discrimination of Hunner's lesions in interstitial cystitis from urinary cytokines, diagnosis of urinary incontinence, presence of lower urinary tract symptoms from urine metabolomics, as well as voiding dysfunction in women with multiple sclerosis (**Table 6**). Wang and colleagues[16] also evaluated 799 urodynamic studies with manifold learning to accurately identify detrusor overactivity with an AUC of 0.84.

Men's health

Men's health remains a nascent field in respect to the application of AI and ML. Xu and colleagues[17] evaluated 69 patients with MRI and used a support vector machine trained on functional connectivity features to differentiate patients with lifelong premature ejaculation from controls with an accuracy of 0.85. The 2 other studies diagnosed erectile dysfunction from penile ultrasound examination and MRI, hypogonadism via questionnaires (**Table 7**).

Kidney stones

Grosse Hokamp and associates[18] diagnosed the composition of kidney stones from CT scans with a shallow neural network with an accuracy ranging from 87.1% to 90.4%. De Perrot and colleagues[19] trained an algorithm based on AdaBoost to differentiate a kidney stone from a phlebolith on low-dose CT with an AUC of 0.902 (**Table 8**).

Outcome Prediction

The task of predicting patient outcomes is an excellent match for AI and ML algorithms. because complex models can account for complicated interactions between large number of variables within medical databases (nature outcome prediction). Our review of the literature identified 37 publications looking at outcome prediction in urology.

Prostate cancer

The treatment of prostate cancer results in a multitude of measured outcomes. Seventeen articles were found to predict urinary continence, biochemical recurrence, lower urinary tract symptoms, mortality, and progression of cancer. Hung and colleagues[20] trained a deep learning neural network, DeepSurv, on automated performance metrics and clinicopathologic data to predict return of urinary continence with a C-index of 0.6. Feature ranking demonstrated automated performance metrics as the top 10 drivers of the model. Wong and colleagues[21] evaluated biochemical recurrence after robotic-assisted prostatectomy and found superiority in 3 ML algorithms, k-nearest neighbors, logistic regression, and random forest over traditional Cox regression analysis (AUCs of 0.903, 0.924, 0.940, and 0.865, respectively). Lower urinary tract symptoms were also evaluated after radiation therapy. Lee and colleagues[22] used a random forest model trained on genome-wide single nucleotide polymorphisms to predict a number of genitourinary toxicities with the ability to determine postprocedural weak stream with an AUC of 0.70. Hanson and colleagues[23] trained a random forest model using the Surveillance, Epidemiology, and End Results database to assess the important factors in predicting prostate cancer specific mortality with the finding that tumor characteristics were the most important factor with race only attributing 5% as much to the projected outcome of the model. The remaining articles were as identified in **Table 9**.

Bladder cancer

Nine articles evaluated predictions of recurrence of bladder cancer, mortality, readmission, and response to immune checkpoint inhibitors (**Table 10**). Hasnain and colleagues[24] evaluated a

Table 3
Kidney Cancer Diagnosis

Study	Application	Category	Subcategory	Algorithms/ Models (List)	Neural Network: Architecture	Preprocessing Methodology Disclose (Y/N)	Reporting Size of Dataset (n)	No. of Features	Train/ Test Explanation (Y/N)	Train-Test Split	Cross-Validation or Monte Carlo Runs (Y/N)	Lay Term Explanation of AI Methodology	Performance Metrics	Implications/ Significance Discussion of How AI/ML Advances the Field (Y/N)	Comparison to Traditional Method (Y/N)	Feature Ranking (Y/N)
Sun 2019	Identification of benign vs malignant solid renal masses with radiomics	Diagnosis	Kidney cancer	Support vector machine	N/A	Y	288	17	Y	N/A	Y	N	AUC Sensitivity Specificity F-1 score PPV NPV Accuracy	Y	Y	N
Pedersen 2020	Diagnosing oncocytoma on CT scan	Diagnosis	Kidney cancer	Convolutional neural network	Y	N	369	Not explained	Y	70:20	N	N	AUC Accuracy Sensitivity Specificity	Y	N	N
Uhlig 2020	Diagnosing malignant renal masses on CT scan	Diagnosis	Kidney cancer	k-Nearest neighbor s Random forest Extreme gradient boosting Support vector machine Neural network	N/A	Y	94	120	Y	N/A	Y	N	AUC Accuracy Sensitivity Specificity	Y	Y	N
Zheng 2016	Detecting RCC from serum metabolomics before and after nephrectomy	Diagnosis	Kidney cancer	Clustering Artificial neural network Artificial neural network	Y	Y	104	16	Y	83–21	Y	Y	Accuracy	Y	N	N
Kocak 2019	Diagnosing 3 major subtypes of RCCs on CT scan	Diagnosis	Kidney cancer	Artificial neural network Support vector machine	N/A	Y	68	275	Y	N/A	Y	Y	Accuracy Sensitivity Specificity	Y	Y	N
Haifler 2018	Diagnosing malignant renal masses with infrared Raman spectroscopy	Diagnosis	Kidney cancer	Sparse multinomial logistic regression	N/A	Y	12	11	Y	N/A	Y	Y	AUC Accuracy	Y	N	Y
Kanapuli 2018	Diagnosing malignant renal	Diagnosis	Kidney cancer	Relational functional gradient	N/A Y Y	N	150	40	Y	N/A	Y	Y	Accuracy F1 score AUC	Yes	Y	N

(continued on next page)

Table 3
(*continued*)

Study	Application	Category	Subcategory	Algorithms/ Models (List)	Neural Network: Architecture	Preprocessing Methodology Disclose (Y/N)	Reporting Size of Dataset (n)	No. of Features	Train/ Test Explanation (Y/N)	Train-Test Split	Cross-Validation or Monte Carlo Runs (Y/N)	Lay Term Explanation of AI Methodology	Performance Metrics	Implications/ Significance Discussion of How AI/ML Advances the Field (Y/N)	Comparison to Traditional Method (Y/N)	Feature Ranking (Y/N)
	masses on CT scan			boosting Artificial neural network Artificial neural network Support vector machine Support vector machine Support vector machine Logistic regression Decision trees Ensemble (RF) Ensemble (Bagging) Naive Bayesian	N/A N/A N/A N/A N/A N/A N/A N/A											

Abbreviations: NPV, negative predictive value; PPV, positive predictive value.

Table 4
Testicular Cancer Diagnosis

Study	Application	Category	Subcategory	Algorithms/ Models (List)	Neural Network: Architecture (Descriptor) (Y, N, N/A)	Preprocessing Methodology Disclose (Y/N)	Reporting Size of Dataset (n)	No. of Features	Train/Test Explanation (Y/N)	Train-Test Split	Cross-Validation or Monte Carlo Runs (Y/N)	Lay Term Explanation of AI Methodology	Performance Metrics	Implications/ Significance Discussion of How AI/ML Advances the Field (Y/N)	Comparison with Traditional Method (Y/N)	Feature Ranking (Y/N)
Baessler et al 2019	Predict histopathology of lymph nodes patients with nonseminomatous germ cell tumors treated with chemotherapy from CT scan	Diagnosis	Testicular cancer	Gradient boosted t ree	N/A	Y	80	97	Y	120:23	Y	Y	Accuracy, sensitivity, specificity, AUC	Y	Y	Y

Table 5
Pediatric Urology Diagnosis

Study	Application	Category	Subcategory	Algorithms/ Models (List)	Neural Network: Architecture	Preprocessing Methodology Disclose (Y/N)	Reporting Size of Dataset (n)	No. of Features	Train/ Test Explanation (Y/N)	Train-Test Split	Cross-Validation or Monte Carlo Runs (Y/N)	Lay Term Explanation of AI Methodology	Performance Metrics	Implications/ Significance Discussion of How AI/ML Advances the Field (Y/N)	Comparison to Traditional Method (Y/N)	Feature Ranking (Y/N)
Smail 2020	Grade hydronephrosis from ultrasound	Diagnosis	Pediatrics	Convolutional neural network	Y	Y	2420	N/A	Y	N/A	Y	Y	Accuracy Sensitivity Specificity Positive predictive value F-score	Y	N	Y
Logvinenko 2015	Diagnose voiding cystourethrogram findings based on RBUS findings	Diagnosis	Pediatrics	Artificial neural network	Y	Y	3995	10	N	N/A	Y	Y	Sensitivity Specificity AUC	Y	Y	N
Blum 2017	Detection of clinically significant hydronephrosis caused by ureteropelvic junction obstruction	Diagnosis	Pediatrics	Support vector machine	N/A	N	55	45	Y	N/A	Y	N	AUC Accuracy Sensitivity Specificity	Y	Y	Y
Cerrolaza 2014	Detect obstruction from hydronephrosis and ultrasound	Diagnosis	Pediatrics	Support vector machine Support vector machine Logistic regression Logistic regression	N/A	Y	45	10	Y	N/A	Y	Y	AUC Accuracy Sensitivity Specificity	Y	N	Y

Table 6
General Urology Diagnosis

Study	Application	Category	Subcategory	Algorithms/ Models (List)	Neural Network: Architecture	Preprocessing Methodology Disclose (Y/N)	Reporting Size of Dataset (n)	No. of Features	Train/ Test Explanation (Y/N)	Train-Test Split	Cross-Validation or Monte Carlo Runs (Y/N)	Lay Term Explanation of AI Methodology	Performance Metrics	Implications/ Significance Discussion of How AI/ML Advances the Field (Y/N)	Comparison to Traditional Method (Y/N)	Feature Ranking (Y/N)
Wang 2020	Detect detrusor overactivity on urodynamic studies	Diagnosis	General	Manifold learning	N/A	Y	799	Not specified	N	N/A	Y	Y	AUC Accuracy Sensitivity Specificity	Y	N	N
Chancellor 2018	Detect Hunner's lesions in patients with interstitial cystitis with evaluation of urinary cytokines	Diagnosis	General	Bladder Permeability Defect Risk Score	N/A	Y	153	Not specified	Y	53:393	N	N	Accuracy	Y	N	N
Hao 2016	Diagnose lower urinary tract symptoms with urine metabolomics	Diagnosis	General	Support vector machine	N/A	Y	46	63	Y	N/A	Y	Y	AUC	Y	N	N
Lopes 2013	Diagnose different types of urinary incontinence and urinary retention from cases of altered urinary elimination	Diagnosis	General	FCM	N	N	195	36	Y	N/A	N	Y	Sensitivity Specificity	Y	Y	N
Karmonik 2019	Diagnose neurogenic voiding dysfunction in women with multiple sclerosis	Diagnosis	General	Random forest Neural network Generalized linear model Partial Least Squares	N/A	N	27	Not specified	Y	50:50	Y	Y	AUC Accuracy	Y	N	N Y

Abbreviations: FCM, fuzzy c-means clustering.

Table 7
Men's Health Diagnosis

Study	Application	Category	Subcategory	Algorithms/ Models (List)	Neural Network: Architecture (Descriptor) (Y, N, N/A)	Preprocessing Methodology Disclose (Y/N)	Reporting Size of Dataset (n)	No. of Features	Train/ Test Explanation (Y/N)	Train-Test Split	Cross-Validation or Monte Carlo Runs (Y/N)	Lay Term Explanation of AI Methodology	Performance Metrics	Implications/ Significance Discussion of How AI/ML Advances the Field (Y/N)	Comparison to Traditional Method (Y/N)	Feature Ranking (Y/N)
Li et al. 2018	Predict venous erectile dysfunction from penile ultrasound examination and MRI of the brain	Diagnosis	Men's health	Logistic regression	N/A	Y	95	200	N	Not disclosed	Y	N	Accuracy, sensitivity, specificity	Y	Y	Y
	Predict venous erectile dysfunction from penile ultrasound examination and MRI of the brain	Diagnosis	Men's health	Support vector machine	N/A	Y	95	200	N	Not disclosed	Y	N	Accuracy, sensitivity, specificity	Y	Y	Y
Lu et al. 2016	Identify late-onset hypogonadism in elderly men from questionnaire	Diagnosis	Men's health	Decision tree	N/A	Y	772	17	Y	Not disclosed	Y	Y	Accuracy, sensitivity, specificity	Y	N	N
	Identify late-onset hypogonadism in elderly men from questionnaire	Diagnosis	Men's health	AdaBoost decision tree	N/A	Y	772	17	Y	Not disclosed	Y	Y	Accuracy, sensitivity, specificity	Y	N	N
	Identify late-onset hypogonadism in elderly men from questionnaire	Diagnosis	Men's health	Local Gaussian regression	N/A	Y	772	17	Y	Not disclosed	Y	Y	Accuracy, sensitivity, specificity	Y	N	N
	Identify late-onset hypogonadism in elderly men from questionnaire	Diagnosis	Men's health	Adaboost local Gaussian regression	N/A	Y	772	17	Y	Not disclosed	Y	Y	Accuracy, sensitivity, specificity	Y	N	N
	Identify late-onset hypogonadism in elderly men from questionnaire	Diagnosis	Men's health	AMS	N/A	Y	772	17	Y	Not disclosed	Y	Y	Accuracy, sensitivity, specificity	Y	N	N
	Identify late-onset hypogonadism in elderly men from questionnaire	Diagnosis	Men's health	ADAM	N/A	Y	772	17	Y	Not disclosed	Y	Y	Accuracy, sensitivity, specificity	Y	N	N

Xu Z 2019	Detect patients with lifelong premature ejaculation from controls analyzing MRI and functional connectivity	Diagnosis	Men's health	Support vector machine	N/A	Y	69	4005	Y	N/A	Y	N	AUC, Accuracy, sensitivity, specificity	N	N	Y

Abbreviation: ADAM, androgen deficiency in the aging male; AMS, aging male's symptoms; N/A, not applicable.

Table 8
Kidney Stone Diagnosis

Study	Application	Category	Subcategory	Algorithms/ Models (List)	Neural Network: Architecture	Preprocessing Methodology Disclose (Y/N)	Reporting Size of Dataset (n)	No. of Features	Train/Test Explanation (Y/N)	Train-Test Split	Cross-Validation or Monte Carlo Runs (Y/N)	Lay Term Explanation of AI Methodology	Performance Metrics	Implications/ Significance Discussion of How AI/ML Advances the Field (Y/N)	Comparison to Traditional Method (Y/N)	Feature Ranking (Y/N)
Hokamp 2019	Diagnosing stone composition from CT scan	Diagnosis	Kidney stone	Artificial neural network	Y	Y	200	75,735	Y	70% training, 15% test, 15% validation	Y	Y	Accuracy	Y	N	N
De Perrot 2019	Diagnosing kidney stones and differentiating from phleboliths on CT scan	Diagnosis	Kidney stone	AdaBoost	N/A	Y	416	1,47,029	Y	369–47	Y	Y	AUC	Y	N	N

Table 9
Prostate Cancer Outcome Prediction

Study	Application	Category	Subcategory	Algorithms/ Models (List)	Neural Network: Architecture (Descriptor) (Y, N, N/A)	Preprocessing Methodology Disclose (Y/N)	Reporting Size of Dataset (n)	No. of Features	Train/Test Explanation (Y/N)	Train-Test Split	Cross-Validation or Monte Carlo Runs (Y/N)	Lay Term Explanation of AI Methodology	Performance Metrics	Implications/ Significance Discussion of How AI/ML Advances the Field (Y/N)	Comparison to Traditional Method (Y/N)	Feature Ranking (Y/N)
Hung et al. 2018	Predict hospital length of stay after RARP with automated performance metrics and clinical data	Outcome prediction	Prostate cancer	Random forest	N/A	N	78	25	Y	N/A	Y	Y	Accuracy	Y	N	Y
	Predict hospital length of stay after RARP with automated performance metrics and clinical data	Outcome prediction	Prostate cancer	Random forest	N/A	N	78	25	Y	N/A	Y	Y	Accuracy	Y	N	Y
	Predict hospital length of stay after RARP with automated performance metrics and clinical data	Outcome prediction	Prostate cancer	Support vector machine	N/A	N	78	25	Y	N/A	Y	Y	Accuracy	Y	N	Y
	Predict hospital length of stay after RARP with automated performance metrics and clinical data	Outcome prediction	Prostate cancer	Logistic regression	N/A	N	78	25	Y	N/A	Y	Y	Accuracy	Y	N	Y
Harder 2018	Predict progression of prostate cancer with tissue phenomics	Outcome prediction	Prostate cancer	Naïve Bayes classifier	N/A	Y	90	20	Y	N/A	Y	Y	Accuracy, sensitivity, specificity	Y	N	Y
	Predict progression of prostate cancer with tissue phenomics	Outcome prediction	Prostate cancer	Naïve Bayes classifier	N/A	Y	90	8	Y	N/A	Y	Y	Accuracy, sensitivity, specificity	Y	N	Y
					N/A	Y	90	20	Y	N/A	Y	Y		Y	N	Y

(continued on next page)

Table 9
(continued)

Study	Application	Category	Subcategory	Algorithms/ Models (List)	Neural Network: Architecture (Descriptor) (Y, N, N/A)	Preprocessing Methodology Disclose (Y/N)	Reporting Size of Dataset (n)	No. of Features	Train/Test Explanation (Y/N)	Train-Test Split	Cross-Validation or Monte Carlo Runs (Y/N)	Lay Term Explanation of AI Methodology	Performance Metrics	Implications/ Significance Discussion of How AI/ML Advances the Field (Y/N)	Comparison to Traditional Method (Y/N)	Feature Ranking (Y/N)
	Predict progression of prostate cancer with tissue phenomics	Outcome prediction	Prostate cancer	Classification and regression trees									Accuracy, sensitivity, specificity			
	Predict progression of prostate cancer with tissue phenomics	Outcome prediction	Prostate cancer	Classification and regression trees	N/A	Y	90	8	Y	N/A	Y	Y	Accuracy, sensitivity, specificity	Y	N	Y
	Predict progression of prostate cancer with tissue phenomics	Outcome prediction	Prostate cancer	k-Nearest neighbors	N/A	Y	90	20	Y	N/A	Y	Y	Accuracy, sensitivity, specificity	Y	N	Y
	Predict progression of prostate cancer with tissue phenomics	Outcome prediction	Prostate cancer	k-Nearest neighbors	N/A	Y	90	8	Y	N/A	Y	Y	Accuracy, sensitivity, specificity	Y	N	Y
	Predict progression of prostate cancer with tissue phenomics	Outcome prediction	Prostate cancer	Linear predictor	N/A	Y	90	20	Y	N/A	Y	Y	Accuracy, sensitivity, specificity	Y	N	Y
	Predict progression of prostate cancer with tissue phenomics	Outcome prediction	Prostate cancer	Linear predictor	N/A	Y	90	8	Y	N/A	Y	Y	Accuracy, sensitivity, specificity	Y	N	Y
	Predict progression of prostate cancer with tissue phenomics	Outcome prediction	Prostate cancer	Support vector machine (linear kernel)	N/A	Y	90	20	Y	N/A	Y	Y	Accuracy, sensitivity, specificity	Y	N	Y
	Predict progression of prostate cancer with tissue phenomics	Outcome prediction	Prostate cancer	Support vector machine (linear kernel)	N/A	Y	90	8	Y	N/A	Y	Y	Accuracy, sensitivity, specificity	Y	N	Y
	Predict progression of prostate cancer with tissue phenomics	Outcome prediction	Prostate cancer	Support vector machine (radial kernel)	N/A	Y	90	20	Y	N/A	Y	Y	Accuracy, sensitivity, specificity	Y	N	Y
	Predict progression of prostate cancer with tissue phenomics	Outcome prediction	Prostate cancer	Support vector machine (radial kernel)	N/A	Y	90	8	Y	N/A	Y	Y	Accuracy, sensitivity, specificity	Y	N	Y

	Predict progression of prostate cancer with tissue phenomics	Outcome prediction	Prostate cancer	Hierarchical clustering	N/A	Y	90	20	N	N/A	N	Y	Accuracy, sensitivity, specificity	Y	N	Y
	Predict progression of prostate cancer with tissue phenomics	Outcome prediction	Prostate cancer	Hierarchical clustering	N/A	Y	90	8	N	N/A	N	Y	Accuracy, sensitivity, specificity	Y	N	Y
Lalonde 2014	Predict prostate cancer biochemical recurrence with genomic and micro-environmental indices	Outcome prediction	Prostate cancer	Hierarchical clustering	N/A	N	126	Not explained	Y	126:154 126:117	N	No	Not reported	N	N	N
	Predict prostate cancer biochemical recurrence with genomic and micro-environmental indices	Outcome prediction	Prostate cancer	Random forest	N/A	N	126	Not explained	Y	126:154 126:117	N	No	AUC, other	N	N	N
Lee 2018	Predict frequency after radiation with genomic analysis	Outcome prediction	Prostate cancer	Random forest	N/A	Y	324	14	Y	119:60	Y	Y	AUC	Y	N	Y
	Predict urgency after radiation with genomic analysis	Outcome prediction	Prostate cancer	Random forest	N/A	Y	324	14	Y	161:81	Y	Y	AUC	Y	N	Y
	Predict nocturia after radiation with genomic analysis	Outcome prediction	Prostate cancer	Random forest	N/A	Y	324	14	Y	111:56	Y	Y	AUC	Y	N	Y
	Predict intermittency after radiation with genomic analysis	Outcome prediction	Prostate cancer	Random forest	N/A	Y	324	14	Y	164:82	Y	Y	AUC	Y	N	Y
	Predict weak stream after radiation with genomic analysis	Outcome prediction	Prostate cancer	Random forest	N/A	Y	324	14	Y	149:75	Y	Y	AUC	Y	N	Y
	Predict straining after radiation with genomic analysis	Outcome prediction	Prostate cancer	Random forest	N/A	Y	324	14	Y	196:98	Y	Y	AUC	Y	N	Y
	Predict incomplete emptying after radiation with genomic analysis	Outcome prediction	Prostate cancer	Random forest	N/A	Y	324	14	Y	168:84	Y	Y	AUC	Y	N	Y

(continued on next page)

Table 9
(*continued*)

Study	Application	Category	Subcategory	Algorithms/ Models (List)	Neural Network: Architecture (Descriptor) (Y, N, N/A)	Preprocessing Methodology Disclose (Y/N)	Reporting Size of Dataset (n)	No. of Features	Train/Test Explanation (Y/N)	Train-Test Split	Cross-Validation or Monte Carlo Runs (Y/N)	Lay Term Explanation of AI Methodology	Performance Metrics	Implications/ Significance Discussion of How AI/ML Advances the Field (Y/N)	Comparison to Traditional Method (Y/N)	Feature Ranking (Y/N)
Zhang 2016	Biochemical recurrence after radical prostatectomy with MRI radiomics	Outcome prediction	Prostate cancer	Support vector machine	N/A	N	205	12	N	N/A	N	Y	AUC, Accuracy, sensitivity, specificity	Y	Y	N
	Biochemical recurrence after radical prostatectomy with MRI radiomics	Outcome prediction	Prostate cancer	Support vector machine	N/A	N	205	8	N	N/A	N	Y	AUC, Accuracy, sensitivity, specificity	Y	Y	N
Zhang 2017	Predict biochemical recurrence with somatic mutation	Outcome prediction	Prostate cancer	Support vector machine	N/A	Y	424	43	Y	283:141	Y	N	AUC, Accuracy	N	Y	N
	Predict tumor status with somatic mutation	Outcome prediction	Prostate cancer	Support vector machine	N/A	Y	388	43	Y	283:141	Y	N	AUC, Accuracy	N	Y	N
Suh 2020	Prediction of clinically significant prostate cancer after biopsy with clinical factors in a decision support tool	Outcome prediction	Prostate cancer	Extreme gradient boosting	N/A	Y	2843	11	Y	75%:25%	Y	N	AUC, Accuracy, F-1	Y	N	Y
Bhambhvani 2020	Prediction 5 y survival in pediatric genitourinary rhabdo-myosarcoma	Outcome prediction	Prostate cancer	Deep neural network	Y	N	277	9	Y	80%:20%	Y	N	AUC	Y	Y	N
Sumitomo 2020	Feature selection for prediction urinary continence after RARP	Outcome prediction	Prostate cancer	Convolutional neural network	Y	Y	400	4096	Y	Not disclosed	N	N	Not disclosed	Y	N	Y

	Prediction urinary continence after RARP using MRI	Outcome prediction	Prostate cancer	Naïve Bayes classifier	N/A	Y	400	30	N	Not disclosed	N	N	AUC, Accuracy, sensitivity, specificity	Y	N	Y
	Prediction urinary continence after RARP using MRI	Outcome prediction	Prostate cancer	Random forest	N/A	Y	400	30	N	Not disclosed	N	N	AUC, Accuracy, sensitivity, specificity	Y	N	Y
	Prediction urinary continence after RARP using MRI	Outcome prediction	Prostate cancer	Support vector machine	N/A	Y	400	30	N	Not disclosed	N	N	AUC, Accuracy, sensitivity, specificity	Y	N	Y
	Prediction urinary continence after RARP using MRI	Outcome prediction	Prostate cancer	Artificial neural network	N/A	Y	400	30	N	Not disclosed	N	N	AUC, Accuracy, sensitivity, specificity	Y	N	Y
	Prediction urinary continence after RARP using MRI	Outcome prediction	Prostate cancer	AdaBoost	N/A	Y	400	30	N	Not disclosed	N	N	AUC, Accuracy, sensitivity, specificity	Y	N	Y
Shiradkar et al. 2018	Predict biochemical recurrence on MRI	Outcome prediction	Prostate cancer	Linear discriminant analysis	N/A	Y	120	5 groups	Y	70:50	Y	N	AUC	Y	Y	Y
	Predict biochemical recurrence on MRI	Outcome prediction	Prostate cancer	Support vector machine	N/A	Y	120	5 groups	Y	70:50	Y	N	AUC	Y	Y	Y
	Predict biochemical recurrence on MRI	Outcome prediction	Prostate cancer	Random forest	N/A	Y	120	5 groups	Y	70:50	Y	N	AUC	Y	Y	Y
	Predict biochemical recurrence on MRI	Outcome prediction	Prostate cancer	Support vector machine	N/A	Y	120	5 groups	Y	70:50	Y	N	AUC	Y	Y	Y
	Predict biochemical recurrence on MRI	Outcome prediction	Prostate cancer	Support vector machine	N/A	Y	120	5 groups	Y	70:50	Y	N	AUC	Y	Y	Y
	Predict biochemical recurrence on MRI	Outcome prediction	Prostate cancer	Support vector machine	N/A	Y	120	5 groups	Y	70:50	Y	N	AUC	Y	Y	Y
Abdollahi et al 2019	Predict early intensity-modulated radiation therapy response, Gleason	Outcome prediction	Prostate cancer	Support vector machine	N/A	Y	33	1135	Y	1021:114	Y	N	AUC	Y	Y	Y

(*continued on next page*)

Table 9
(continued)

Study	Application	Category	Subcategory	Algorithms/ Models (List)	Neural Network: Architecture (Descriptor) (Y, N, N/A)	Preprocessing Methodology Disclose (Y/N)	Reporting Size of Dataset (n)	No. of Features	Train/Test Explanation (Y/N)	Train-Test Split	Cross-Validation or Monte Carlo Runs (Y/N)	Lay Term Explanation of AI Methodology	Performance Metrics	Implications/ Significance Discussion of How AI/ML Advances the Field (Y/N)	Comparison to Traditional Method (Y/N)	Feature Ranking (Y/N)
	scores and prostate cancer stages using MRI															
	Predict early intensity-modulated radiation therapy response, Gleason scores and prostate cancer stages using MRI	Outcome prediction	Prostate cancer	Linear Regression	N/A	Y	33	1135	Y	1021:114	Y	N	AUC	Y	Y	Y
	Predict early intensity-modulated radiation therapy response, Gleason scores and prostate cancer stages using MRI	Outcome prediction	Prostate cancer	BENB	N/A	Y	33	1135	Y	1021:114	Y	N	AUC	Y	Y	Y
	Predict early intensity-modulated radiation therapy response, Gleason scores and prostate cancer stages using MRI	Outcome prediction	Prostate cancer	Stochastic Gradient Descent - Classifier	N/A	Y	33	1135	Y	1021:114	Y	N	AUC	Y	Y	Y
	Predict early intensity-modulated radiation therapy response, Gleason	Outcome prediction	Prostate cancer	k-Nearest neighbors	N/A	Y	33	1135	Y	1021:114	Y	N	AUC	Y	Y	Y

	scores and prostate cancer stages using MRI														
	Predict early intensity-modulated radiation therapy response, Gleason scores and prostate cancer stages using MRI	Outcome prediction	Prostate cancer	Decision tree	N/A	Y	33	1135	Y	1021:114	Y	N	AUC	Y	Y	Y
	Predict early intensity-modulated radiation therapy response, Gleason scores and prostate cancer stages using MRI	Outcome prediction	Prostate cancer	Random forest	N/A	Y	33	1135	Y	1021:114	Y	N	AUC	Y	Y	Y
	Predict early intensity-modulated radiation therapy response, Gleason scores and prostate cancer stages using MRI	Outcome prediction	Prostate cancer	ADBO	N/A	Y	33	1135	Y	1021:114	Y	N	AUC	Y	Y	Y
	Predict early intensity-modulated radiation therapy response, Gleason scores and prostate cancer stages using MRI	Outcome prediction	Prostate cancer	GANB	N/A	Y	33	1135	Y	1021:114	Y	N	AUC	Y	Y	Y
Connell et al 2019	providing diagnostic information on disease status prior to biopsy, and prognostic information for men on active surveillance with post-DRE urine sample	Outcome prediction	Prostate cancer	Least absolute shrinkage and selection operator	N/A	Y	535	17	Y	358:177	Y	N	AUC	Y	N	N

(continued on next page)

Table 9
(*continued*)

Study	Application	Category	Subcategory	Algorithms/ Models (List)	Neural Network: Architecture (Descriptor) (Y, N, N/A)	Preprocessing Methodology Disclose (Y/N)	Reporting Size of Dataset (n)	No. of Features	Train/Test Explanation (Y/N)	Train-Test Split	Cross-Validation or Monte Carlo Runs (Y/N)	Lay Term Explanation of AI Methodology	Performance Metrics	Implications/ Significance Discussion of How AI/ML Advances the Field (Y/N)	Comparison to Traditional Method (Y/N)	Feature Ranking (Y/N)
Hung et al 2019	Predict urinary continence recovery after RARP using a deep learning model	Outcome prediction	Prostate cancer	DeepSurv	N/A	Y	161	508	Y	Not disclosed	Y	N	Other	Y	Y	Y
Auffenburg 2019	Predict treatment decisions for prostate cancer based on patients with similar characteristics	Outcome prediction	Prostate cancer	Random forest	N/A	N	7543	8	Y	5029:2514	N	Y	AUC	Y	N	N
Hanson 2019	Predict cancer specific mortality with analysis of contributing factors including race, socioeconomic status and clinical factors	Outcome prediction	Prostate cancer	Random forest	N/A	N	5,14,878	15		70%:30%	N	Y	Other	Y	N	Y
Hectors 2019	Predict prostate cancer aggressiveness with multiparametric MRI	Outcome prediction	Prostate cancer	Logistic regression	N/A	N	64	226	Y	N/A	Y	No	AUC	Y	N	N
Wong 2019	Compare ML algorithm with traditional regression for predicting early biochemical recurrence of prostate cancer	Outcome prediction	Prostate cancer	Cox regression	N/A	N	338	19	Y	70%:30%	Y	Y	AUC, accuracy	Y	Y	N
					N/A	N	338	19	Y	70%:30%	Y	Y		Y	Y	N

Compare ML algorithm with traditional regression for predicting early biochemical recurrence of prostate cancer	Outcome prediction	Prostate cancer	k-Nearest neighbors									AUC, accuracy			
Compare ML algorithm with traditional regression for predicting early biochemical recurrence of prostate cancer	Outcome prediction	Prostate cancer	Linear regression	N/A	N	338	19	Y	70%:30%	Y	Y	AUC, accuracy	Y	Y	N
Compare ML Algorithm with traditional regression for predicting early biochemical recurrence of prostate cancer	Outcome prediction	Prostate cancer	Random forest	N/A	N	338	19	Y	70%:30%	Y	Y	AUC, Accuracy	Y	Y	N

Abbreviations: ABDO, adaptive boosting; GNB gaussian naive bayes; N/A. not applicable; RARP, robotic-assisted radical prostatectomy.

Table 10
Bladder Cancer Outcome Prediction

Study	Application	Category	Subcategory	Algorithms/Models (List)	Neural Network: Architecture	Preprocessing Methodology Disclose (Y/N)	Reporting Size of Dataset (n)	No. of Features?	Train/Test Explanation (Y/N)	Train-Test Split?	Cross-Validation or Monte Carlo Runs (Y/N)	Lay Term Explanation of AI Methodology	Performance Metrics	Implications/Significance Discussion of How AI/ML Advances the Field (Y/N)	Comparison to Traditional Method (Y/N)	Feature Ranking (Y/N)
Bartsch 2016	Recurrence of non-muscle invasive bladder cancer after transurethral resection of a bladder tumor with genome profiling	Outcome prediction	Bladder cancer	Genetic programming	N/A	Y	100	21	Y	100:83	Y	Y	Sensitivity Specificity	Y	N	N
Lam 2014	Predict mortality after radical cystectomy	Outcome prediction	Bladder cancer	Artificial neural network	Y	N	117	5	Y	82:18	Y	Y	AUC	Y	Y	N
Sapre 2016	Predict urothelial carcinoma recurrence with urine microRNA	Outcome prediction	Bladder cancer	Support vector machine	N/A	Y	131	6	Y	81:50	Y	N	AUC	Y	N	Y
Wang 2015	Predict mortality after radical cystectomy	Outcome prediction	Bladder cancer	Back propagation network Radial basis function network Extreme learning machine Regularized extreme learning machine Support vector machine k-Nearest neighbors Naïve Bayes classifier	Y N/A	Y	117	10	Y	N/A	Y Y Y Y Y Y Y	Y	Accuracy Sensitivity Specificity Precision	Y	Y	N
Song 2019	Prediction of response to immune checkpoint inhibitor with molecular analysis	Outcome prediction	Bladder cancer	Hierarchical clustering	N/A	Y	165	786	Y	165:884	Y	N	N/A	Y	N	Y

Kirk 2020	Predicting readmission after radical cystectomy	Outcome prediction	Bladder cancer	Support vector machine	N/A	N	996	21	N	N/A	N	N	c-Index AUC	Y	N	Y
				Logistic regression	N/A				Y	50:50	N	N				
				Random forest					N	N/A	N	N				
Song 2020	Predicting overall survival from clinical and molecular features in bladder cancer	Outcome prediction	Bladder cancer	Logistic regression	N/A	Y	525	12	Y	525:286	Y	N	AUC Accuracy Sensitivity Specificity F-1 score	Y	N	Y
Hasnain 2019	Forecasting cancer recurrence and survival after radical cystectomy	Outcome prediction	Bladder cancer	Support vector machine Random forest Gradient boosting Adaboost	N/A	Y	3499	54	Y	N/A	Y	Y	Accuracy	Y	Y	N
Yao 2019	Predicting overall survival in patients with brain metastasis and bladder cancer	Outcome prediction	Bladder cancer	Least absolute shrinkage and selection operator	N/A	N	234	18	Y	169:65	Y	N	AUC	Y	N	Y

Abbreviation: N/A. not applicable.

database with 3499 patients who had undergone radical cystectomy with a random forest model and was able to predict recurrence at 1 year and survival at years 1, 3, and 5, with a greater than 70% sensitivity and specificity. Kirk and colleagues[25] trained 2 AI models using a support vector machine for feature selection, with logistic regression and random forest models to predict readmission in patients with bladder cancer with an AUC of 0.62 and 0.68, respectively.

Kidney cancer

There were 2 publications identified that predicted outcomes in kidney cancer in our review of the literature (**Table 11**). Bhandari and colleagues[26] used logistic regression, random forest, and neural network models trained on patient demographics and preoperative data to predict intraoperative events and postoperative events. The random forest model was found to be the best performing with an AUC under the receiver operating characteristic of 0.858 and 0.875, respectively.[26] Khene and colleagues[27] used radiomics to predict the response of patients with metastatic RCC to immunotherapy. Logistic regression obtained the highest AUC with 0.92 with k-nearest neighbor, random forest, and support vector machine obtaining values of 0.79, 0.67, and 0.71, respectively.[27]

Pediatric urology

The MIT ORC Personalized Medicine Group trained an optimal classification tree to predict recurrent urinary tract infection and vesicoureteral reflux in children after an initial urinary tract infection. The model predicted recurrent urinary tract infection–associated vesicoureteral reflux with AUC at 0.761.[28] Lorenzo and colleagues[29] trained a boosted decision tree model and a neural network model to create an optimized model that was able to predict surgical intervention in patients from a prenatal hydronephrosis database with an AUC of 0.9 (**Table 12**).

Kidney stones

Extracorporeal shock wave lithotripsy and percutaneous nephrolithotomy were the most common procedural outcomes evaluated. Five articles predicted postoperative success with 1 assessing quality of life metrics from clinical datasets. Aminsharifi and colleagues[30] examined patients undergoing percutaneous nephrolithotomy and were able to use a support vector machine model to predict stone free status with an AUC of 0.915, a value much higher than the Guy's Stone Score (0.615) or the Clinical Research Office of Endourological Society nomogram (0.621). In regards to extracorporeal shock wave lithotripsy, Choo and colleagues[31] trained a decision tree model on 1803 patients with clinical and radiographic data to predict stone-free status after a single session of extracorporeal shock wave lithotripsy. They were able to achieve 92.29% accuracy and an AUC of 0.951.[31] Additionally, Nguyen and colleagues[32] trained 2 models, gradient boosting and a neural network, to predict health-related quality of life from demographic and clinical data with an AUC of 0.62 and 0.59, respectively (**Table 13**).

General urology

One publication in outcome prediction was noted in general urology (**Table 14**). Sheyn and colleagues[33] trained a total of 5 AI models to predict treatment failure to anticholinergic medications in overactive bladder patients: support vector machine, random forest, naïve Bayes, logistic regression, and an artificial neural network. Both the logistic regression and artificial neural network performed no better than chance. The random forest resulted in the highest AUC in the external validation group (0.78). The overall accuracy was 80.3% for random forest and 71.9% and 71.3% for support vector machine and naïve Bayes models, respectively.[33]

Surgical Skill

The field of surgical skills assessment is growing because patient outcomes have been linked to surgical skill.[34] Our review of the literature identified 2 publications assessing surgical skill with the assistance of ML algorithms (**Table 15**). French and colleagues[35] were able to determine surgical skill ex vivo in the laboratory with greater than 80% accuracy with linear discriminant analysis, quadratic discriminant analysis, support vector machine, and logistic regression.[35] Shafiei and colleagues[36] examined electroencephalogram records from an attending surgeon observing trainee performances and was able to use a support vector machine to differentiate "trustworthy" from "concerning" performances with a classification accuracy of 98.81% and 93.97% for the urethrovesical anastomosis and the lymph node dissection, respectively.

Artificial Intelligence Reporting Standards

There was a total of 331 algorithms used in the 112 articles listed. The most common classifiers used were support vector machine (n = 71), followed by random forest (n = 53), logistic regression (n = 24), and artificial neural network (n = 24), with the remainder as shown in **Box 2**.

Table 11
Kidney Cancer Outcome Prediction

Study	Application	Category	Subcategory	Algorithm Categories (List)	Algorithms/ Models (List)	Neural Network: Architecture	Preprocessing Methodology Disclose (Y/N)	Reporting Size of Dataset (n)	No. of Features?	Train/Test Explanation (Y/N)	Train-Test Split?	Cross-Validation or Monte Carlo Runs (Y/N)	Lay Term Explanation of AI Methodology	Performance Metrics	Implications/ Significance Discussion of How AI/ML Advances the Field (Y/N)	Comparison to Traditional Method (Y/N)	Feature Ranking (Y/N)
Khene 2020	Predict tumor response to immunotherapy from radiomics	Outcome prediction	Kidney cancer	Classification	k-Nearest neighbors Support vector machine Random forest Logistic regression	N/A	Y	48	5	N	N/A	N	N	AUC Accuracy Sensitivity Specificity	N	N	N
Bhandari 2020	Predicting intraoperative and postoperative events from clinical data in patients undergoing robotic-assisted partial nephrectomy	Outcome prediction	Kidney cancer	Classification	Logistic regression Random forest Artificial neural network	N/A Y	Y	1406	59	Y	N/A	Y	Y	AUC	Y	Y	Y

Abbreviation: N/A. not applicable.

Table 12
Pediatric Urology Outcome Prediction

Study	Application	Category	Subcategory	Algorithms/ Models (List)	Neural Network: Architecture	Preprocessing Methodology Disclose (Y/N)	Reporting Size of Dataset (n)	No. of Features?	Train/Test Explanation (Y/N)	Train-Test Split?	Cross-Validation or Monte Carlo Runs (Y/N)	Lay Term Explanation of AI Methodology	Performance Metrics: _x000 B_	Implications/ Significance Discussion of How AI/ML Advances the Field (Y/N)	Comparison to Traditional Method (Y/N)	Feature Ranking (Y/N)
Advanced Analytics Group 2019	Predict probability of both recurrent urinary tract infection and vesicoureteral reflux ("recurrent urinary tract infection–associated vesicoureteral reflux") among children after initial urinary tract infection	Outcome prediction	Pediatrics	Optimal classification tree	N/A	Y	500	42	Y	440:79	Y	Y	AUC	Y	N	N
Lorenzo 2018	Predict surgical intervention in infants with prenatal hydronephrosis	Outcome prediction	Pediatrics	Decision tree Artificial neural network	N/A N	N	557	9	Y	70:30	N	N	AUC Accuracy Precision	Y	N	N

Table 13
Kidney Stone Outcome Prediction

Study	Application	Category	Subcategory	Algorithms/ Models (List)	Neural Network: Architecture (Descriptor) _x000 B_	Preprocessing Methodology Disclose (Y/N)	Reporting Size of Dataset (n)	No. of Features?	Train/Test Explanation (Y/N)	Train-Test Split?	Cross-Validation or Monte Carlo Runs (Y/N)	Lay Term Explanation of AI Methodology	Performance Metrics: _x000 B_	Implications/ Significance Discussion of How AI/ML Advances the Field (Y/N)	Comparison to Traditional Method (Y/N)	Feature Ranking (Y/N)
Aminsharifi 2017	Predict postoperative outcome of percutaneous nephrolithotomy	Outcome prediction	Kidney stone	Artificial neural network	Y	Y	454	18	Y	200:254	Y	Y	True positive False positive Accuracy Precision	Y	N	Y
Mannil 2018	Predict success of extracorporeal shock wave lithotripsy	Outcome prediction	Kidney stone	Random forest Random forest k-Nearest neighbors Back propagation network Random forest Sequential minimal optimization J48	N/A N N/A	Y	51	6 3 224	N Y	N/A 2:1	N N	N N	AUC AUC Sensitivity Specificity	Y Y	N N	Y Y
Nguyen 2020	Predicting quality of life from clinical data features in patients with kidney stones	Outcome prediction	Kidney stone	Gradient boosting Neural network	N/A Y	N N	3206	Supplementary table	Y	70:20	Y	N	AUC	Y	N	Y N
Yang 2020	Predicting stone free rate after extracorporeal shock wave lithotripsy	Outcome prediction	Kidney stone	Extreme gradient boosting Random forest Light gradient boosting	N/A	N	358	42	Y	80:20	Y	N	AUC Sensitivity Specificity Positive predictive value	Y	N	Y
Aminsharifi 2020	Predicting outcome of percutaneous nephrolithotomy	Outcome prediction	Kidney stone	Support vector machine	N/A	N	146	Supplementary table	N	N/A	N	N	AUC	Y	Y	Y

(continued on next page)

Table 13
(continued)

Study	Application	Category	Subcategory	Algorithms/ Models (List)	Neural Network: Architecture (Descriptor) _x000 B_	Preprocessing Methodology Disclose (Y/N)	Reporting Size of Dataset (n)	No. of Features?	Train/Test Explanation (Y/N)	Train-Test Split?	Cross-Validation or Monte Carlo Runs (Y/N)	Lay Term Explanation of AI Methodology	Performance Metrics: _x000 B_	Implications/ Significance Discussion of How AI/ML Advances the Field (Y/N)	Comparison to Traditional Method (Y/N)	Feature Ranking (Y/N)
Choo 2019	Assessing stone-free status after single session of shockwave lithotripsy	Outcome prediction	Kidney stone	Decision tree	N/A	N	791	15	Y	N/A	Y	Y	AUC	Y	N	Y

Abbreviation: N/A. not applicable.

Table 14
General Urology Outcome Prediction

Study	Application	Category	Subcategory	Algorithms/Models (List)	Neural Network: Architecture	Preprocessing Methodology Disclose (Y/N)	Reporting Size of Dataset (n)	No. of Features?	Train/Test Explanation (Y/N)	Train-Test Split?	Cross-Validation or Monte Carlo Runs (Y/N)	Lay Term Explanation of AI Methodology	Performance Metrics	Implications/Significance Discussion of How AI/ML Advances the Field (Y/N)	Comparison to Traditional Method (Y/N)	Feature Ranking (Y/N)
Sheyn 2019	Predict response to anticholinergic medications in patients with overactive bladder	Outcome prediction	General	Random forest Support vector machine Naïve Bayes classifier Artificial neural network Logistic regression	N/A Y N/A	Y	559	8	Y	559:82	Y	Y N	AUC Sensitivity Specificity	Y	N	N

Abbreviation: N/A. not applicable.

Table 15
Surgical Skill Analysis

Study	Application	Category	Subcategory	Algorithms/ Models (List)	Neural Network: Architecture (Descriptor) (Y, N, N/A)	Preprocessing Methodology Disclose (Y/N)	Reporting Size of Dataset (n)	No. of Features	Train/Test Explanation (Y/N)	Train-Test Split	Cross-Validation or Monte Carlo Runs (Y/N)	Lay Term Explanation of AI Methodology	Performance Metrics	Implications/ Significance Discussion of How AI/ML Advances the Field (Y/N)	Comparison to Traditional Method (Y/N)	Feature Ranking (Y/N)
Shafiei 2018	Identify trustworthy performance on urethrovesical anastomosis	Surgical skill	Prostate cancer	Support vector machine with kernel target alignment	N/A	Y	87	3	Y	N/A	Y	N	Accuracy	N	N	Y
	Identify trustworthy performance on urethrovesical anastomosis	Surgical skill	Prostate cancer	Support vector machine with kernel target alignment	N/A	Y	87	3	Y	N/A	Y	N	Accuracy, F-score	N	N	Y
	Identify trustworthy performance on lymph node dissection	Surgical skill	Prostate cancer	Support vector machine with kernel target alignment	N/A	Y	83	9	Y	N/A	Y	N	Accuracy	N	N	Y
	Identify trustworthy performance on lymph node dissection	Surgical skill	Prostate cancer	Support vector machine with kernel target alignment	N/A	Y	83	9	Y	N/A	Y	N	Accuracy, F-score	N	N	Y
French 2017	Identification of surgical skill from dry-lab laparoscopy	Surgical skill	Other	Logistic regression	N/A	Y	98	4	Y	N/A	Y	N	Accuracy	Y	N	Y
	Identification of surgical skill from dry-lab laparoscopy	Surgical skill	Other	Support vector machine	N/A	Y	98	4	Y	N/A	Y	N	Accuracy	Y	N	Y
	Identification of surgical skill from dry-lab laparoscopy	Surgical skill	Other	Linear discriminant analysis	N/A	Y	98	4	Y	N/A	Y	N	Accuracy	Y	N	Y
	Identification of surgical skill from dry-lab laparoscopy	Surgical skill	Other	Quadratic discriminant analysis	N/A	Y	98	4	Y	N/A	Y	N	Accuracy	Y	N	Y

Abbreviation: N/A. not applicable.

Box 2
AI reporting standards

Algorithm	Count
Support vector machine	71
Random forest	53
Logistic regression	24
Artificial neural network	24
k-Nearest neighbors	15
Convolutional neural network	13
Gradient boosting	12
Neural network	12
Naïve Bayesian	8
AdaBoost	8
Clustering	8
Decision tree	7
Linear discriminant analysis	6
Other	70

In total, 48 algorithms were classified as a form of neural network with 37 (77.1%) reporting the architecture of the neural network. A similar proportion of articles (70 of 112 [62.5%]) disclosed their methodology of pre∖processing data.

All articles (n = 112) detailed the size of their dataset, ranging from 5 to 514,878. Of the 112 article, 98 (87%) reported the number of features used to train their algorithm. Most articles detailed the training and testing methodology (n = 103). Ninety-three algorithms reported their train:test split.

Of the 112 articles, 92 (82.1%) used cross-validation or Monte Carlo random runs. There was heterogeneity in reporting of model performance: accuracy, sensitivity, specificity, precision, recall, negative predictive value, positive predictive value, variable importance measure, an AUC receiver operating characteristic curve, c-index, F-1 score, Rand index, true positive, and false-positive rate.

Of the 112 articles, 68 (60.7%) explained ML concepts and ideas in layman's terms. Within the discussion, the majority of articles (94 of 112 [83.9%]) described the significance of the findings specifically in regards to AI and/or ML. Only 48 of the 112 articles (42.9%) compared the AI/ML algorithm to a non-AI form of evaluation (traditional statistical approach). And fewer than one-half of the investigations (52 of 112 [46.4%]) performed feature ranking or feature importance.

DISCUSSION

Modern machine-learning models use complex calculations beyond the human level by processing large amounts of high dimensional data, without any particular guiding hypothesis, to directly uncover unseen connections and knowledge.[37] Owing to this ability, it is paramount to ensure that results and methodologies reported in the field of AI are not lost in translation. We hope to create a standardized checklist for reporting outcomes that improves readability and reproducibility.

Considerations for Reporting Artificial Intelligence Methodology

We begin with a clear description of the algorithm and model. From our data, it is evident that there are a number of classifiers to choose from in designing an experiment. A clear explanation of the algorithm would help the general readership to understand the relevant nuances and permutations of AI algorithms.

Of the many classifiers available, neural networks (implying deep learning) remain one of the more popular. Although neural networks are powerful models that have improved state-of-the-art speech recognition, image recognition, and other medical applications, the methods behind their ability to learn abstract representations of data input can be opaque. Because of the difficulty in determining feature importance and variability in construction of the neural network, an explanation of the architecture gives the reader a sense of the learnable parameters. Explanation allows for comparisons between different neural networks and to assess and possibly build on the published work.

With the growth of Big Data, in theory, more data would lead to better predictive power and insight. However, these data must first be preprocessed because the real-world data may be incomplete, noisy, and inconsistent. This process includes data cleaning, deduplication (removal of duplicates), imputation (substitution of estimated value for missing data), category mapping (translating input data for the algorithm), and feature selection (finding those features that contribute most to the output).[38] Although we are in a time of ever-growing data, tasks such as imputation remain important to maximizing all available data sources.[39] Because many articles use shared national databases and datasets, this important step of preprocessing can change the reported outcomes, even if the remaining analysis and algorithms remain the same. Data preprocessing is necessary to generate quality data and should be disclosed to improve reproducibility and provide transparency for critical review.

Research in other disciplines has demonstrated the importance in the size of the dataset on performance. For example, in natural language processing, a messier dataset with more errors that is 1 million times larger than a well-annotated dataset can be far more effective if used the right way.[40] On the other end, having too few training samples has been shown to degrade the performance of a classifier.[41] Although all articles in the review disclosed the size of their dataset, not all were able to take advantage of Big Data. In our review of the literature, there were datasets reporting a number as low as 5.

Similarly, there exists an optimal number of features that improves performance of algorithms and models. Inclusion of too many features in some cases can increase classification error and be counterproductive to the stated goal.[41] On the other end of the spectrum is a lack of features, which can result in underfitting. Surprisingly, although all articles reported the size of the dataset, we find that only 87% of the listed articles reported the number of features used in the associated algorithm. Features ranged from 3 to 10,000.

AI and ML algorithms are first trained on a dataset to develop a predictive model. This model is then evaluated on a test set of data, which is the reported outcome of the investigation. Therefore, the explanation of model training and testing, with or without validation, is necessary to assess the performance of the algorithm. To this end, reporting of the train and test split is helpful to evaluate reliability of the result as well extrapolation of the algorithm to external test sets. A large proportion of reviewed articles (92.0%) reported the training and testing methodology and a train:test split. Cross-validation, a technique to tune hyperparameters and assess model performance on previously unseen data, partitions a dataset into subsets, comprising a training set and a test set. Hyperparameter tuning affects the speed and quality of the learning of the algorithm. Cross-validation is usually performed in multiple rounds on different partitions to decrease performance variability in the target application. It is considered the gold standard to avoid selection bias and to avoid overfitting.[42] We find that a large proportion of algorithms in our review (82.1%) used cross-validation. This finding is likely due to the prevalence of smaller datasets, which limit the ability to generate unbiased training and testing sets.

Last, the most important disclosure in the methodology for readability is the layman's explanation of which algorithm and why it was selected by the authors. Because we are focusing on clinician-facing research, it is imperative to do so in nontechnical terms. We expect a diverse readership with varying levels of fluency with AI and ML terminology in urology. With the variability and nuance in selecting different algorithms, it is important to explain how each algorithm operates and why the algorithm was selected. There can be subtle differences that affect outcomes even within classifiers. A brief explanation as to why the support vector machine with linear kernel classifier was selected as compared with the random forest would be helpful to the reader and other clinicians hoping to advance the field of AI. The aforementioned reporting standards serve to provide a foundation for an explanation of the methodology in layman's terms. In this review, only 68 of the 112 articles (60.7%) reported their methodology in such a fashion. Both insufficient background information as well as overly technical discussion limited the generalizability of the articles.

Considerations for Reporting Artificial Intelligence Results

This literature review also revealed large-scale heterogeneity in the reporting of results. Although there are many acceptable methods to report model performance, certain metrics have been found to be more accurate and revealing. In particular, the AUC and F-1 score have been found to be more accurate than reporting sensitivity and specificity alone especially when data are imbalanced.[43] Imbalanced datasets, a common occurrence in medical data, occur when the target variable (eg, a rare disease) is poorly represented on the training sample. Other reporting options gaining traction include net benefit. Although none of the articles reviewed listed net benefit as an outcome, there is evidence to support its advantages compared with current reporting methodologies. The use of the net benefit should be considered, because it incorporates prevalence and misclassification costs in assessing clinical impact.[44]

Discussion of the Implications and Significance of Artificial Intelligence and Machine Learning Work

As AI and ML grows in popularity and demonstrates superiority over traditional methods, it is important to consider that AI may not always result in improved prediction or projection of outcome or ground truth. Many AI algorithms reported outcomes in terms of AUC without a comparison. Although an evaluation of the discriminatory ability of an algorithm with an AUC is possible, a lack of comparison with traditional methods inhibits the clinical application of newly developed AI models.[45] For example, there is little reason to use a new AI model for prediction if there is no improvement in performance as compared with current Cox proportional hazard models.[46] In this regard, reporting ML results in comparison with traditional methods will ensure a healthy baseline level of performance to truly hone and advance the field of AI.

As a final reported metric, feature importance is essential to extrapolating conclusions from AI and ML. Although humans may not be able to match the discriminatory ability of AI in large datasets, knowledge of the major contributors in classification can serve both as a means of education and of validation. Previously overlooked features may illuminate new avenues and directions for research. Additionally, features that seem incongruent or counterintuitive to established heuristics could indicate overfitting or some other flaw in the algorithm. When possible, feature importance should be reported to increase trust and allow for future research to build on current methodologies.[47]

SUMMARY

The field of AI continues to grow in medicine. The aforementioned review of the literature and proposal of reporting standard serve as methods to improve AI literacy for urologic clinicians. We hope that this would serve as a starting point in improving foundational knowledge to make AI and ML accessible to all participants.

FUNDING

Research reported in this publication was supported in part by the National Cancer Institute under Award No. R01CA251579-01A1.

REFERENCES

1. He J, Baxter SL, Xu J, et al. The practical implementation of artificial intelligence technologies in medicine. Nat Med 2019;25(1):30–6.
2. Luo W, Phung D, Tran T, et al. Guidelines for developing and reporting machine learning predictive models in biomedical research: a multidisciplinary view. J Med Internet Res 2016;18(12):e323.
3. Kolachalama VB, Garg PS. Machine learning and medical education. NPJ Digit Med 2018;1(1):1–3.
4. Chen J, Remulla D, Nguyen JH, et al. Current status of artificial intelligence applications in urology and their potential to influence clinical practice. BJU Int 2019;124(4):567–77.
5. Briganti G, Le Moine O. Artificial intelligence in medicine: today and tomorrow. Front Med 2020;7:27.
6. Long D, Magerko B. What is AI literacy? Competencies and design considerations. In: Paper presented at: Proceedings of the 2020 CHI Conference on Human Factors in Computing Systems. 2020.
7. Connell SP, O'Reilly E, Tuzova A, et al. Development of a multivariable risk model integrating urinary cell DNA methylation and cell-free RNA data for the detection of significant prostate cancer. Prostate 2020;80(7):547–58.
8. Leyh-Bannurah SR, Tian Z, Karakiewicz PI, et al. Deep learning for natural language processing in urology: state-of-the-art automated extraction of detailed pathologic prostate cancer data from narratively written electronic health records. JCO Clin Cancer Inform 2018;2:1–9.
9. Sugano D, Sanford D, Abreu A, et al. Impact of radiomics on prostate cancer detection: a systematic review of clinical applications. Curr Opin Urol 2020;30(6):754–81.
10. Varghese B, Chen F, Hwang D, et al. Objective risk stratification of prostate cancer using machine learning and radiomics applied to multiparametric magnetic resonance images. Sci Rep 2019;9(1): 1570.
11. Shkolyar E, Jia X, Chang TC, et al. Augmented bladder tumor detection using deep learning. Eur Urol 2019;76(6):714–8.
12. Pedersen M, Andersen MB, Christiansen H, et al. Classification of renal tumour using convolutional neural networks to detect oncocytoma. Eur J Radiol 2020;133:109343.
13. Zheng H, Ji J, Zhao L, et al. Prediction and diagnosis of renal cell carcinoma using nuclear magnetic resonance-based serum metabolomics and self-organizing maps. Oncotarget 2016;7(37):59189–98.
14. Baessler B, Nestler T, Pinto Dos Santos D, et al. Radiomics allows for detection of benign and malignant histopathology in patients with metastatic testicular germ cell tumors prior to post-chemotherapy retroperitoneal lymph node dissection. Eur Radiol 2020;30(4):2334–45.
15. Smail LC, Dhindsa K, Braga LH, et al. Using deep learning algorithms to grade hydronephrosis severity: toward a clinical adjunct. Front Pediatr 2020;8:1.
16. Wang HHS, Cahill D, Panagides J, et al. Pattern recognition algorithm to identify detrusor overactivity on urodynamics. Neurourol Urodyn 2021;40(1): 428–34.
17. Xu Z, Yang X, Gao M, et al. Abnormal resting-state functional connectivity in the whole brain in lifelong premature ejaculation patients based on machine learning approach. Front Neurosci 2019;13:448.
18. Grosse Hokamp N, Lennartz S, Salem J, et al. Dose independent characterization of renal stones by means of dual energy computed tomography and

machine learning: an ex-vivo study. Eur Radiol 2020; 30(3):1397–404.
19. De Perrot T, Hofmeister J, Burgermeister S, et al. Differentiating kidney stones from phleboliths in unenhanced low-dose computed tomography using radiomics and machine learning. Eur Radiol 2019; 29(9):4776–82.
20. Hung AJ, Chen J, Ghodoussipour S, et al. A deep-learning model using automated performance metrics and clinical features to predict urinary continence recovery after robot-assisted radical prostatectomy. BJU Int 2019;124(3):487–95.
21. Wong NC, Lam C, Patterson L, et al. Use of machine learning to predict early biochemical recurrence after robot-assisted prostatectomy. BJU Int 2019; 123(1):51–7.
22. Lee S, Kerns S, Ostrer H, et al. Machine learning on a genome-wide association study to predict late genitourinary toxicity after prostate radiation therapy. Int J Radiat Oncol Biol Phys 2018;101(1): 128–35.
23. Hanson HA, Martin C, O'Neil B, et al. The relative importance of race compared to health care and social factors in predicting prostate cancer mortality: a random forest approach. J Urol 2019;202(6): 1209–16.
24. Hasnain Z, Mason J, Gill K, et al. Machine learning models for predicting post-cystectomy recurrence and survival in bladder cancer patients. PLoS One 2019;14(2):e0210976.
25. Kirk PS, Liu X, Borza T, et al. Dynamic readmission prediction using routine postoperative laboratory results after radical cystectomy. In: Paper presented at: Urologic Oncology: Seminars and Original Investigations. 2020.
26. Bhandari M, Nallabasannagari AR, Reddiboina M, et al. Predicting intra-operative and postoperative consequential events using machine-learning techniques in patients undergoing robot-assisted partial nephrectomy: a Vattikuti Collective Quality Initiative database study. BJU Int 2020;126(3):350–8.
27. Khene ZE, Mathieu R, Peyronnet B, et al. Radiomics can predict tumour response in patients treated with nivolumab for a metastatic renal cell carcinoma: an artificial intelligence concept. World J Urol 2020;1–3.
28. Advanced Analytics Group of Pediatric U, Group ORCPM. Targeted workup after initial febrile urinary tract infection: using a novel machine learning model to identify children most likely to benefit from voiding cystourethrogram. J Urol 2019;202(1):144–52.
29. Lorenzo AJ, Rickard M, Braga LH, et al. Predictive analytics and modeling employing machine learning technology: the next step in data sharing, analysis, and individualized counseling explored with a large, prospective prenatal hydronephrosis database. Urology 2019;123:204–9.
30. Aminsharifi A, Irani D, Tayebi S, et al. Predicting the postoperative outcome of percutaneous nephrolithotomy with machine learning system: software validation and comparative analysis with Guy's Stone Score and the CROES Nomogram. J Endourol 2020;34(6):692–9.
31. Choo MS, Uhmn S, Kim JK, et al. A prediction model using machine learning algorithm for assessing stone-free status after single session shock wave lithotripsy to treat ureteral stones. J Urol 2018; 200(6):1371–7.
32. Nguyen DD, Luo JW, Lu XH, et al. Estimating the health-related quality of life of kidney stone patients: initial results from the Wisconsin Stone Quality of Life Machine-Learning Algorithm (WISQOL-MLA). BJU Int 2021 Jul;128(1):88–94.
33. Sheyn D, Ju M, Zhang S, et al. Development and validation of a machine learning algorithm for predicting response to anticholinergic medications for overactive bladder syndrome. Obstet Gynecol 2019;134(5):946–57.
34. Birkmeyer JD, Finks JF, O'reilly A, et al. Surgical skill and complication rates after bariatric surgery. N Engl J Med 2013;369(15):1434–42.
35. French A, Lendvay TS, Sweet RM, et al. Predicting surgical skill from the first N seconds of a task: value over task time using the isogony principle. Int J Comput Assist Radiol Surg 2017;12(7): 1161–70.
36. Shafiei SB, Hussein AA, Muldoon SF, et al. Functional brain states measure mentor-trainee trust during robot-assisted surgery. Sci Rep 2018;8(1): 3667.
37. Cleophas TJ, Zwinderman AH. Machine learning in medicine-a complete overview. Cham, Switzerland: Springer; 2015.
38. Taleb I, Dssouli R, Serhani MA. Big data preprocessing: a quality framework. In: Paper presented at: 2015 IEEE international congress on big data. 2015.
39. Jerez JM, Molina I, García-Laencina PJ, et al. Missing data imputation using statistical and machine learning methods in a real breast cancer problem. Artif intelligence Med 2010;50(2):105–15.
40. Halevy A, Norvig P, Pereira F. The unreasonable effectiveness of data. IEEE Intell Syst 2009;24(2): 8–12.
41. Raudys SJ, Jain AK. Small sample size effects in statistical pattern recognition: recommendations for practitioners. IEEE Trans Pattern Anal Mach Intell 1991;13(3):252–64.
42. Stone M. Cross-validatory choice and assessment of statistical predictions. J R Stat Soc Ser B Methodol 1974;36(2):111–33.
43. Huang J, Ling CX. Using AUC and accuracy in evaluating learning algorithms. IEEE Trans Knowledge Data Eng 2005;17(3):299–310.

44. Halligan S, Altman DG, Mallett S. Disadvantages of using the area under the receiver operating characteristic curve to assess imaging tests: a discussion and proposal for an alternative approach. Eur Radiol 2015;25(4):932–9.
45. Hosmer DW Jr, Lemeshow S, Sturdivant RX. Applied logistic regression, Vol 398. New Jersey, USA: John Wiley & Sons; 2013.
46. Kattan MW. Comparison of Cox regression with other methods for determining prediction models and nomograms. J Urol 2003;170(6 Pt 2):S6–9.discussion S10.
47. Ribeiro MT, Singh S, Guestrin C. "Why should I trust you?" Explaining the predictions of any classifier. In: Paper presented at: Proceedings of the 22nd ACM SIGKDD international conference on knowledge discovery and data mining. 2016.

The Life and Death of Percutaneous Stone Removal

"Looking Back—Looking Forward"

Pengbo Jiang, MD*, Andrew Brevik, MS, Ralph V. Clayman, MD

KEYWORDS

• Urolithiasis • Kidney stones • Percutaneous nephrolithotomy • Ureteroscopy • Lithotripsy

KEY POINTS

- Percutaneous nephrolithotomy has risks of significant complications, has a long learning curve, and results in reduction of functioning renal parenchyma.
- The evolving technology for flexible ureteroscopy is robust at this time. These advances include alterations in ureteral access sheaths, new laser technology, improvement in methods for stone fragment evacuation, and development of multifunctional ureteroscopes.
- Compared with holmium lasers, the superpulse thulium fiber laser energy can be transmitted through fibers as small as 50µ, thereby facilitating irrigant flow and deflection of the ureteroscope. Second, it provides more efficient energy transmission while allowing for lower pulse energies and higher frequencies. Lastly, the thulium unit has greater portability and lower voltage requirements, allowing usage in any operating room.
- Advances in our knowledge regarding ureteral physiology combined with technical developments applied to ureteral access sheath deployment and size, along with the advent of the thulium laser and better technology for fragment evacuation and newer ureteroscopes, may well propel retrograde intrarenal surgery to the forefront of kidney stone removal, regardless of stone size or location.

HISTORY AND BACKGROUND

The ability to access the kidney via a percutaneous approach was first reported in the 1950s by Dr Willard Goodwin, with the placement of a nephrostomy tube.[1] It was more than 2 decades before Drs Fernström and Johansson, in 1976, expanded the percutaneous nephrostomy tract beyond a method of drainage to become a route of access for the removal of renal calculi and thereby brought percutaneous nephrolithotomy (PCNL) into the urologist's realm.[2] Through collaborative efforts of urologists and radiologists, favorable PCNL success rates began to be widely reported by the mid-1980s.[1,3,4] Refinements in fluoroscopy and renal ultrasonography, novel methods for rapid dilation of the nephrostomy tract, and the development of efficient lithotripsy devices (eg, ultrasonic, pneumatic, and laser) elevated PCNL to today's standard of care.[3–5] In 2021, the need for an open surgical procedure to treat urolithiasis is a rare event.

PROCEDURE LIMITATIONS: ACCESS AND COMPLICATIONS

Percutaneous Renal Access

As the widespread adoption of PCNL ensued, the steep learning curve for percutaneous renal access became more evident. Gaining renal access

Department of Urology, University of California - Irvine, 333 City Boulevard West, Suite 2100, Orange, CA 92868, USA
* Corresponding author.
E-mail address: pengboj@hs.uci.edu

Urol Clin N Am 49 (2022) 119–128
https://doi.org/10.1016/j.ucl.2021.07.010

became the most challenging step of PCNL for the urologist. As such, access is often achieved by an interventional radiologist a day or more before the actual removal of the stone; thereby, creating a 2-step procedure that is less efficient.

Despite urologists becoming more involved in gaining their own renal access during PCNL, as of 2017, interventional radiologists continue to gain access in nearly two-thirds of cases.[6] For urologists willing to learn this skill, the learning curve is often too steep and the cases too few, as competency does not begin to plateau until 60 PCNLs have been performed; indeed, it may take as many as 115 cases before screening time and radiation dose level off.[7,8] Because of concerns of radiation exposure, ultrasonography-guided PCNL has also been studied; however, even with this radiation-free approach, the learning curve ranges from 20 to 60 cases.[9,10] Accordingly, for a urologist to become proficient in access requires a minimum case load of 2 to 5 PCNL cases/month.

Advances in renal access include both endoscopic and robotic techniques. The addition of endoscopic-assisted nephrostomy tract placement mitigates fluoroscopic screening time and the number of nephrostomy needle passes, but this approach entails the use of a flexible ureteroscope and of an assistant (eg, partner, resident, or operating room OR nurse) capable of maintaining the endoscopic view of the desired calyceal point of entry.[11] On the horizon is the use of robotic needle placement controlled by electromagnetic guidance such that the ureteroscope or a retrograde catheter carries the homing device and once in place and activated, the needle passes directly into the identified calyx, stopping at the tip of the ureteroscope or catheter. The advantages include real-time, 3-dimensional targeting without radiation exposure.[12]

Percutaneous Nephrolithotomy Complications

PCNL complications span the gamut of minor to fatal (0.3%).[13] In part, the risk of the procedure is further complicated by the comorbidities common among the urolithiasis population. Many urolithiasis patients suffer from the metabolic syndrome, creating a challenging surgical problem due to obesity along with diabetes, hypertension, and hyperlipidemia.[14,15]

Intraoperative complications during PCNL occur in upward of 15% of patients.[13] These problems include injury to the pleura with associated pneumothorax/hydrothorax (16% for supracostal access or 4.5% for infracostal access), extravasation from the collecting system (7.2%), and intraoperative hemorrhage requiring transfusion (5%–7%) or procedural abandonment (1.7%).[13,16,17] More rare is injury to ipsilateral organs such as the liver, spleen, or colon (0.2%–0.8%).[14,18]

Postoperative adverse events are as or more common than intraoperative complications. In a review of 300 PCNL patients, postoperative systemic inflammatory response syndrome developed in 27%; sepsis developed in 8%.[19] In a multicenter review completed by the Clinical Research Office of the Endourological Society (CROES) from 2007 to 2009, among 5800 PCNLs submitted for review, 15% had a complication. As the single institution study of Koras and colleagues, the CROES study found postoperative fever to be the most common complication (10.5%), followed by bleeding (7.8%), transfusion (5.7%), perforation of the renal pelvis (3.4%), procedural abandonment (1.7%), and hydrothorax (1.8%).[13] In other studies, immediate postoperative (<24 hours) urine leakage from the nephrostomy site occurred in 7% to 15%, whereas persistent leakage occurred in 1.5% to 3% of patients.[17,20–22] Mild perioperative pain and discomfort is quite common; however, long-term postoperative pain persists in less than 1% of patients.[17,23–25]

In addition to intraoperative and perioperative adverse events, late or delayed complications of PCNL are similarly concerning. Infundibular stenosis, although rare, occurs due to iatrogenic tearing of the infundibular urothelium during the procedure and may result in the eventual obliteration of the infundibulum with attendant loss of function of that portion of the kidney.[26] In a systematic review of the impact on renal function following PCNL, Reeves and colleagues noted risk factors for worse postoperative renal function: multiple percutaneous nephrostomy tracts, poor preoperative renal function, diabetes, postoperative urinary tract infection, and complicated/lengthy procedures.[27] Indeed, recent studies recorded a 21% decline in ipsilateral renal parenchymal volume after PCNL.[28] Using nuclear renal scans before and after PCNL, Aguiar and colleagues demonstrated regional renal function decreases in the accessed portion of the kidney in most patients.[29] In a randomized controlled trial of 75 patients undergoing PCNL with before and after technetium-99m-dimercaptosuccinic acid scans, Ünsal and colleagues found that although immediate renal function was preserved or improved, new focal cortical defects occurred in 18% of patients.[30] Whether these parenchymal losses will have an impact on long-term (ie, >/ = 1 year) postoperative renal function has yet to be determined.

MINIATURIZED PERCUTANEOUS NEPHROLITHOTOMY: "LESS IS LESS"

One approach to mitigate complications from the traditional 30F nephrostomy tract for PCNL is to reduce the diameter of the nephrostomy tract. The miniaturization of PCNL has led to the development of mini-PCNL (tract sizes ranging from 15 to 24F). The utilization of these smaller tracts has reduced the rate of complications (7.9% vs 20.5% in standard PCNL) and lowered transfusion rates (3.7% vs 7.9% in standard PCNL) while providing for a shorter hospital stay and less need for placing a postoperative nephrostomy tube; however, with these improvements, there has been a decrease in stone-free rates.[23,31] Proponents of mini-PCNL have countered that although these SFRs are less than with traditional PCNL, they are better than ureteroscopy for similar sized stones.[23]

Further miniaturization of access tracts has brought on the development of the ultramini-PCNL (tract size of 11–13Fr) and the micro-PCNL (tract size of 4.8–10Fr).[32] Despite this massive decrease in the tract size, a comparison with ureteroscopy/retrograde intrarenal surgery (RIRS) revealed that micro-PCNL was associated with greater blood loss, more pain, and greater analgesic use.[33–35] Nonetheless, one proposed niche indication for mini-PCNL is the treatment of lower pole renal stones that may otherwise be inaccessible with retrograde ureteroscopy.[36]

Flexible Ureteroscopy: The Challenge to Percutaneous Nephrolithotomy

Although miniaturized PCNL tracts may have lower rates of complication compared with traditional tracts, they still remain higher than those of flexible ureteroscopy (FUS) (ie, RIRS or natural orifice transendoscopic surgery for the genitourinary tract). However, FUS has clear limitations, most notably lower stone-free rates than PCNL. Indeed, the current stone-free rates with FUS are not dissimilar to shock wave lithotripsy (SWL) albeit with FUS being a more invasive and more morbid approach than SWL.

The key question is: "Can FUS success rates be improved by new technology until they rival or exceed success rates with traditional PCNL?" The evolving technology for FUS is robust at this time. These advances include alterations in ureteral access sheaths, new laser technology, improvement in methods for stone fragment evacuation, and development of multifunctional ureteroscopes. Should these advances realize their full potential, PCNL may well go the way of open stone surgery and become part of the rich history of Urology.

Ureteral access sheaths—how big, so big?

The advent of ureteral access sheaths (UAS) provides easy, repeated access to the renal pelvis. Use of UAS improves irrigation flow and decreases intrarenal pressure. Even with irrigation pressure set to 200 cm H_2O, the UAS maintains the intrapelvic renal pressure at less than 30 cm H_2O.[37] In addition, studies have shown that deployment of a UAS expands the "life" of the flexible ureteroscope while expediting stone extraction by upward of 10 minutes per case, an estimated cost savings of $700/procedure.[38,39] There was one area in which UAS deployment to date has not been shown to be beneficial: improved SFR.[40,41]

Despite the advantages of deploying a UAS, due to fear of acute ureteral injury or delayed ureteral stricture formation, upward of one-fourth of urologists do not use a UAS, whereas most of the remaining urologists selected the smallest UAS necessary for the procedure. Although fears of acute ureteral trauma are certainly justified by recent reports of 26% high-grade injury (ie, partial of full-thickness splitting of the ureter), concerns over ureteral stricture formation seem unjustified.[42–44] Of note, despite prior animal studies showing decreased ureteral perfusion with ischemia and even focal ureteral necrosis following UAS placement, the clinical use of a UAS has not led to a higher incidence of postureteroscopic ureteral strictures.[40,45] In a series of 130 patients, Delvecchio and colleagues found that only one patient developed a stricture on follow-up imaging (1.4%).[46] Similarly, in the CROES study on ureteroscopy as well as in other reports, the incidence of ureteral strictures following ureteroscopy was similar, whether a UAS was or was not used: 1% to 1.4% and 0.35% to 1%, respectively.[47–51]

In contradistinction to the approach of placing the smallest (ie, 11–12Fr) UAS possible, emerging studies reveal that placement of the largest UAS possible (ie, 16Fr) might be desirable. Studies in this regard have revealed that the largest UAS provides for more efficient stone extraction and, in contradistinction to earlier UAS studies, higher stone-free rates.[52–54] Given the desire to safely deploy a larger UAS, it was hypothesized that use of a ureteral wall relaxing agent, such as an alpha blocker, might be beneficial. Indeed, in a retrospective study of 72 unstented patients, patients treated with 1 week of tamsulosin had an 87% successful deployment of a 16Fr UAS compared with 43% in the nontamsulosin group.[55] Subsequently, in a prospective randomized controlled trial of 135 patients, Koo and colleagues found that maximal UAS insertion force was significantly lower in the alpha blocker group compared with control and concluded that preoperative alpha blockade and slow deployment of the UAS may reduce the force needed to deploy a larger UAS.[56] Indeed, Koo and colleagues noted that up to 600g (5.88N) could be safely applied during UAS insertion without ureteral injury. In a similar work, albeit in the porcine ureter, using a purpose built UAS force sensor, capable of measuring force in hundredths of a Newton, Kaler and colleagues found that significant ureteral injury (PULS >/ = 3) can be routinely avoided if the applied force is less than 6 N, thereby corroborating the findings of Koo and colleagues; high-grade injury (PULS >/ = 3) was only noted if the applied force exceeded 8.1 N[55] Armed with this information, the same investigators embarked on a clinical study of 200 patients among whom the recommendation was to not exceed 6N of UAS deployment force. In these patients, a 16Fr UAS was deployed in 61% of cases with a mean peak force of 5.7N. No high-grade ureteral injuries were encountered when the maximal force applied was less than 6N. Factors that were predictors of successful passage of 16Fr UAS included prior stone surgery, prestenting and tamsulosin, and recently treated bacteriuria. Furthermore, in patients without prior surgery or an indwelling stent, preoperative tamsulosin favored deployment of a 16Fr UAS. On follow-up, there were no strictures that developed as a result of UAS deployment.[57] Presently, at our institution, efforts are underway to create an inexpensive, easily deployable force sensing device to be used in conjunction with UAS deployment, which would inform the urologist when the deployment force reached 6N. With a device of this nature, it is thought that more urologists would feel comfortable using a larger UAS knowing that ureteral injury would be avoided.

If greater than 60% of patients can accept a 16Fr UAS without exceeding the safety threshold of 6N, the question arises: "How many patients might accept deployment of an 18Fr or even 20Fr UAS?". In an attempt to answer this question, an in vivo porcine investigation was completed, using a week of ureteral prestenting to promote ureteral relaxation. After a week of an indwelling 4.7Fr or 7Fr ureteral stent, there was nearly a 4Fr (1.33 mm) increase in luminal circumference. In 25% of prestented porcine ureters an 18Fr dilator could be passed to the renal pelvis, whereas in 12.5% a 20Fr or larger (maximum of 24Fr) dilator could be deployed (Jiang, P., Afyouni A., King T., et al.: The Impact of One Week of Pre-stenting on Porcine Ureteral Diameter – accepted for presentation - American Urologic Association National Meeting: Sept. 2021, Las Vegas). At 18F, the UAS rivals a mini-PCNL. The question arises: will an 18F UAS produce stone-free rates equivalent to an 18F PCNL?

Laser technology for lithotripsy

Given the size constraints of flexible ureteroscopes, laser lithotripsy has become the primary method for stone fragmentation. The holmium:YAG laser (Ho:YAG) has become the standard for laser lithotripsy since its introduction in the 1990s.[58] Although the Ho:YAG is able to fragment all stones, problems persist with regard to either evacuating all of the fragments or reducing the stone to sufficiently small particles (ie, dust: <100 μ) that could be flushed from the system. To this end various "dusting" settings have been used; however, these settings more commonly result in "sand" (ie, 100–1000μ), which can neither be flushed from the system nor removed with current basket technology.[59]

To more efficiently perform laser lithotripsy, the Ho:YAG laser has been expanded to include MOSES technology (Lumenis Ltd, Yokneam, Israel). The MOSES effect uses an initial pulse of energy to create a bubble to disperse the liquid between the tip of the probe and the stone; as such, the near immediate firing of a second pulse allows it to travel through the gaseous bubble, thereby affecting the stone with a greater, more effective amount of energy.[58] In a double-blind prospective randomized controlled trial, Ibrahim and colleagues demonstrated that the MOSES effect resulted in a significantly shorter time for lithotripsy as well as shorter procedural time. In addition, activation of the Moses mode resulted in significantly less retropulsion.[60] To date, to the best of our knowledge, there have been no studies to evaluate whether the MOSES effect creates an increased amount of dustlike particles that can be more easily evacuated, thereby enhancing stone free rates.

The latest advance in laser lithotripsy is the superpulse thulium fiber laser (sTFL). Lithotripsy with sTFL has several major advantages. First, the laser energy can be transmitted through fibers as small as 50μ, thereby facilitating irrigant flow and deflection of the ureteroscope. At present the smallest fibers that are available for routine use with sTFL are 200 μm from tip to shaft; this is smaller than the smallest Ho:YAG laser fibers, which although only 272 μm at the tip, the attendant cladding results in upsizing the probe to as large as 445 μm.[61,62] Second, sTFL for laser lithotripsy operates at 1940 nm, a wavelength that approximates water's absorption peak; this results in more efficient energy transmission to the target and may aid fragmentation, given that there are commonly water interfaces within the stone itself. Indeed, the nearly 4-fold increase in absorption coefficient versus Ho:YAG means that a lower threshold and higher ablation efficiency can be achieved at equivalent pulse energies. As such, the sTFL can use lower pulse energies (as low as 0.025 J) with higher frequencies (up to 2000 Hz). Studies in our laboratory have shown that at equivalent power output, sTFL routinely produces stone fragments all less than 2 mm; whereas Ho:YAG as well as Ho:YAG MOSES produced stone fragments less than or equal to 4 mm and less than or equal to 3.5 mm, respectively. (Jiang P., Peta A., Arada R., et al. Superpulse Thulium, Holmium, and Holmium MOSES Laser Lithotripsy: An ex vivo Laboratory Evaluation on the Effectiveness of "Dusting" Coupled with Ureteroscopic Fragment Aspiration. accepted for presentation - American Urologic Association National Meeting: Sept. 2021, Las Vegas). Third, the sTFL laser unit weighs 38 kg, providing a more than 6-fold decrease in weight and greater transportability when compared with other currently available laser devices.[63] Fourth, sTFL has lower voltage requirements and thus can be used with outlets present in any operating room. Lastly, the diode assembly is simpler than Ho:YAG, resulting in lower maintenance costs.[64]

Given the foregoing attributes, it is not surprising that in vitro studies have shown sTFL to be significantly better than Ho:YAG at reducing stones to dustlike particles.[65,66] Further, Blackmon and colleagues showed that the stone vaporization rate with sTFL was nearly 10-fold more rapid than with Ho:YAG. Chiron and colleagues demonstrated that a single firing of the sTFL was able to ablate 3 times more stone volume than Ho:YAG. In addition, stone clearance was 5 times faster with sTFL compared with Ho:YAG.[67]

A major concern with sTFL is its potential to generate high temperatures within the collecting system. To assess this risk, Okhunov and colleagues used 4-point temperature sensing probes deployed in vivo in the porcine kidney in order to evaluate the temperature of the irrigant/urine in the area of the calyces as well as the temperature at the level of the urothelium and throughout the renal parenchyma. The sTFL when deployed without a 14F UAS produced intracalyceal temperatures capable of causing tissue damage (ie, > 44°C) during both fragmentation and dusting mode; however, when sTFL was used with a UAS in place via a dual lumen ureteroscope, there were no temperatures recorded greater than 39°C. Furthermore, despite intracalyceal temperatures as high as 70°C in the non-UAS situation, the temperature recorded within the renal papilla and the renal parenchyma never exceeded 42°C, suggesting a protective heat-sink effect.[68]

The question arises as to what is the true potential of sTFL? Will it enable the urologist to rapidly render stones larger than 2 cm to dustlike particles that can be cleared from the collecting system via the UAS? If this proves to be the case, the need for PCNL might possibly be largely eliminated.

Stone fragment retrieval and evacuation

Rendering the kidney stone free by technological means remains an ongoing challenge for the urologist. Traditional means have revolved around stone baskets with more recent forays into the areas of actively aspirating fragments from the collecting system or introducing substances that would alter the stone fragments and thereby render them more amenable to removal. Possibly, one or more of these approaches could provide an effective and efficient means of cleansing the kidney of all stone remnants.

Stone baskets have been the most common means available to the urologist for removing small calculi. First described in 1948 and used blindly and later under fluoroscopic control, stone baskets have evolved in both design and materials.[69] Today, there are varying shapes of stone retrieval baskets: tipless (4-wire round), tipless (end-engaging), tipless (meshed), as well as with an extended tip. Over recent years, tipless 4-wire nitinol baskets have replaced the older metal baskets, becoming the primary stone retrieval basket for urologists given the relative atraumatic tip and ease of entrapping stones.[70] In addition, these newer baskets allow the urologist to release a stone if it proves too large to safely extract in contrast to the older metal baskets, which once secured on a stone would often kink and could not be reopened. Recently, Cordes and colleagues described a spring-actuated fixating nitinol stone basket, which allows for automatic stone grasping as well as the ability to disassemble the basket handle and remove the ureteroscope completely but still keep the stone in the basket. In addition, the basket incorporates a color-coded scale to measure stone size.[71] Still what remains most vexing is the inability of any stone basket to remove fragments smaller than 1 mm; hence even in the hands of the very best ureteroscopist, sand and dust remain in the kidney, serving as potential nidi for future stone formation, which remains the major drawback to ureteroscopy as indeed the stone-free rate fails to rival PCNL (≥90% stone-free rate).

Other means of stone fragment evacuation include attempts to aspirate stone fragments via the UAS or the ureteroscope itself. Zeng and colleagues described a modified UAS with a side port that would allow for suction to be applied in order to clear fragments during ureteroscopy (ie, ClearPetra System [Well Lead Medical Co, Guangzhou, China]). Zeng and colleagues used the ClearPetra UAS in 74 patients undergoing ureteroscopic stone removal; SFR (determined solely by abdominal radiographs) was uniquely high at 97%, the mean operative time was 27 minutes, and there were 3 (4%) postoperative complications.[72] Further studies, including postoperative computed tomography scans with 2 mm cuts to define SFR are needed to corroborate these encouraging results. A prior attempt at creating a suction and irrigation system was described in a case report by Cadeddu and Jarrett in 1998 in which a 10Fr Salem sump nasogastric tube was inserted coaxially over a guidewire under fluoroscopic guidance into the target calyx and stone fragments were blindly irrigated and aspirated.[73]

Aspiration via the flexible ureteroscope has also been attempted. An in vitro assessment of stone fragment suctioning via the working channel of the flexible ureteroscope demonstrated frequent clogging and required time-consuming clearance of the working channel. The investigators noted that suction was hampered by the size of the working channel as well as the angulation of the port as it exited the handle of the endoscope.[74] More recently, creative attempts to improve complete stone evacuation from the kidney have revolved around alteration of the stone fragments themselves to enhance their removal. In one iteration, Tracy and colleagues incubated calcium oxalate stones with iron-oxide microparticles that rendered the stones paramagnetic, thereby allowing for their extraction with a magnetic tool. Since the initial publication in 2010, there has been only one other in vitro study reported.[75] Other efforts at fragment entrapment and clearance have been based on the coagulum pyelolithotomy as pioneered by Dees for open stone surgery.[76] Cloutier and colleagues described the feasibility of using an autologous venous blood sample to create an in vivo blood clot (ie, "*glue-clot*") to instill into the renal collecting system as a means to agglutinate stone fragments for subsequent removal. Hein and colleagues subsequently developed a polysaccharide-based adhesive that could be delivered through the ureteroscope, which would form a blue gel at body temperature without adhering to the collecting system. In an ex vivo porcine model, the investigators noted 100% SFR as well as a reduction in stone retrieval time.[77] In their subsequent in vivo porcine model, they were able to remove 80% to 90% of stone fragments with their blue gel.[78] To date, there have been no clinical reports with this approach.

Advances in ureteroscope design

The most recent advance in ureteroscope design is the delivery of the Wolf Cobra ureteroscope, which provides the urologist with 2 lumens for the flow of irrigant and the passage of instrumentation. The working ports in the initial iteration were both 3.3Fr; however, in the most recent rendition the working ports are 2.4Fr and 3.6Fr, allowing for a dedicated laser port and a larger channel for the passage of stone baskets. In vitro studies have shown significant improvements in irrigant flow when using the second channel, including a 37-fold increase in flow with a 2.4Fr N-Compass basket (Cook Urologic, Spencer, IN) in place.[79,80] One drawback is that these endoscopes are slightly larger than other flexible ureteroscopes, having a shaft size of 9.9Fr.[81]

The other major shift in ureteroscope technology has been the move toward disposable ureteroscopes. Because of the fragile nature of reusable endoscopes and concerns over resterilization and decontamination, the market has now been flooded with myriad disposable ureteroscopes.[60] Studies comparing the technical aspects of disposable and reusable ureteroscopes have demonstrated that single-use ureteroscopes have comparable optical capabilities, deflection, and flow to the reusable ureteroscopes.[82,83]

Sadly, at this time, to the best of the investigators' knowledge, there have been no major advances in disposable ureteroscope design, despite the low threshold for rapid iteration of prototypes. In this regard, Karani and colleagues described the first female-specific ureteroscope that simply resulted from shortening the ureteroscope from its traditional 65 to 70 cm length (necessary for male ureteroscopy) to 45 cm, ideal for ureteroscopy in women. Not surprisingly, shortening the endoscope by 20 cm resulted in an average increase in flow rate by up to 17% when a stone basket was passed.[84]

It is the opinion of the investigators that with the advent of disposable flexible ureteroscopes, industry has the opportunity to develop endoscopes that would be "personalized." Similar to ureteral stents and ureteral access sheaths, the length and diameter of the ureteroscope used would depend on the gender of the patient and the size of the UAS deployed. In the latter case, a 16Fr UAS would allow passage of a 13Fr ureteroscope with perhaps multiple channels and a larger working channel for effective aspiration of stone sand/

dust. In sum, the surgeon could tailor the ureteroscope to the patient and procedure as opposed to the current one-size-fits-all armamentarium.

SUMMARY

Advances in our knowledge regarding ureteral physiology combined with technical developments applied to ureteral access sheath deployment and size, along with the advent of the thulium laser and better technology for fragment evacuation and newer ureteroscopes, may well propel retrograde intrarenal surgery to the forefront of kidney stone removal, regardless of stone size or location. As these abilities expand, PCNL will accordingly shrink until it, as with its open surgical predecessor, becomes part of the rich history of Urology. Primum non nocere.

CLINICS CARE POINTS

- For a urologist to become proficient in access requires a minimum case load of 2 to 5 PCNL cases/month.
- The use of ureteral access sheath is not associated with an increase in the rate of ureteral stricture after ureteroscopy.
- Kaler and colleagues found that significant ureteral injury while inserting an ureteral access sheath can be routinely avoided if the applied force is limited to less than 6 N of force.
- Prestenting allows for ureteral relaxation and accommodation of larger ureteral access sheaths, and this has been proved in a porcine model and further suggested by retrospective clinical studies.
- Superpulse thulium fiber laser allows for use of smaller laser fibers, more efficient energy transmission, lower pulse energies, higher frequencies, and smaller stone fragments (ie, dust).

DISCLOSURE

The authors have nothing to disclose.

REFERENCES

1. Patel SR, Nakada SY. The modern history and evolution of percutaneous nephrolithotomy. J Endourol 2015;29:153–7.
2. Fernström I, Johansson B. Percutaneous pyelolithotomy: a new extraction technique. Scand J Urol Nephrol 1976;10:257–9.
3. Yuhico MP, Ko R. The current status of percutaneous nephrolithotomy in the management of kidney stones. Minerva Urol Nefrol 2008;60:159–75.
4. Dasgupta P, Rose K, Wickham JEA. Percutaneous renal surgery: a pioneering perspective. J Endourol 2006;20:167–9.
5. Sampaio FJB, Zanier JFC, AragãO AHM, et al. Intrarenal access: 3-dimensional anatomical study. J Urol 1992;148:1769–73.
6. Metzler IS, Holt S, Harper JD. Surgical trends in nephrolithiasis: increasing *De Novo* renal access by urologists for percutaneous nephrolithotomy. J Endourol 2021;35:769–74.
7. Allen D, O'Brien T, Tiptaft R, et al. Defining the learning curve for percutaneous nephrolithotomy. J Endourol 2005;19:279–82.
8. Tanriverdi O, Boylu U, Kendirci M, et al. The learning curve in the training of percutaneous nephrolithotomy. Eur Urol 2007;52:206–12.
9. Usawachintachit M, Masic S, Allen IE, et al. Adopting ultrasound guidance for prone percutaneous nephrolithotomy: evaluating the learning curve for the experienced surgeon. J Endourol 2016;30:856–63.
10. Song Y, Ma Y, Song Y, et al. Evaluating the learning curve for percutaneous nephrolithotomy under total ultrasound guidance. Edited by RK Hills. PLoS One 2015;10:e0132986.
11. Khan F, Borin JF, Pearle MS, et al. Endoscopically guided percutaneous renal access: "Seeing Is Believing". J Endourol 2006;20:451–5.
12. Borofsky MS, Rivera ME, Dauw CA, et al. Electromagnetic guided percutaneous renal access outcomes among surgeons and trainees of different experience levels: a pilot study. Urology 2020;136:266–71.
13. de la Rosette J, Assimos D, Desai M, et al. The clinical research office of the endourological society percutaneous nephrolithotomy global study: indications, complications, and outcomes in 5803 patients. J Endourol 2011;25:11–7.
14. Michel MS, Trojan L, Rassweiler JJ. Complications in percutaneous nephrolithotomy. Eur Urol 2007;51:899–906.
15. Sharbaugh A, Morgan Nikonow T, Kunkel G, et al. Contemporary best practice in the management of staghorn calculi. Ther Adv Urol 2019;11. 175628721984709.
16. Lee W, Smith A, Cubelli V, et al. Complications of percutaneous nephrolithotomy. Am J Roentgenol 1987;148:177–80.
17. Shin TS, Cho HJ, Hong S-H, et al. Complications of percutaneous nephrolithotomy classified by the modified clavien grading system: a single center's experience over 16 years. Korean J Urol 2011;52:769.
18. Ganpule AP, Vijayakumar M, Malpani A, et al. Percutaneous nephrolithotomy (PCNL) a critical review. Int J Surg 2016;36:660–4.

19. Koras O, Bozkurt IH, Yonguc T, et al. Risk factors for postoperative infectious complications following percutaneous nephrolithotomy: a prospective clinical study. Urolithiasis 2015;43:55–60.
20. Tefekli A, Karadag MA, Tepeler K, et al. Classification of percutaneous nephrolithotomy complications using the modified clavien grading system: looking for a standard. Eur Urol 2008;53:184–90.
21. Agrawal MS, Agrawal M, Gupta A, et al. A randomized comparison of tubeless and standard percutaneous nephrolithotomy. J Endourology 2008;22:439–42.
22. Liatsikos E, Kapoor R, Lee B, et al. "Angular Percutaneous Renal Access". Multiple tracts through a single incision for staghorn calculous treatment in a single session. Eur Urol 2005;48:832–7.
23. Thapa BB, Niranjan V. Mini PCNL Over Standard PCNL: What Makes it Better? Surg J 2020;06:e19–23.
24. Labate G, Modi P, Timoney A, et al. The percutaneous nephrolithotomy global study: classification of complications. J Endourol 2011;25:1275–80.
25. Wagenius M, Borglin J, Popiolek M, et al. Percutaneous nephrolithotomy and modern aspects of complications and antibiotic treatment. Scand J Urol 2020;54:162–70.
26. Gadzhiev N, Malkhasyan V, Akopyan G, et al. Percutaneous nephrolithotomy for staghorn calculi: troubleshooting and managing complications. Asian J Urol 2020;7:139–48.
27. Reeves T, Pietropaolo A, Gadzhiev N, et al. Role of endourological procedures (PCNL and URS) on renal function: a systematic review. Curr Urol Rep 2020;21:21.
28. Wang M, Bukavina L, Mishra K, et al. Kidney volume loss following percutaneous nephrolithotomy utilizing 3D planimetry. Urolithiasis 2020;48:257–61.
29. Aguiar P, Pérez-Fentes D, Garrido M, et al. A method for estimating DMSA SPECT renal function for assessing the effect of percutaneous nephrolithotripsy on the treated pole. Q J Nucl Med Mol Imaging 2016;60:154–62.
30. Ünsal A, Koca G, Reşorlu B, et al. Effect of percutaneous nephrolithotomy and tract dilatation methods on renal function: assessment by quantitative single-photon emission computed tomography of technetium-99m–dimercaptosuccinic acid uptake by the kidneys. J Endourol 2010;24:1497–502.
31. Zhu W, Liu Y, Liu L, et al. Minimally invasive versus standard percutaneous nephrolithotomy: a meta-analysis. Urolithiasis 2015;43:563–70.
32. Ruhayel Y, Tepeler A, Dabestani S, et al. Tract sizes in miniaturized percutaneous nephrolithotomy: a systematic review from the european association of urology urolithiasis guidelines panel. Eur Urol 2017;72:220–35.
33. Ghani KR, Andonian S, Bultitude M, et al. Percutaneous nephrolithotomy: update, trends, and future directions. Eur Urol 2016;70:382–96.
34. Sabnis RB, Ganesamoni R, Doshi A, et al. Micropercutaneous nephrolithotomy (Microperc) vs retrograde intrarenal surgery for the management of small renal calculi: a randomized controlled trial: Microperc vs RIRS for small renal calculi. BJU Int 2013;112:355–61.
35. De S, Autorino R, Kim FJ, et al. Percutaneous nephrolithotomy versus retrograde intrarenal surgery: a systematic review and Meta-analysis. Eur Urol 2015;67:125–37.
36. Aldoukhi AH, Black KM, Ghani KR. Emerging Laser Techniques for the Management of Stones. Urol Clin North Am 2019;46:193–205.
37. Rehman J, Monga M, Landman J, et al. Characterization of intrapelvic pressure during ureteropyeloscopy with ureteral access sheaths. Urology 2003;61:713–8.
38. Breda A, Territo A, López-Martínez JM. Benefits and risks of ureteral access sheaths for retrograde renal access. Curr Opin Urol 2016;26:70–5.
39. Kourambas J, Byrne RR, Preminger GM. Does a ureteral access sheath facilitate ureteroscopy? J Urol 2001;165:789–93.
40. Wong VKF, Aminoltejari K, Almutairi K, et al. Controversies associated with ureteral access sheath placement during ureteroscopy. Investig Clin Urol 2020;61:455.
41. Huang J, Zhao Z, AlSmadi JK, et al. Use of the ureteral access sheath during ureteroscopy: a systematic review and meta-analysis. Edited by X Gao. PLoS One 2018;13:e0193600.
42. Fulla J, Prasanchaimontri P, Rizk A, et al. Ureteral diameter as predictor of ureteral injury during ureteral access sheath placement. J Urol 2021;205:159–64.
43. Loftus CJ, Ganesan V, Traxer O, et al. Ureteral wall injury with ureteral access sheaths: a randomized prospective trial. J Endourol 2020;34:932–6.
44. Traxer O, Thomas A. Prospective evaluation and classification of ureteral wall injuries resulting from insertion of a ureteral access sheath during retrograde intrarenal surgery. J Urol 2013;189:580–4.
45. Lildal SK, Sørensen FB, Andreassen KH, et al. Histopathological correlations to ureteral lesions visualized during ureteroscopy. World J Urol 2017;35:1489–96.
46. Delvecchio FC, Auge BK, Brizuela RM, et al. Assessment of stricture formation with the ureteral access sheath. Urology 2003;61:518–22.
47. Cooper JL, François N, Sourial MW, et al. The impact of ureteral access sheath use on the development of abnormal postoperative upper tract imaging after ureteroscopy. J Urol 2020;204:976–81.
48. Adiyat KT, Meuleners R, Monga M. Selective postoperative imaging after ureteroscopy. Urology 2009;73:490–3.
49. Sofer M, Watterson JD, Wollin TA, et al. Holmium: YAG laser lithotripsy for upper urinary tract calculi in 598 patients. J Urol 2002;167:31–4.

50. Weizer AZ, Auge BK, Silverstein AD, et al. Routine postoperative imaging is important after ureteroscopic stone manipulation. J Urol 2002;168:46–50.
51. de la Rosette J, Denstedt J, Geavlete P, et al. The clinical research office of the endourological society ureteroscopy global study: indications, complications, and outcomes in 11,885 patients. J Endourology 2014;28:131–9.
52. L'esperance JO, Ekeruo WO, Scales CD, et al. Effect of ureteral access sheath on stone-free rates in patients undergoing ureteroscopic management of renal calculi. Urology 2005;66:252–5.
53. Patel RM, Jefferson FA, Owyong M, et al. Characterization of intracalyceal pressure during ureteroscopy. World J Urol 2021;39:883–9.
54. Tracy CR, Ghareeb GM, Paul CJ, et al. Increasing the size of ureteral access sheath during retrograde intrarenal surgery improves surgical efficiency without increasing complications. World J Urol 2018;36:971–8.
55. Kaler KS, Lama DJ, Safiullah S, et al. Ureteral access sheath deployment: how much force is too much? Initial studies with a novel ureteral access sheath force sensor in the porcine ureter. J Endourol 2019;33:712–8.
56. Koo KC, Yoon J-H, Park N-C, et al. The impact of preoperative α-adrenergic antagonists on ureteral access sheath insertion force and the upper limit of force required to avoid ureteral mucosal injury: a randomized controlled study. J Urol 2018;199:1622–30.
57. Tapiero S, Kaler KS, Jiang P, et al. Determining the safety threshold for the passage of a ureteral access sheath in clinical practice using a purpose-built force sensor. J Urol 2021. https://doi.org/10.1097/JU.0000000000001719. JU.0000000000001719.
58. Ventimiglia E, Traxer O. What is moses effect: a historical perspective. J Endourology 2019;33:353–7.
59. Nazif OA, Teichman JMH, Glickman RD, et al. Review of laser fibers: a practical guide for urologists. J Endourol 2004;18:818–29.
60. Ibrahim A, Elhilali MM, Fahmy N, et al. Double-blinded prospective randomized clinical trial comparing regular and moses modes of holmium laser lithotripsy. J Endourol 2020;34:624–8.
61. Kronenberg P, Traxer O. The truth about laser fiber diameters. Urology 2014;84:1301–7.
62. Mues AC, Teichman JMH, Knudsen BE. Evaluation of 24 holmium:YAG laser optical fibers for flexible ureteroscopy. J Urol 2009;182:348–54.
63. Martov AG, Ergakov DV, Guseynov M, et al. Clinical comparison of super pulse thulium fiber laser and high-power holmium laser for ureteral stone management. J Endourol 2021;35:795–800.
64. Gao B, Bobrowski A, Lee J. A scoping review of the clinical efficacy and safety of the novel thulium fiber laser: the rising star of laser lithotripsy. Can Urol Assoc J 2021;15:56–66.
65. Andreeva V, Vinarov A, Yaroslavsky I, et al. Preclinical comparison of superpulse thulium fiber laser and a holmium:YAG laser for lithotripsy. World J Urol 2020;38:497–503.
66. Blackmon RL, Irby PB, Fried NM. Holmium:YAG (λ = 2,120 nm) versus Thulium Fiber (λ = 1,908 nm) Laser Lithotripsy. Lasers Surg Med 2010;42:232–6.
67. Chiron* P, Berthe L, Haddad M, et al. PD59-06 In vitro comparison of efficiency between superpulsed thulium fiber laser and Ho:YAG laser for endocorporeal lithotripsy. J Urol 2019;201:e1093.
68. Okhunov Z, Jiang P, Afyouni AS, et al. Caveat Emptor: The Heat Is "ON": An in vivo evaluation of the thulium fiber laser and temperature changes in the porcine kidney during dusting and fragmentation modes. J Endourol 2021. end.2021.0206.
69. Morton WP. A new ureteral stone basket. J Urol 1948;60:242–3.
70. Khaleel SS, Borofsky MS. Innovations in disposable technologies for stone management. Urol Clin North Am 2019;46:175–84.
71. Cordes J, Nguyen F, Pinkowski W, et al. A new automatically fixating stone basket (2.5 F) Prototype with a nitinol spring for accurate ureteroscopic stone size measurement. Adv Ther 2018;35:1420–5.
72. Zeng G, Wang D, Zhang T, et al. Modified access sheath for continuous flow ureteroscopic lithotripsy: a preliminary report of a novel concept and technique. J Endourol 2016;30:992–6.
73. Cadeddu JA, Jarrett T. Use of a nasogastric tube to evacuate stone debris after ureteroscopic holmium lithotripsy. Urology 1998;52:882–4.
74. Schneider D, Abedi G, Larson K, et al. In vitro evaluation of stone fragment evacuation by suction. J Endourol 2021;35:187–91.
75. Tan YK, Pearle MS, Cadeddu JA. Rendering stone fragments paramagnetic with iron-oxide microparticles to improve the efficiency of endoscopic stone fragment retrieval. Curr Opin Urol 2012;22:144–7.
76. Dees JE. The use of a fibrinogen coagulum in pyelolithotomy. J Urol 1946;56:271–83.
77. Hein S, Schoenthaler M, Wilhelm K, et al. Novel biocompatible adhesive for intrarenal embedding and endoscopic removal of small residual fragments after minimally invasive stone treatment in an ex vivo porcine kidney model: initial evaluation of a prototype. J Urol 2016;196:1772–7.
78. Hein S, Schoeb DS, Grunwald I, et al. Viability and biocompatibility of an adhesive system for intrarenal embedding and endoscopic removal of small residual fragments in minimally-invasive stone treatment in an in vivo pig model. World J Urol 2018;36:673–80.
79. Bach T, Netsch C, Herrmann TRW, et al. Objective assessment of working tool impact on irrigation

flow and visibility in flexible ureterorenoscopes. J Endourol 2011;25:1125–9.
80. Haberman K, Ortiz-Alvarado O, Chotikawanich E, et al. A dual-channel flexible ureteroscope: evaluation of deflection, flow, illumination, and optics. J Endourol 2011;25:1411–4.
81. Lusch A, Okhunov Z, del Junco M, et al. Comparison of optics and performance of single channel and a novel dual-channel fiberoptic ureteroscope. Urology 2015;85:268–72.
82. Dale J, Kaplan AG, Radvak D, et al. Evaluation of a novel single-use flexible ureteroscope. J Endourol 2021;35:903–7.
83. Scotland KB, Chan JYH, Chew BH. Single-use flexible ureteroscopes: how do they compare with reusable ureteroscopes? J Endourology 2019;33:71–8.
84. Karani R, Arada RB, Ayad M, et al. Evaluation of a novel female gender flexible ureteroscope: comparison of flow and deflection to a standard flexible ureteroscope. J Endourol 2021;35:840–6.

Evolution of Focal Therapy in Prostate Cancer

Past, Present, and Future

Rohith Arcot, MD*, Thomas J. Polascik, MD

KEYWORDS

• Prostate cancer • Localize • Focal therapy • Nomenclature • Ablation

KEY POINTS

- The evolution of patient selection for FT has migrated from men with GGG 1 to GGG $\geq$ 2 PCa, but may have limited value in high-risk disease.
- Presently, mpMRI/US fusion biopsy systems have replaced traditional TRUS biopsy to identify biopsy-concordant lesions suspicious of cancer on mpMRI and provide a roadmap for the pattern of ablation.
- Despite IFF being occasionally identified, retreatment with FT may prevent transition to radical treatment, but the functional implications of FT retreatment are still not well described.
- The future of patient selection for FT will rely on advanced imaging that improves NPV for GGG $\geq$ 2 PCa.
- Uniform definitions, data collection, and standardized FT outcome metrics demonstrating favorable long-term functional and oncologic outcomes will be paramount to support FT adoption in the community.

INTRODUCTION

Since the late 1980s, the widespread use of prostate-specific antigen (PSA) screening has led to the increased detection of prostate cancer (PCa) with low malignant potential.[1,2] This rise in low-grade and early-stage disease has been met with a rise in the use of radiation therapy and radical prostatectomy (RP). Despite effective oncologic outcomes, whole gland (WG) treatments can result in considerable patient morbidity attributed to erectile dysfunction and urinary incontinence.[3–5] These findings coupled with longitudinal outcomes highlighting the limited mortality of observation in low-risk cohorts has called into question the timing and need for WG treatment in patients thought to harbor otherwise indolent disease[6,7]

To rectify inadvertent overtreatment in some and potential undertreatment in others, urologists have sought new avenues in the form of active surveillance (AS) and minimally invasive, focal ablative therapies to manage low and intermediate-risk, localized PCa.[8,9] The goal of focal therapy (FT) is to improve functional outcomes without sacrificing oncologic control afforded by WG treatment or lost with AS.

The earliest description of FT for PCa is credited to Gary Onik in 2002 when he described the use of hemigland cryoablation, later coining the term the "male lumpectomy."[10,11] Since that time, the evolution of FT from past to present for the management of clinically localized PCa has followed the technological advancements that have improved the reliable detection and ablation of PCa. Herein, we present a historical perspective on patient

Funding: None.

Division of Urology, Duke University Medical Center, Duke University, Duke Cancer Center, 20 Duke Medicine Circle, Durham, NC 27710, USA
* Corresponding author.
E-mail address: rohith.arcot@duke.edu

Urol Clin N Am 49 (2022) 129–152
https://doi.org/10.1016/j.ucl.2021.07.011

selection, ablation approach, and follow-up that have evolved over the last two decades.

INITIAL YEARS

The initial foray into FT of PCa relied on anatomic boundaries to construct regional patterns of ablation (eg, hemigland ablation) as described by Onik and colleagues.[10] Patient selection followed and was largely limited to those with unilaterally detected PCa, and specifically targeting low-risk disease in whom ablation would have the lowest risk of long-term progression.

Pathologic Basis for Focal Therapy

Unilateral and unifocal cancer

The basis for the application of FT to a region of the prostate stemmed from RP cohorts highlighting the stage migration of PCa in the PSA era toward the diagnosis of more small volume, unifocal and/or unilateral disease. Considered contemporary at the time, retrospective RP studies have shown unifocal PCa to be present in 13% to 38% and unilateral PCa in 19% to 63% of RP specimens.[12–15] Furthermore, over a 20-year period, Stamey and colleagues found the mean volume of the largest foci of cancer to decrease in size from 5.3 cc to 2.4 cc.[16] In a separate study examining the frequency of unilateral cancers across PSA eras, Polascik and colleagues had identified an increase in the proportion of patients diagnosed with pT2a disease from 2.8% in 1988 to 1995 to 13% in 2001 to 2006.[17] These findings highlight a select group of patients who, if identified, could potentially be managed by an organ-sparing approach.

Index lesion

Although the majority of PCa is multifocal, proponents of FT have cited studies concluding the index lesion drives the biology of disease. The index lesion is often considered the largest, highest grade tumor, and/or the tumor with extraprostatic extension (EPE), whereas secondary lesions comprise the converse.[18] In multiple RP series, most patients harbor multifocal disease, but in these same studies, secondary lesions were very small (average 0.3–0.63 cm^3) and potentially insignificant.[12,19,20] When comparing patients with multifocal PCa consisting of secondary lesions greater than 0.5 cc (group 1) and less than 0.5 cc (group 2), Noguchi and colleagues found that secondary lesions less than 0.5 cc had little impact on PSA failure after RP.[21] Finally, investigators claim 80% of the total tumor volume within the prostate could be eradicated with ablation of the index tumor, and that 92% of lesions with EPE are derived from the index lesion.[12,19] Although the pathologic processing has varied among these studies, together they suggest that in select patients with localized disease, the ablation of the index lesion, if identified, could provide oncologic control similar to WG treatment.

Patient Selection

Diagnostic approach

Before the advent of multiparametric MRI (mpMRI) of the prostate, accurately identifying patients with an index lesion, or even unifocal or unilateral cancer, remained a challenge. Clinicians have been limited to the regional localization of unifocal and unilateral PCa by transrectal ultrasound (TRUS)-guided biopsy and transperineal mapping biopsy (TMB). However, at the time of many early ablation series, consensus did not yet exist as to the number of cores necessary, nor which biopsy method was best to select suitable FT candidates. The sextant and standard 10 to 12 core TRUS biopsy is associated with a sampling error of 10% to 30% when compared with WG pathology.[22,23] When examining an RP cohort, Tsivian and colleagues showed that extended TRUS (10–20 core) when compared with standard TRUS (6–9 cores) biopsy improved specificity for predicting unilateral cancer from 37.1% to 53.9%, but overall specificity remained low.[24] These authors concluded that a 12-core biopsy was not the ideal diagnostic test to select FT candidates. To overcome the limitations of TRUS biopsy, clinicians explored the use of TMB described by Barzell and Melamed in 2007 using a transperineal 5-mm biopsy grid. In a study of 80 patients, TRUS biopsy had a false negative rate of 47%, and 54% of patients deemed suitable for FT were unsuitable by TMB.[25] Using an autopsy study, Crawford and colleagues found that 5 mm spacing using computer modeling improved the detection of all cancer and provided 95% sensitivity and negative predictive value (NPV) for the detection of clinically significant cancer compared to whole-mount pathology.[26] Though early FT series relied on extended TRUS biopsy for localization, later studies converted to TMB to improve the detection of unilateral disease that could be completely eradicated using FT.

Approach to Ablation

Ablation energy source

Although many ablative technologies currently exist for the destruction of prostate tissue, early studies primarily incorporated cryoablation (CRYO) and high-intensity focused ultrasound (HIFU). A list of commonly used ablative technologies and their mechanism of action is described in **Table 1**.[27–30]

Early focal ablation series

As described in **Table 2**, many of the early FT series made use of various biopsy techniques and inclusion criteria. Altogether, the goal of ablation was eradication of all known PCa using anatomic boundaries for the pattern of ablation: hemigland, dog-leg (for example, $^{3}/_{4}$ gland ablation), and subtotal. Most patients included in the early series had been D'Amico low and intermediate-risk candidates.[31]

Metastasis-free survival (MFS) and cancer-specific survival (CSS) after short follow-up was nearly 100% in all studies. Functional outcomes defined by pad-free continence was greater than 93% in all studies, and erectile function, defined by ability to achieve erection sufficient for penetration, was preserved in greater than 70% of patients ± phosphodiesterase type 5 inhibitor (PDE5I) use. Overall, functional outcomes were better with FT compared with traditional WG treatment[3–5] (see **Table 2**).

Follow-up Postablation

Early FT series lacks uniformity in postablation follow-up protocols because no long-term follow-up data had existed to set precedent, and consensus opinion did not exist. Nevertheless, most agreed at the time that patients should be followed with AS protocols and undergo pre-protocol follow-up biopsy. Onik and colleagues reported a negative biopsy result in 6 of 9 patients who had follow-up data.[11] Ellis and colleagues reported that only 35 of 60 patients underwent post-treatment biopsy of whom 14 of 35 patients (40%) were positive for any cancer, but only 1 from the treated lobe.[32] Bahn and colleagues reported that 48 of 70 patients (69%) had follow-up biopsy per protocol or due to rising PSA, that was positive in 12 of 48 patients (25%)—1 in the treated lobe and 11 in the untreated lobe.[33] Muto and colleagues describe per-protocol biopsies being negative in 76.5% at 12 months.[34] Ahmed and colleagues state per-protocol biopsy had only been performed of the ablation site at 6 months and completed in 39 of 41 patients (95%) of whom 9 of 39 (23%) had evidence of cancer with 3 of 39 (8%) having clinically significant cancer[35] (see **Table 2**). Together, these early FT studies support the potential for short-term cancer control within the treatment zone.

PRESENT

Men most suitable for FT primarily include National Comprehensive Cancer Network (NCCN) intermediate-risk, some localized higher volume low-risk, and targetable higher risk lesions, the latter of whom are recommended to be treated under protocol or clinical trial.[36] The identification of candidates now relies on improved diagnostic modalities, mpMRI, and ultrasound (US) fusion biopsy platforms, affording clinicians the ability to visualize, accurately diagnose, and plan image-targeted ablation. Until long-term follow-up data become available, the current basis for patient selection, ablation approach, and surveillance following FT continue to be based on consensus opinion from several international multidisciplinary consensus committees using the modified Delphi method along with short-term to mid-term published outcome data.

Patient Selection

Early in the development of FT, patients with low Gleason grade PCa were felt to benefit the least from WG treatment and most from an organ-sparing approach.[6,37] However, in 2015, Klotz and colleagues and Tosoian and colleagues published on the safety of AS in NCCN low-risk and very-low patients showing the CSS to be 98.1% and 99.9% at 10 years, respectively.[38,39] In the same year, Donaldson and colleagues reported from a consensus meeting that offering FT to men with well-characterized low-risk PCa may represent overtreatment.[40] In these same AS cohorts, at greater than 10 years of follow-up, at least 50% of men on AS transitioned to active treatment due to disease progression, reclassification, or anxiety. Regardless of the reason, in a recent interdisciplinary consensus conference, Tan and colleagues noted that experts in the field of FT believe that an organ-sparing approach might be appropriate for those discontinuing AS for a solitary focus of Gleason 3 + 4 cancer as an alternative to WG treatment.[41]

As familiarity with AS grows, attempts have been made to expand the inclusion criteria to men with NCCN low volume, intermediate-risk cancer. However, studies have continually suggested that this strategy results in higher rates of adverse pathology at delayed RP, biochemical recurrence, eventual metastasis, and decreased overall survival.[42–44] Thus, the potential role of FT may find itself uniquely positioned to provide patients, who fall just outside the eligibility for AS, the opportunity to enter an AS protocol after successful ablation of their intermediate-risk disease.

Based on consensus opinion, the position of FT within the treatment spectrum of localized PCa continues to shift away from NCCN and/or D'Amico low-risk PCa. The "ideal" candidate likely represents an individual with greater than 10 years

Table 1
Ablation energy sources[27–30]

Therapy	Ablation Energy	Mechanism of Cell Death	Approach	Intraoperative Monitoring	Advantages	Disadvantages
CRYO	Freezing/mechanical	Cell membrane rupture, biochemical changes, ischemia, apoptosis	Transperineal	TRUS, CT, MRI, thermocouples	Familiar approach, real-time TRUS monitoring of ablation zone	Limited precision
HIFU	Heat/mechanical	Coagulative necrosis at the focal point of transducer, acoustic cavitation	Transrectal	TRUS	Least invasive, precise ablation zone	Ablation limited by device focal length, limited ability to target anterior tumors
FLA	Heat	Coagulative necrosis	Transperineal	MRI-thermometry	Potentially office-based procedure	Requires precise overlapping of treatment zones
IRE	Electrical/mechanical	Short pulses of direct electrical current cause pores in cell membranes = irreversible cell death	Transperineal	MRI, TRUS	Ability to destroy tumors near vital structures with limited collateral damage	No long-term follow-up data
VTP	Nonthermal; vascular targeting	Interaction between light, photosensitizer, and oxygen; ROS lead to apoptosis, destruction of tumor vasculature inflammatory response	Transperineal	TRUS	Photosensitizer preferentially accumulates in malignant cells; level 1 evidence	Oxygen and photosensitizer dependent; lack of reliable treatment planning

Abbreviations: CT, computed tomography; FLA, focal-laser ablation; IRE, irreversible electroporation; ROS, reactive oxygen species; VTP, vascular-targeted photodynamic therapy.

Data from Gardner TA, Koch MO. Prostate cancer therapy with high-intensity focused ultrasound. Clin Genitourin Cancer. 2005;4(3):187-192; and Ganzer R, Arthanareeswaran VKA, Ahmed HU, et al. Which technology to select for primary focal treatment of prostate cancer?-European Section of Urotechnology (ESUT) position statement. Prostate Cancer Prostatic Dis. 2018;21(2):175-186; and Bozzini G, Colin P, Nevoux P, Villers A, Mordon S, Betrouni N. Focal therapy of prostate cancer: energies and procedures. Urol Oncol. 2013;31(2):155-167; and Lodeizen O, de Bruin M, Eggener S, et al. Ablation energies for focal treatment of prostate cancer. World J Urol. 2019;37(3):409-418.

Table 2
Early focal therapy series

Reference	Design	N	Biopsy Type	Inclusion	Median Follow-up	Ablation Template	D'Amico Risk Group	Metastasis-Free Survival	Cancer-Specific Survival	Urinary Continence	Erectile Function	Biopsy Outcomes Postablation
CRYO												
Onik,[11] 2004	R	9	TRUS, repeat biopsy on negative lobe	Cancer confined to one lobe	3 y	Hemiablation or Subtotal	Low: 66% Intermediate: 22% High: 11%	100%	100%	100%	78%	6 patients had biopsy and all negative
Ellis et al,[32] 2007	R	60	Unknown	Localized cancer by biopsy, T1-T3	1.36 y	Dog-leg	Low: 66% Intermediate: 23.5% High: 10%	100%	100%	93.4%	70.6%	Positive biopsy rate 23.3% at 1 y
Bahn et al,[33] 2012	R	73	TRUS sextant w/single core of any lesion visible on TRUS	Unilateral, low-intermediate risk cancer	3.7 y	Hemiablation	Low: 33% Intermediate: 67%	100%	100%	100%	88.9%	Positive biopsy in 12/48 (25%)
HIFU												
Muto et al,[34] 2008	P	29	TRUS extended (>12 core)	Biopsy or MRI proven localized disease	~2 y	Dog-leg	Low: 55.2 Intermediate: 20.7 High 17.2	NR	100%	94%	NR	Biopsy positive rate at 12 mo—23.5%

(*continued on next page*)

Table 2
(continued)

Reference	Design	N	Biopsy Type	Inclusion	Median Follow-up	Ablation Template	D'Amico Risk Group	Metastasis-Free Survival	Cancer-Specific Survival	Urinary Continence	Erectile Function	Biopsy Outcomes Postablation
Ahmed et al,[35] 2012	P	41	TMB	Localized disease after biopsy and MRI	1 y	Focal operator dependent	*NCCN* risk Low: 27% Intermediate: 63% High: 10%	100%	100%	100%	89% 9% use of PDE5I	Biopsy positive for any cancer 9/39 (23%) Biopsy positive for GGG $\geq$ 2 3/39 (8%)

Abbreviations: "Dog-leg" = ¾ gland ablation; NR, not recorded; P, prospective; PDE5I, phosphodiesterase-five inhibitor; R, retrospective; TMB, transperineal-mapping biopsy.

life-expectancy, a single or multiple well-delineated mpMRI-visible, biopsy-proven Gleason 3 + 4 cancer(s) in a location(s) amenable to ablation with a treatment margin not likely to injury the neurovascular bundle, urethra, or sphincter. What continues to remain unknown is if there is a limit to the volume of Gleason 3 + 3 PCa that can remain untreated at the time of FT. The evolution of patient selection for FT is described in **Table 3**.[40,41,45–48]

Diagnostic Approach

Today, the identification of men with NCCN intermediate-risk PCa suitable for FT relies on commercially available mpMRI/US fusion biopsy platforms that not only allow image-targeted biopsy but also creates a similar pathway to perform image-targeted PCa ablation. Although the first MRI of the prostate was described in 1982, it was not until the early 2000s that mpMRI combined multiple imaging sequences—T1-weighted and T2-weighted, diffusion-weighted imaging, dynamic contrast enhancement (DCE)—that would be described for the localization of PCa.[49,50] The ability to visualize lesions steered the development of targeted biopsy techniques that used image coregistration software to integrate the mpMRI image with real-time US for image-guided mpMRI/US fusion prostate biopsy.[51] In 2011, Pinto and colleagues were one of the first to show the increased cancer detection rates with a targeted biopsy approach using a fusion-biopsy system when compared with standard 12-core TRUS.[52] In 2015, Siddiqui and colleagues showed that targeted mpMRI/US fusion biopsy when compared with TRUS biopsy preferentially increased the detection of high-risk (Gleason $\geq$ 4 + 3) over low-risk (Gleason 3 + 3, low volume Gleason 3 + 4) cancers with improved sensitivity (77% vs 53%) for the detection of intermediate (Gleason 3 + 4 with >50% core involvement) and high-risk cancers at RP.[53] Two clinical trials supported these results. The PROMIS trial showed that mpMRI had improved sensitivity to detect Gleason $\geq$ 3 + 4 cancer (87% vs 60%) compared to TRUS biopsy (TMB as the reference standard).[54] The PRECISION trial showed targeted biopsy alone preferentially increases the detection of Gleason $\geq$ 3 + 4 cancer when compared to TRUS biopsy alone.[55] Despite the ability of targeted biopsy to increase the detection of Gleason $\geq$ 3 + 4 cancer over standard TRUS biopsy, mpMRI has several limitations most important of which include the underestimation of lesion size at final pathology by up to 10 mm and understaging since mpMRI may miss anywhere from 5% to 28% of "invisible" Gleason $\geq$ 3 + 4 cancers.[56–58] At present, the selection of FT candidates should include either mpMRI/US fusion targeted biopsy plus 12 systematic cores or TMB before FT planning (see **Table 3**).

Ablation Approach

Ablation energy source

Over the last decade, the armamentarium for personalized FT treatment planning has grown. The most recent clinical trials have included a number of technologies listed in **Table 1**.[27–30] At present, no one modality has superior oncologic outcomes, each with its own limitations, and each is chosen based on clinician familiarity, cost/reimbursement, and individual patient tumor characteristics.[40,59]

Definition of Focal Ablation

As the number of FT series for localized PCa grows, there is an increasing need to standardize the definition of FT. In the most recent multidisciplinary consensus conference, Lebtaschi and colleagues report that FT is meant to describe image-guided ablation of image-defined, biopsy-concordant, cancerous lesions with a safety margin (up to 10 mm). Furthermore, all biopsy-concordant MRI-visible lesions of Gleason grade group (GGG) $\geq$ 2 should be targeted for FT. For lesions that are not image-identified and whose destruction by an ablation pattern relies on anatomic boundaries to provide an organ-sparing approach, the descriptive term should be partial gland ablation (PGA)[48] (**Fig. 1**).

Present Focal Ablation Series

Although several thermal and nonthermal ablative technologies are available, CRYO and HIFU still remain the most well-studied therapeutic modalities for FT. Over the last decade, several single-arm FT series have reported short-term and medium-term follow-up showing greater than 98% MFS and greater than 99% CSS. Among these series, the efficacy of FT has most commonly been defined by failure-free survival (FFS)—defined as freedom from transition to WG, systemic therapy, metastasis, cancer-specific mortality—or treatment-free survival (TFS) defined by transition to WG, RP, or radiation. Overall, the rate of FFS ranges from 85% to 96.8% and TFS as reported in one study was 81%. Subgroup analysis showed FFS tends to be worse in those with D'Amico high-risk compared with intermediate-risk disease, suggesting patient selection be limited to the latter

Table 3
Evolution of patient selection

Date	2010	2014	2015	2017	2021
Lead Author	de la Rosette[45]	van den Bos[46]	Donaldson[40]	Tay[47]	Tan[41]
Goal of FT	Eradication of all known cancer	Eradication of clinically significant disease (tumor >0.5 mL)	Eradication of dominant or index lesion	Eradication of cancer by targeted, quadrant or hemiablation	Eradication of surveillance biopsy-proven disease progression
D'Amico Risk Group	Low to intermediate risk	Low to intermediate risk	Intermediate	Intermediate	NR
Diagnostic Approach	Ideally TMB	mpMRI/TRUS fusion biopsy + systematic biopsy	mpMRI/TRUS fusion biopsy + systematic or TMB when mpMRI unavailable	mpMRI/US fusion + systematic biopsy or No agreement on type of biopsy to use if mpMRI unavailable	mpMRI/TRUS fusion + systematic biopsy or TMB when mpMRI unavailable
Disease factors	Unilateral disease; GGG1 Low vol. GGG 2 Clinical $\leq$ T2a Radiographic $\leq$ T2b	PSA < 15 GGG 1 GGG 2 T1c-T2a	Ideally GGG 2 Not GGG 1 No max lesion size	PSA $\leq$ 10 Ideally GGG 2 Max GGG 3 Lesion vol 1.5 mL or 3 mL if considering hemigland ablation	Localized, unifocal PSA < 10 GGG 2
Residual Disease Permissible	No measurable disease allowed	NR	3 + 3 up to 5 mm	3 + 3 up to 1 mm	NR

Abbreviations: GGG, Gleason grade group; mpMRI, multiparametric MRI; NR, not recorded; TMB, transperineal-mapping biopsy; vol., volume.

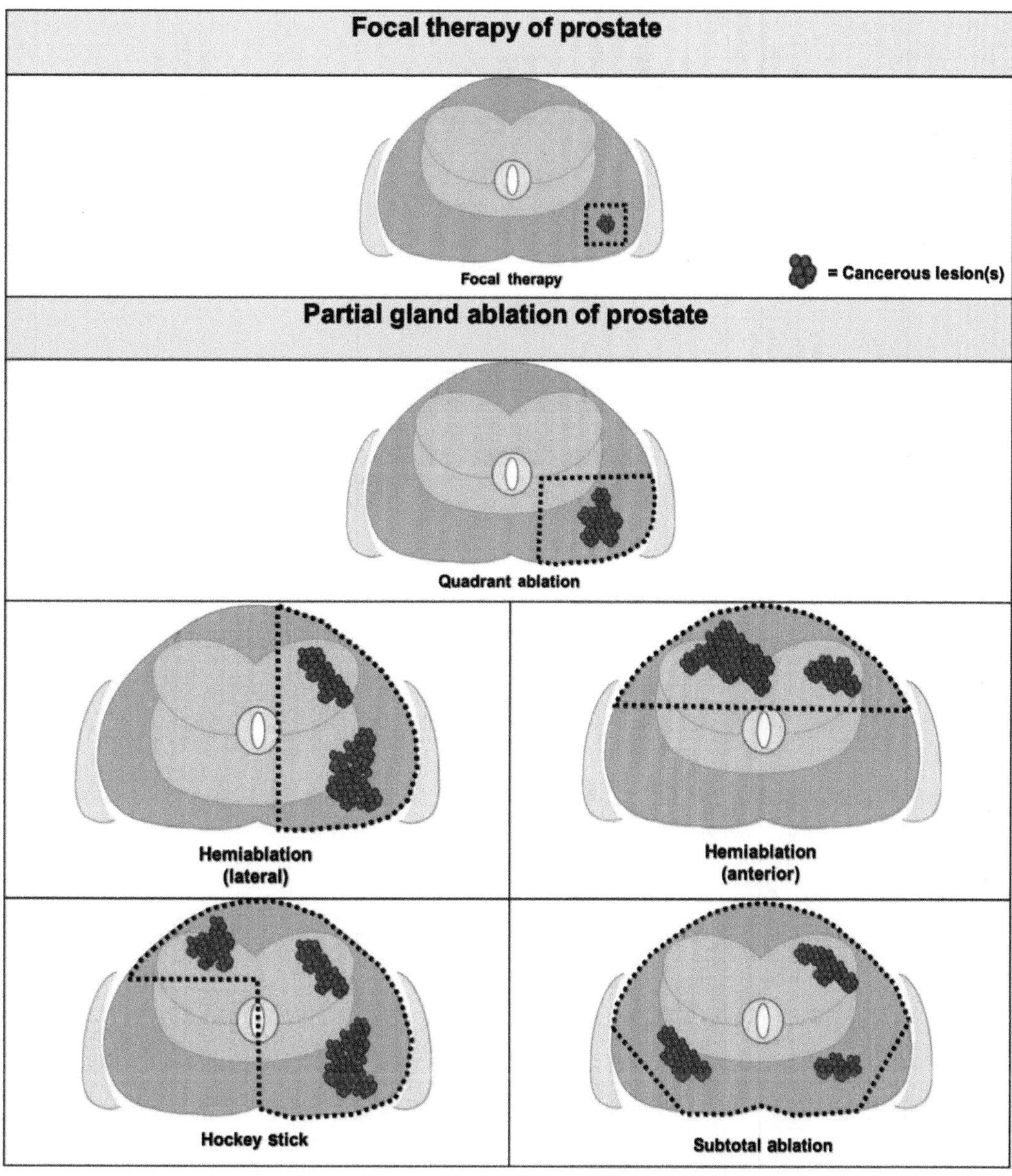

Fig. 1. Focal therapy versus partial gland ablative procedures. Graphics demonstrating distinction between focal therapy and templated organ-preserving partial gland ablations. Focal therapy: image-guided focused ablation of image-visible, biopsy-confirmed malignant lesion(s) plus an adequate safety margin. Quadrant ablation: destruction of all prostate tissue within a quadrant of the prostate. Hemiablation: destruction of all prostate tissue within a lateralized hemisphere of the prostate or the anterior half of the prostate. Hockey stick: destruction of all prostate tissue within a lateralized hemisphere plus anterior contralateral region. Subtotal ablation: destruction of most of the prostate tissue with preservation of a posterior lateral region (unilaterally or bilaterally). The goal intended is to preserve at least one neurovascular bundle during ablation. (*From* Lebastchi AH, George AK, Polascik TJ, et al. Standardized Nomenclature and Surveillance Methodologies After Focal Therapy and Partial Gland Ablation for Localized Prostate Cancer: An International Multidisciplinary Consensus. Eur Urol. 2020;78(3):371-378; with permission.)

group. Functional outcomes remain excellent across series with pad-free continence of 97% to 100% and preserved erectile function in 76% to 100%. The oncologic and functional outcomes for the aforementioned trials are summarized in **Table 4**.[60–65]

In a randomized controlled trial (RCT) evaluating FT, Azzouzi and colleagues allocated 413 men

Table 4
Present focal therapy series

Reference	Design	n	Biopsy Type	Inclusion/ Exclusion	Median Follow-up	Ablation Plan	Risk Group	Metastasis-Free Survival	Cancer-Specific Survival	Urinary Continence (Pad Free)	Erectile Function (Persevered)	Primary Outcome
CRYO												
Shah et al,[60] 2019	P	122	mpMRI/ TRUS fusion targeted + syste-matic or TMB	Concordant MRI lesion and site of biopsy; T2a-T3a Median PSA: 10.8 GGG 1 $\geq$ 6 mm GGG 2 GGG 3 Excluded: Lesion abutting the sphincter	2.31 y	Anterior only (65.6%) Anterior/ Posterior (19.7%) Posterior only (1.6%) Missing (13%)	*NCCN* Intermediate: 71% High: 28.7%	98% at 3 y	100% at 3 y	100%	83.8%	FFS at 3 y Overall: 90.5% Inter-mediate-risk: 93.3% High-risk: 84.7%
Oishi et al,[61] 2019	R	160	Unknown	Unilateral disease; no GGG or PSA restrictions; bilateral low volume disease (GGG 2 or less) 29 patients received ADT before FT	3.3 y	Hemi-ablation	*D'Amico* Low: 18% Intermediate: 66% High: 16%	100% at 5 y	100% at 5 y	97%	73%	FFS at 5 y Overall: 85% Low-risk: 95% Inter-mediate-risk: 83% High-risk: 78%

HIFU												
Guillaumier et al,[62] 2018	P	625	mpMRI/TRUS fusion targeted + systematic or TMB	Concordant MRI lesion and site of biopsy; T1c-T3b PSA ≤30 GGG 1 > 4 mm GGG 2–5	4.6 y	Hemi-ablation or Wide-local ablation	*D'Amico* Low: 13% Intermediate: 53% High: 32%	98% at 5 y	100% at 5 y	98%	NR	FFS at 5 y Overall: 88% Low-risk: 96% Inter-mediate-risk: 88% High-risk: 84%
Stabile et al,[63] 2019	P	1032	mpMRI/TRUS fusion targeted + systematic or TMB	Concordant MRI lesion and site of biopsy; T1-T3 No PSA restriction GGG 1–4	3 y	Hemi-ablation or Ablation of index lesion	*Gleason score* 3 + 3: 19.7% 3 + 4: 63.4% 4 + 3: 15.4% 4 + 4: 1.6%	NR	NR	NR	NR	TFS at 8 y Overall: 81% Freedom from biopsy failure (GGG ≥2) at 8 y: 54% OS at 8 y: 97%
FLA												
Chao et al,[64] 2018	P	34	Unknown	Concordant MRI lesion and site of biopsy; T1c or T2a PSA <10 GGG < 4	2 y	Focal ablation	*Gleason score* 3 + 3: 47% 3 + 4: 47% 4 + 3: 6%	NR	NR	100%	No significant change in SHIM at 3 mo	FFS NR 53% post-FT recurrence GGG 1 or GGG 2 Biopsy failure (GGG >2): 28%

(*continued on next page*)

Table 4
(*continued*)

Reference	Design	n	Biopsy Type	Inclusion/ Exclusion	Median Follow-up	Ablation Plan	Risk Group	Metastasis-Free Survival	Cancer-Specific Survival	Urinary Continence (Pad Free)	Erectile Function (Persevered)	Primary Outcome
IRE												
Blazevski et al,[65] 2019	P	123	mpMRI/ TRUS fusion targeted + systematic or TMB	Concordant MRI lesion and site of biopsy; No T stage listed PSA <15 GGG 1 >4 mm GGG 2 GGG 3	3 y	Focal ablation	*G score* 3 + 3: 10% 3 + 4: 71% 4 + 3: 19% *D'Amico* Low 9% Intermediate 91%	98.5% at 3 y	100% at 3 y	98.8%	76% no change in potency	FFS at 3 y Overall: 96.8%
VTP												
Azzouzi et al,[66] 2017 Gill et al,[67] 2018	RCT	413 AS: 207 VTP: 206	TRUS biopsy	Low risk, localized cancer Gleason 3 + 3 T1a-T2a PSA ≤ 10	2 y	Focal ablation	*D'Amico* Low 100%	AS: 99% at 4 y VTP: 99% at 4 y	100% at 4 y	99%	AS 89% VTP: 62%	TF at 24 mo AS: 58% VTP: 28% Negative Bx at 24 mo AS: 14% VTP: 49% Conversion to radical treatment: AS: 53% at 4 y VTP: 24% at 4 y

FFS: absence of need to transition to radical, whole gland, systemic therapy, metastasis, or prostate cancer morality.
TFS: absence of need for whole gland treatment, radical prostatectomy, or radiation.
Treatment failure (TF) histologic progression of cancer from low to moderate or high risk or prostate cancer-related death at 24 mo.
Abbreviations: Bx, biopsy; FLA, focal-laser ablation; IRE, irreversible electroporation; mpMRI, multiparametric MRI; NR, not recorded; P, prospective; R, retrospective.

with Gleason 3 + 3 PCa to AS (206) or FT (207) using vascular-targeted photodynamic (VTP) therapy to compare treatment failure defined by biopsy progression from low to moderate or high-risk cancer and the absence of definitive cancer therapy at 24 months (see **Table 4**). The VTP group had a lower rate of progression on follow-up biopsy (28% vs 59%, *P* <.0001) and a higher rate of negative biopsy compared with AS (49% vs 14%, *P* <.0001).[66] With extended follow-up at 4 years, Gill and colleagues reported conversion to radical treatment was 53% in the AS arm versus 24% for VTP. The authors suggest the utility of VTP compared to AS is evident by the limited conversion to radical treatment. However, VTP was associated with increased treatment morbidity compared with AS regarding erectile function (37% vs 11%).[66,67]

One advantage of FT over WG is the ability to retreat areas of persistence within the ablation zone deemed in-field failure (IFF) or to areas of de novo cancer termed out-of-field failure (OFF) on follow-up biopsy, the later representing patient selection failure in contrast to true ablation failure. The most current consensus opinion defines IFF or OFF as any biopsy-proven GGG $\geq$ 2, and experts agree that if amenable, these can be managed with repeat ablation, respectively.[48,68] Among the present trials, IFF and OFF were not always reported or accurately defined and retreatment of these failures with FT ranged from 6% to 20% when recorded.[60–66] Though biopsy-proven recurrence of any GGG $\geq$ 2 ranged from ~16 to 60% among the present series, the overall FFS or TFS remained high suggesting some recurrences can be successfully salvaged with focal retreatment. The impact of retreatment on functional outcomes has not been clearly elucidated, but a recent retrospective review of a HIFU registry noted a second HIFU compared to a single treatment had only minor worsening of urinary and erectile function scores.[69] A summary of recurrences for the aforementioned trials is presented in **Table 5**.

Postablation Follow-up

Evolution in the goals of FT, post-treatment monitoring, and definitions of ablation failure have paralleled the changes that have occurred in patient selection. The progression of current consensus opinion on postablation follow-up is listed in **Table 6**.[40,45,46,48,68]

The appeal of FT relies on its superior functional outcomes when compared to WG treatment. Thus, long-term outcomes should strive to include both oncologic and functional measures. Patient-reported functional outcomes can be measured with various validated survey instruments, but at a minimum urinary and sexual function should be periodically measured until stabilization, and resumed following each additional intervention, if applicable.

Monitoring oncologic outcomes following FT involves periodic PSA evaluation at frequencies similar to WG treatment; however, there is no consensus biochemical definition of recurrence. In a recent study, %PSA reduction following HIFU was inversely associated with additional treatment.[70] This retrospective, hypothesis-generating study will require a prospective study to determine any benefit of %PSA reduction and thresholds for intervention following FT.

Owing to the possibility of understaging, follow-up biopsy of the ablation zone and untreated areas are paramount to surveillance following FT. Following a multidisciplinary Delphi consensus project in 2014, Muller and colleagues concluded that mpMRI is the most suitable imaging technology for FT monitoring. Persistence is marked by enhancement in the DCE sequence within the ablated region and targeted biopsies should be taken to verify suspicious areas.[71] In the 2020 international FT symposium, consensus was reached that mpMRI-guided biopsies of targets plus systematic biopsy of untreated sectors should occur between 6 and 12 months post-treatment, and repeated for-cause such as rising PSA, abnormal mpMRI, or DRE. When persistence is identified, current consensus opinion is that GGG 1 cancers can be managed by AS and GGG 2 cancers may be retreated with FT or PGA depending on tumor characteristics, but WG therapies may be appropriate.[48]

FUTURE

The future of FT is bright, but much work is needed to improve upon patient selection, approach to ablation, and long-term monitoring of oncologic outcomes.

Patient Selection

If the success of FT rests on the ability to eradicate or control clinically significant cancer, then appropriate patient selection relies on the ability to accurately identify this disease. Although mpMRI has significantly improved the detection of GGG $\geq$ 2 PCa, it is not perfect. In a recent meta-analysis, mpMRI had a pooled NPV to detect GGG $\geq$ 2 PCa of 90.8% (IQR, 88.1-93.1).[72] The clinical need is to optimize image identification of multifocal and small (<5 mm) GGG$\geq$2 lesions that are missed by mpMRI.[56]

On the horizon lie a number of promising technologies to improve cancer detection—increased

Table 5
Biopsy outcomes in present focal therapy series

Reference	Design	n	Time to Oncologic Follow-up	Retreatment Rate	Reason for Post-FT Biopsy	Patients Undergoing Follow-up Biopsy n (%)	Patients with Positive Biopsy (n)	Any In-Field Failure (n)	Any Out-of-Field Failure (n)	Any In-Field + Out-of-Field Failure (n)	Absence of Any Prostate Cancer n (%)	Presence of (GGG ≥ 2) n (%)
CRYO												
Shah et al,[60] 2019	P	122	12 mo	8 (6.5%)	For cause: rising PSA and/or suspicious MRI	29 (23.7%)	21	9	9	3	8/29 (27%)	20/29 (68%)
Oishi et al,[61] 2019	R	160	12 mo	14%	Per protocol Or For cause: rising PSA and/or suspicious MRI	104 (65%)		NR	NR	NR	47% at 5 y	37% at 5 y
HIFU												
Guillaumier et al,[62] 2018	P	625	12 mo	112 (18%) one repeat HIFU 9 (1.4%) two repeat HIFU	Per protocol Or For cause: rising PSA and/or suspicious MRI	222(35%) 111 per protocol 111 for cause	56	29	11	16	166/222 (75%)	NR
Stabile et al,[63] 2019	P	1032	6–12 mo	205 (20%)	Per protocol Or For cause: rising PSA and/or suspicious MRI	424/1032 (41%)	325	NR	NR	NR	NR	255/424 (60%)

FLA												
Chao et al,[64] 2018	P	34	6 mo	NR	Per protocol Or For cause: rising PSA and/or suspicious MRI	32 8 for suspicious MRI 24 without suspicious MRI	17	NR	NR	NR	5/32 (14.7%)	9/32 (28%)
IRE												
Blazevski et al,[65] 2019	P	123	12 mo	18/123 (14.6%)	Per protocol	102	23	10	13	NR	79/102 (77.5%)	23/102 (22.5%)
VTP												
Azzouzi et al,[66] 2017 Gill et al,[67] 2018	RCT	AS: 207 VTP: 206	24 mo	13/206 (6%)	Per protocol	NR	NR	NR	NR	NR	NR	PDT: 25% AS: 44%

Abbreviations: FLA, focal-laser ablation; IRE, irreversible electroporation; NR, not recorded; P, prospective; R, retrospective.

Table 6
Evolution of outcomes and follow-up

Date	2010	2012	2015	2019	2020
Lead Author	de la Rosette[45]	van den Bos[46]	Donaldson[40]	Tay[68]	Lebastchi[48]
Goal of FT	Eradication of all known cancer	Eradication of clinically significant disease (tumor >0.5 mL)	Eradication of dominant or index lesion	Eradication of cancer by targeted, quadrant, or hemiablation	FT: Eradication of all biopsy confirmed MRI "visible" GGG 2 cancer PGA: Eradication of all biopsy confirmed GGG 2
Disease monitoring	PSA per common practice for standard therapy Biopsy 6–12 mo post-treatment by TMB	PSA every 3 mo in year 1 PSA every 6 mo in year 2 PSA yearly at year 3 Then PSA at discretion of physician targeted + systematic biopsy 6–12 mo post-treatment	Monitoring by PSA not evaluated Optimal timing for post-treatment biopsy 1 y or earlier for rising PSA or MRI suspicion Targeted biopsy of ablation area preferred; no consensus on biopsy of untreated areas	PSA monitoring per standard of care, insufficient evidence to define the use of PSA mpMRI recommended at least once 6–12 mo after initial treatment targeted biopsy: 4–6 core from the treated zone alone at 3–6 mo and/or nontreated areas suspicious on mpMRI targeted + 12 core systematic biopsy of the treated and untreated zone at 12–24 mo >24 mo, the gland should be biopsied only if there is suspicious change in MRI, PSA, or clinical findings	PSA every 3 mo in year 1 PSA every 6 mo thereafter PSA alone cannot predict failure mpMRI at 6 mo, 12 mo, then yearly per institutional surveillance protocol (early enhancement in ablation zone suggest failure) Targeted biopsy of ablation zone 6–12 mo after treatment; systematic biopsy of untreated zone 6–12 mo after treatment Repeat biopsy for triggering factors: rising PSA, MRI abnormalities, abnormal DRE

Focal Retreatment	NR	One time focal retreatment acceptable for any IFF or OFF recurrence	Focal retreatment rates ≤20% are acceptable	NR	NR
Functional Outcomes	IIEF ICIQ FACT-P Short Form-36 EuroQoL EORTC QoL	No guidance for which PRO to use	Not described	Not described	Urinary, bowel, and sexual function should be assessed q3-6 mo until stable No pads = satisfactory urinary control No consensus was reached for sexual function success
Oncologic Failures	Biopsy-proven cancer in treatment area	IFF: Cancer of higher grade; persistent cancer of the same grade or lower grade after repeat focal; Whole gland treatment OFF: ≥3 + 3 of 3 mm equal selection	IFF: any vol or grade of cancer higher than original cancer; any whole gland treatment Accurate definition of biochemical failure cannot be made	IFF: No decrease in volume of Gleason 3 + 3 or significant volume (≥0.2 cc or ≥ 7 mm in diameter) of Gleason 3 + 4 OFF: foci of clinically significant cancer requiring further therapy	IFF: any GGG ≥ 2 *IFF may be managed with repeat FT/PGA OFF: any GGG ≥ 2 *OFF may be managed with repeat FT/PGA Low grade, GGG 1 tumors should be managed by active surveillance per institutional protocols

Abbreviations: DRE; digital rectal exam; FACT-P, Functional Assessment of Cancer Therapy-Prostate; ICIQ, international incontinence scale of urinary incontinence; IFF, in-field failure; IIEF, international index of erectile function; mpMRI, multiparametric MRI; NR, not recorded; OFF, out-of-field failure; PGA, partial-gland ablation; PRO, patient-reported outcome; TMB, transperineal-mapping biopsy.

Table 7
Future comparator trials in focal therapy

PI and Site	Name, Identifier	Trial Design	Participants (n)	Inclusion	Status	Primary Outcome	End Date
Ahmed[80] UK Multicenter	CHRONOS NCT04049747	Open-label Phase II RCT CHRONOS-A: FT (HIFU, CRYO) vs RT (EBRT, Brachy) or RP CHRONOS-B: multiarm RCT focal vs focal + neoadjuvant (12 wk) Finasteride or Bicalutamide	Estimated enrollment: 2450 Parallel assignment CHRONOS-A or CHRONOS-B	Prebiopsy MRI PSA $\leq$ 20, T $\leq$ 3a GGG 1 $\geq$ 6 mm in any one core GGG 2 or GGG 3 or	Recruiting	A: Progression-free survival: progression to whole gland, systemic therapy, metastasis, or cancer-specific mortality B: Failure-free survival: further focal therapy + progression-free survival	2027
(SITU)[81] UK Multicenter	PART ISRCTN 17249875	Open-label RCT Partial ablation (VTP) vs Radical treatment (RP, EBRT, LD-brachytherapy)	Partial ablation: 400 Radical treatment: 400	Unilateral dominant lesion PSA $\leq$ 20 T $\leq$ 2b GGG 1 >4 mm GGG 2 GGG 3	Recruiting	Oncologic outcomes at 3 y	2027
Baco[82] Oslo University Hospital Single Center	FARP NCT03668652	Open-label RCT FT (HIFU, TULSA-PRO) vs RP	FT: 100 HIFU for lesions <30 mm from rectum; TULSA-PRO for lesions > 30 mm RP: 100	Unilateral PSA $\leq$ 20 T $\leq$ 2b GGG 1 > 5 mm GGG 2 any length	Recruiting	Oncologic outcomes at 36 mo from treatment TF in RP arm: PSA > 0.2, or positive surgical margins and need for EBRT TF in FT arm: need for whole gland treatment	2024

Crouzet[83] Lyon, France Multicenter	HIFUSA NCT03531099	Open-label Phase III RCT FT (HIFU) vs AS	FT: 65 AS: 65	Unilateral PSA $\leq$ 15 T $\leq$ 2a GGG 1 Only one target tumor on MRI or 2 contiguous sextants Tumor 9 mm from external sphincter (for margin) Maximum tumor length > 3 mm	Recruiting	Conversion to radical treatment at 48 mo	2025

Abbreviations: BCR, biochemical recurrence; EBRT, external beam radiation; LD-brachytherapy, low-dose brachytherapy; SITU, surgical trials unit; TULSA-PRO, transurethral ultrasound ablation.

mpMRI magnet strength to 7-Telsa, 29 Hz high-frequency microultrasound, and shear wave elastography, to name a few—but currently limited data exist for any one technology to surpass mpMRI.[73–75] Importantly, advanced US imaging could decrease cost and allow patients to have an in-office diagnostic and therapeutic experience.

Approach to Ablation

The goal to control PCa with minimal disruption to the nonmalignant parenchyma/nontarget organs has led to more precise FT technologies. Increased precision may lead to undertreatment, as IFF remains high even in contemporary series. In the future, using mpMRI alone for precise treatment planning will likely not be sufficient. The utilization of augmented diagnostics to identify the true treatment margin and adjuvants to enhance ablation at the margin will be required.

Recent evidence suggests that without destruction of clonal cell populations within adjacent benign tissue, FT of an index lesion may not be curative.[76] To determine the quantity of "benign" tissue to incorporate, platforms such as ConfirmMDx (MDxHealth, Irvine, California) may be useful. The assay quantifies the methylation of genes (GSPT1, APC, RASSF1 in comparison to reference gene ACTB) from benign cores to predict GGG $\geq$ 2 PCa on repeat biopsy.[77] Further work in this area could lead to decreased IFF.

In addition, there is a clinical need to incorporate adjuvants that increase cell death, particularly, those located within the perimeter of the ablative energy that undergoes apoptosis. However, the selection of a death-inducing agent should be effective but have very low morbidity to preserve functional outcomes.[78]

Follow-up Postablation

The greatest leap forward in the next decade of FT will likely come from effort to improve consistency in reporting of post-treatment outcomes. To achieve this, we collectively should collaborate and participate in multicenter trials, use well-established consensus panel definitions of treatment and success, and use outcomes registries such as the one launched by the Focal Therapy Society.

Despite good functional outcomes following FT, little is known about functional and oncologic outcomes for those who progress from FT to WG treatment. A recent study of 82 patients showed that salvage RP following HIFU was not associated with worse pathologic outcomes at prostatectomy nor increased operative complications when considering historical primary prostatectomy data.[79] More follow-up is needed to determine the potential increased morbidity of salvage treatment that could have been avoided with initial WG therapy.

Finally, to define the true value of FT to treat localized PCa, well-designed RCTs comparing FT to WG are needed. A number of comparative efficacy trials are currently recruiting, these are summarized in **Table 7**.[80–83]

SUMMARY

The evolution of patient selection for FT as a management strategy for GGG $\geq$ 2, localized PCa has paralleled our improved understanding of the low malignant potential of GGG 1 PCa. MP-MRI imaging and fusion systems provide both the target for biopsy and the subsequent ablation. While IFF still remains present in contemporary FT series, FT retreatment may salvage many of these men and prevent conversion to WG treatment. The future of FT will depend on the favorable reports of long-term functional and oncologic outcomes using standardized definitions that allow for comparison across trials using various ablation technologies and treatment templates. Lastly, comparative efficacy trials could provide level 1 evidence necessary to cement FT as a primary management strategy for highly selected patients with localized PCa.

CLINICAL CARE POINTS

- Targeted biopsy of imageable prostate cancer by a mpMRI/US fusion platform or 3D TMB biopsy provides a roadmap for focal prostate cancer ablation.
- Delivery of effective ablative energy to the target tissue with >5+ mm safety margin is more important than type of energy ablation source employed.
- Following ablation patients should be monitored with patient reported outcome surveys for erectile and urinary function until stabilization or following any repeat intervention.
- Oncologic outcomes should be determined by per protocol targeted + systematic biopsy performed between 6-12 months following ablation; if negative, perform repeat biopsy per institutional active surveillance protocols or for triggering factors.

DISCLOSURE

The authors have nothing to disclose.

REFERENCES

1. Cooperberg MR, Lubeck DP, Meng MV, et al. The changing face of low-risk prostate cancer: trends in clinical presentation and primary management. J Clin Oncol 2004;22(11):2141–9.
2. Polascik TJ, Oesterling JE, Partin AW. Prostate specific antigen: a decade of discovery–what we have learned and where we are going. J Urol 1999; 162(2):293–306.
3. Ficarra V, Novara G, Ahlering TE, et al. Systematic review and meta-analysis of studies reporting potency rates after robot-assisted radical prostatectomy. Eur Urol 2012;62(3):418–30.
4. Ficarra V, Novara G, Rosen RC, et al. Systematic review and meta-analysis of studies reporting urinary continence recovery after robot-assisted radical prostatectomy. Eur Urol 2012;62(3):405–17.
5. Resnick MJ, Koyama T, Fan KH, et al. Long-term functional outcomes after treatment for localized prostate cancer. N Engl J Med 2013;368(5):436–45.
6. Albertsen PC, Fryback DG, Storer BE, et al. Long-term survival among men with conservatively treated localized prostate cancer. JAMA 1995;274(8): 626–31.
7. Patel MI, DeConcini DT, Lopez-Corona E, et al. An analysis of men with clinically localized prostate cancer who deferred definitive therapy. J Urol 2004;171(4):1520–4.
8. Eggener SE, Scardino PT, Carroll PR, et al. Focal therapy for localized prostate cancer: a critical appraisal of rationale and modalities. J Urol 2007; 178(6):2260–7.
9. Polascik TJ, Mouraviev V. Focal therapy for prostate cancer. Curr Opin Urol 2008;18(3):269–74.
10. Onik G, Narayan P, Vaughan D, et al. Focal "nerve-sparing" cryosurgery for treatment of primary prostate cancer: a new approach to preserving potency. Urology 2002;60(1):109–14.
11. Onik G. The male lumpectomy: rationale for a cancer targeted approach for prostate cryoablation. A review. Technol Cancer Res Treat 2004;3(4):365–70.
12. Ohori M, Eastham JA, Koh H, et al. Is focal therapy reasonable in patinets with early stage prostate cancer (CAP)? An anlaysis of radical prostatectomy (RP) specimens. [AUA Annual Meeting, Atlanta 2006, Abstract #1574]. J Urol 2006;175:507.
13. Cheng L, Jones TD, Pan CX, et al. Anatomic distribution and pathologic characterization of small-volume prostate cancer (<0.5 ml) in whole-mount prostatectomy specimens. Mod Pathol 2005;18(8): 1022–6.
14. Arora R, Koch MO, Eble JN, et al. Heterogeneity of Gleason grade in multifocal adenocarcinoma of the prostate. Cancer 2004;100(11):2362–6.
15. Mouraviev V, Mayes JM, Sun L, et al. Prostate cancer laterality as a rationale of focal ablative therapy for the treatment of clinically localized prostate cancer. Cancer 2007;110(4):906–10.
16. Stamey TA, Caldwell M, McNeal JE, et al. The prostate specific antigen era in the United States is over for prostate cancer: what happened in the last 20 years? J Urol 2004;172(4 Pt 1):1297–301.
17. Polascik TJ, Mayes JM, Sun L, et al. Pathologic stage T2a and T2b prostate cancer in the recent prostate-specific antigen era: implications for unilateral ablative therapy. Prostate 2008;68(13):1380–6.
18. Sartor AO, Hricak H, Wheeler TM, et al. Evaluating localized prostate cancer and identifying candidates for focal therapy. Urology 2008;72(6 Suppl): S12–24.
19. Wise AM, Stamey TA, McNeal JE, et al. Morphologic and clinical significance of multifocal prostate cancers in radical prostatectomy specimens. Urology 2002;60(2):264–9.
20. Rukstalis DB, Goldknopf JL, Crowley EM, et al. Prostate cryoablation: a scientific rationale for future modifications. Urology 2002;60(2 Suppl 1): 19–25.
21. Noguchi M, Stamey TA, McNeal JE, et al. Prognostic factors for multifocal prostate cancer in radical prostatectomy specimens: lack of significance of secondary cancers. J Urol 2003;170(2 Pt 1):459–63.
22. Bolenz C, Gierth M, Grobholz R, et al. Clinical staging error in prostate cancer: localization and relevance of undetected tumour areas. BJU Int 2009; 103(9):1184–9.
23. Bjurlin MA, Carter HB, Schellhammer P, et al. Optimization of initial prostate biopsy in clinical practice: sampling, labeling and specimen processing. J Urol 2013;189(6):2039–46.
24. Tsivian M, Kimura M, Sun L, et al. Predicting unilateral prostate cancer on routine diagnostic biopsy: sextant vs extended. BJU Int 2010;105(8):1089–92.
25. Barzell WE, Melamed MR. Appropriate patient selection in the focal treatment of prostate cancer: the role of transperineal 3-dimensional pathologic mapping of the prostate–a 4-year experience. Urology 2007;70(6 Suppl):27–35.
26. Crawford ED, Wilson SS, Torkko KC, et al. Clinical staging of prostate cancer: a computer-simulated study of transperineal prostate biopsy. BJU Int 2005;96(7):999–1004.
27. Gardner TA, Koch MO. Prostate cancer therapy with high-intensity focused ultrasound. Clin Genitourin Cancer 2005;4(3):187–92.
28. Ganzer R, Arthanareeswaran VKA, Ahmed HU, et al. Which technology to select for primary focal treatment of prostate cancer?-European Section of

Urotechnology (ESUT) position statement. Prostate Cancer Prostatic Dis 2018;21(2):175–86.
29. Bozzini G, Colin P, Nevoux P, et al. Focal therapy of prostate cancer: energies and procedures. Urol Oncol 2013;31(2):155–67.
30. Lodeizen O, de Bruin M, Eggener S, et al. Ablation energies for focal treatment of prostate cancer. World J Urol 2019;37(3):409–18.
31. D'Amico AV, Whittington R, Malkowicz SB, et al. Biochemical outcome after radical prostatectomy, external beam radiation therapy, or interstitial radiation therapy for clinically localized prostate cancer. JAMA 1998;280(11):969–74.
32. Ellis DS, Manny TB Jr, Rewcastle JC. Focal cryosurgery followed by penile rehabilitation as primary treatment for localized prostate cancer: initial results. Urology 2007;70(6 Suppl):9–15.
33. Bahn D, de Castro Abreu AL, Gill IS, et al. Focal cryotherapy for clinically unilateral, low-intermediate risk prostate cancer in 73 men with a median follow-up of 3.7 years. Eur Urol 2012;62(1):55–63.
34. Muto S, Yoshii T, Saito K, et al. Focal therapy with high-intensity-focused ultrasound in the treatment of localized prostate cancer. Jpn J Clin Oncol 2008;38(3):192–9.
35. Ahmed HU, Hindley RG, Dickinson L, et al. Focal therapy for localised unifocal and multifocal prostate cancer: a prospective development study. Lancet Oncol 2012;13(6):622–32.
36. National Comprehensive Cancer Network. NCCN clinical Practice Guidelines in Oncology: prostate cancer, Vol 2.2021. Plymouth Meeting, PA: National Comprehensive Cancer Network; 2021. Available at: https://www.nccn.org/professionals/physician_gls/pdf/prostate.pdf.
37. Johansson JE, Andren O, Andersson SO, et al. Natural history of early, localized prostate cancer. JAMA 2004;291(22):2713–9.
38. Klotz L, Vesprini D, Sethukavalan P, et al. Long-term follow-up of a large active surveillance cohort of patients with prostate cancer. J Clin Oncol 2015;33(3):272–7.
39. Tosoian JJ, Mamawala M, Epstein JI, et al. Intermediate and Longer-Term Outcomes From a Prospective Active-Surveillance Program for Favorable-Risk Prostate Cancer. J Clin Oncol 2015;33(30):3379–85.
40. Donaldson IA, Alonzi R, Barratt D, et al. Focal therapy: patients, interventions, and outcomes–a report from a consensus meeting. Eur Urol 2015;67(4):771–7.
41. Tan WP, Rastinehad AR, Klotz L, et al. Utilization of focal therapy for patients discontinuing active surveillance of prostate cancer: Recommendations of an international Delphi consensus. Urol Oncol 2021. https://doi.org/10.1016/j.urolonc.2021.01.027.
42. Musunuru HB, Yamamoto T, Klotz L, et al. Active Surveillance for Intermediate Risk Prostate Cancer: Survival Outcomes in the Sunnybrook Experience. J Urol 2016;196(6):1651–8.
43. Balakrishnan AS, Cowan JE, Cooperberg MR, et al. Evaluating the Safety of Active Surveillance: Outcomes of Deferred Radical Prostatectomy after an Initial Period of Surveillance. J Urol 2019;202(3):506–10.
44. Gearman DJ, Morlacco A, Cheville JC, et al. Comparison of Pathological and Oncologic Outcomes of Favorable Risk Gleason Score 3 + 4 and Low Risk Gleason Score 6 Prostate Cancer: Considerations for Active Surveillance. J Urol 2018;199(5):1188–95.
45. de la Rosette J, Ahmed H, Barentsz J, et al. Focal therapy in prostate cancer-report from a consensus panel. J Endourol 2010;24(5):775–80.
46. van den Bos W, Muller BG, Ahmed H, et al. Focal therapy in prostate cancer: international multidisciplinary consensus on trial design. Eur Urol 2014;65(6):1078–83.
47. Tay KJ, Scheltema MJ, Ahmed HU, et al. Patient selection for prostate focal therapy in the era of active surveillance: an International Delphi Consensus Project. Prostate Cancer Prostatic Dis 2017;20(3):294–9.
48. Lebastchi AH, George AK, Polascik TJ, et al. Standardized Nomenclature and Surveillance Methodologies After Focal Therapy and Partial Gland Ablation for Localized Prostate Cancer: An International Multidisciplinary Consensus. Eur Urol 2020;78(3):371–8.
49. Giganti F, Rosenkrantz AB, Villeirs G, et al. The Evolution of MRI of the Prostate: The Past, the Present, and the Future. AJR Am J Roentgenol 2019;213(2):384–96.
50. Turkbey B, Mani H, Shah V, et al. Multiparametric 3T prostate magnetic resonance imaging to detect cancer: histopathological correlation using prostatectomy specimens processed in customized magnetic resonance imaging based molds. J Urol 2011;186(5):1818–24.
51. Kongnyuy M, George AK, Rastinehad AR, et al. Magnetic Resonance Imaging-Ultrasound Fusion-Guided Prostate Biopsy: Review of Technology, Techniques, and Outcomes. Curr Urol Rep 2016;17(4):32.
52. Pinto PA, Chung PH, Rastinehad AR, et al. Magnetic resonance imaging/ultrasound fusion guided prostate biopsy improves cancer detection following transrectal ultrasound biopsy and correlates with multiparametric magnetic resonance imaging. J Urol 2011;186(4):1281–5.
53. Siddiqui MM, Rais-Bahrami S, Turkbey B, et al. Comparison of MR/ultrasound fusion-guided biopsy with ultrasound-guided biopsy for the diagnosis of prostate cancer. JAMA 2015;313(4):390–7.
54. Ahmed HU, El-Shater Bosaily A, Brown LC, et al. Diagnostic accuracy of multi-parametric MRI and

TRUS biopsy in prostate cancer (PROMIS): a paired validating confirmatory study. Lancet 2017; 389(10071):815–22.
55. Kasivisvanathan V, Rannikko AS, Borghi M, et al. MRI-Targeted or Standard Biopsy for Prostate-Cancer Diagnosis. N Engl J Med 2018;378(19): 1767–77.
56. Le JD, Tan N, Shkolyar E, et al. Multifocality and prostate cancer detection by multiparametric magnetic resonance imaging: correlation with whole-mount histopathology. Eur Urol 2015;67(3):569–76.
57. Ahdoot M, Wilbur AR, Reese SE, et al. MRI-Targeted, Systematic, and Combined Biopsy for Prostate Cancer Diagnosis. N Engl J Med 2020; 382(10):917–28.
58. Priester A, Natarajan S, Khoshnoodi P, et al. Magnetic Resonance Imaging Underestimation of Prostate Cancer Geometry: Use of Patient Specific Molds to Correlate Images with Whole Mount Pathology. J Urol 2017;197(2):320–6.
59. Sivaraman A, Barret E. Focal Therapy for Prostate Cancer: An "A la Carte" Approach. Eur Urol 2016; 69(6):973–5.
60. Shah TT, Peters M, Eldred-Evans D, et al. Early-Medium-Term Outcomes of Primary Focal Cryotherapy to Treat Nonmetastatic Clinically Significant Prostate Cancer from a Prospective Multicentre Registry. Eur Urol 2019;76(1):98–105.
61. Oishi M, Gill IS, Tafuri A, et al. Hemigland Cryoablation of Localized Low, Intermediate and High Risk Prostate Cancer: Oncologic and Functional Outcomes at 5 Years. J Urol 2019;202(6):1188–98.
62. Guillaumier S, Peters M, Arya M, et al. A Multicentre Study of 5-year Outcomes Following Focal Therapy in Treating Clinically Significant Nonmetastatic Prostate Cancer. Eur Urol 2018;74(4):422–9.
63. Stabile A, Orczyk C, Hosking-Jervis F, et al. Medium-term oncological outcomes in a large cohort of men treated with either focal or hemi-ablation using high-intensity focused ultrasonography for primary localized prostate cancer. BJU Int 2019; 124(3):431–40.
64. Chao B, Llukani E, Lepor H. Two-year Outcomes Following Focal Laser Ablation of Localized Prostate Cancer. Eur Urol Oncol 2018;1(2):129–33.
65. Blazevski A, Scheltema MJ, Yuen B, et al. Oncological and Quality-of-life Outcomes Following Focal Irreversible Electroporation as Primary Treatment for Localised Prostate Cancer: A Biopsy-monitored Prospective Cohort. Eur Urol Oncol 2020;3(3): 283–90.
66. Azzouzi AR, Vincendeau S, Barret E, et al. Padeliporfin vascular-targeted photodynamic therapy versus active surveillance in men with low-risk prostate cancer (CLIN1001 PCM301): an open-label, phase 3, randomised controlled trial. Lancet Oncol 2017;18(2):181–91.
67. Gill IS, Azzouzi AR, Emberton M, et al. Randomized Trial of Partial Gland Ablation with Vascular Targeted Phototherapy versus Active Surveillance for Low Risk Prostate Cancer: Extended Followup and Analyses of Effectiveness. J Urol 2018;200(4):786–93.
68. Tay KJ, Amin MB, Ghai S, et al. Surveillance after prostate focal therapy. World J Urol 2019;37(3): 397–407.
69. Lovegrove CE, Peters M, Guillaumier S, et al. Evaluation of functional outcomes after a second focal high-intensity focused ultrasonography (HIFU) procedure in men with primary localized, non-metastatic prostate cancer: results from the HIFU Evaluation and Assessment of Treatment (HEAT) registry. BJU Int 2020;125(6):853–60.
70. Stabile A, Orczyk C, Giganti F, et al. The Role of Percentage of Prostate-specific Antigen Reduction After Focal Therapy Using High-intensity Focused Ultrasound for Primary Localised Prostate Cancer. Results from a Large Multi-institutional Series. Eur Urol 2020;78(2):155–60.
71. Muller BG, van den Bos W, Brausi M, et al. Role of multiparametric magnetic resonance imaging (MRI) in focal therapy for prostate cancer: a Delphi consensus project. BJU Int 2014;114(5):698–707.
72. Sathianathen NJ, Omer A, Harriss E, et al. Negative Predictive Value of Multiparametric Magnetic Resonance Imaging in the Detection of Clinically Significant Prostate Cancer in the Prostate Imaging Reporting and Data System Era: A Systematic Review and Meta-analysis. Eur Urol 2020;78(3):402–14.
73. Laader A, Beiderwellen K, Kraff O, et al. 1.5 versus 3 versus 7 Tesla in abdominal MRI: A comparative study. PLoS One 2017;12(11):e0187528.
74. Lughezzani G, Maffei D, Saita A, et al. Diagnostic Accuracy of Microultrasound in Patients with a Suspicion of Prostate Cancer at Magnetic Resonance Imaging: A Single-institutional Prospective Study. Eur Urol Focus 2020. https://doi.org/10.1016/j.euf.2020.09.013.
75. Morris DC, Chan DY, Lye TH, et al. Multiparametric Ultrasound for Targeting Prostate Cancer: Combining ARFI, SWEI, QUS and B-Mode. Ultrasound Med Biol 2020;46(12):3426–39.
76. Cooper CS, Eeles R, Wedge DC, et al. Analysis of the genetic phylogeny of multifocal prostate cancer identifies multiple independent clonal expansions in neoplastic and morphologically normal prostate tissue. Nat Genet 2015;47(4):367–72.
77. Van Neste L, Partin AW, Stewart GD, et al. Risk score predicts high-grade prostate cancer in DNA-methylation positive, histopathologically negative biopsies. Prostate 2016;76(12):1078–87.
78. Baust JM, Rabin Y, Polascik TJ, et al. Defeating cancers' adaptive defensive strategies using thermal therapies: examining cancer's therapeutic resistance, ablative, and computational modeling strategies as a

means for improving therapeutic outcome. Technol Cancer Res Treat 2018;17. 1533033818762207.

79. Marconi L, Stonier T, Tourinho-Barbosa R, et al. Robot-assisted Radical Prostatectomy After Focal Therapy: Oncological, Functional Outcomes and Predictors of Recurrence. Eur Urol 2019;76(1):27–30.

80. Ahmed H. Imperial prostate 4: comparative Health Research outcomes of NOvel Surgery in prostate cancer (IP4-CHRONOS). Imperial College of London; 2019. Available at: https://clinicaltrials.gov/ct2/show/NCT04049747. Accessed May 15, 2021.

81. A randomised controlled trial of Partial prostate Ablation versus Radical Treatment (PART) in intermediate risk, unilateral clinically localised prostate cancer. Surgical Intervention Trials Unit (SITU). 2019. Available at: https://doi.org/10.1186/ISRCTN17249875. Accessed May 15, 2021.

82. Baco E. A randomized control trial of focal prostate ablation versus radical prostatectomy (FARP). Department of Urology Aker, Oslo University Hospital; 2018. Available at: https://clinicaltrials.gov/ct2/show/NCT03668652. Accessed May 15, 2021.

83. Crouzet S. Phase 3, Multicenter, Randomized Study, Evaluating the Efficacy and Tolerability of Focused HIFU Therapy Compared to Active Surveillance in Patients With Significant Low Risk Prostate Cancer (HIFUSA). Hospices Civils de Lyon. 2018. Available at: https://clinicaltrials.gov/ct2/show/NCT03531099. Accessed May 15, 2021.

Disposable Ureteroscopes in Urology

Current State and Future Prospects

Margaret A. Knoedler, MD*, Sara L. Best, MD

KEYWORDS

• Single use • Ureteroscopy • Kidney stone

KEY POINTS

- Reusable ureteroscopes require expensive and time-intensive sterilization and repairs and run the risk of device contamination.
- Single use ureteroscopes were developed to alleviate the need for reprocessing and repairs.
- In terms of performance, environmental impact, and cost, there is not a clear advantage for single use or reusable ureteroscopes.
- Individual- and institutional-level factors should be considered when deciding which ureteroscope to use.

INTRODUCTION

Urolithiasis is a common condition, affecting 1 in 11 people throughout their lifetime. The cost of management has been estimated in excess of $10 billion annually in the United States.[1] The use of ureteroscopy to manage kidney stones continues to increase compared with other stone surgical approaches. Between 2003 and 2013, case logs submitted to the American Board of Urology revealed that the percent of stone surgeries logged that were ureteroscopic increased from 40.9% to 59.6%.[2] The same study found that new urologists certifying for the first time reported 70.9% of their stone cases to be ureteroscopic. A similar trend has been observed in Canada. Ordon and colleagues[3] reported that, although the use of ureteroscopy increased from 25% to 59% (P<.0001) of all stone procedures performed between 1991 and 2010, extracorporeal shock wave lithotripsy use decreased from 69% to 34% (P<.0001). The increased use of these endoscopes however can cause significant wear and tear on these delicate instruments, potentially resulting in decreased deflection capabilities, broken light fibers, punctured working channels, and even disabling of the device altogether.[4] This damage can lead to expensive maintenance and repair costs for facilities offering ureteroscopy and can even lead to cancellation of scheduled procedures if an institution is unable to maintain a large collections of these devices owing to high costs.[5] In addition to cost considerations, the reuse of medical equipment can result in logistical challenges as well as concern for contamination and spread of infection between patients. Factors such as these have resulted in an interest in single use, disposable endoscopes, allowing each patient's surgery to be performed with a new sterile device. This article explores the technical findings such as poor durability and device contamination that have propelled the introduction of disposable ureteroscopes.

DURABILITY AND COST

In 2000, Afane and colleagues[4] assessed the durability of 4 brands of commercially available 9F flexible ureteroscopes and found that they required repair after an average of only 3 to 13 hours of

Department of Urology, University of Wisconsin School of Medicine and Public Health, 1685 Highland Avenue, Madison, WI 53705-2281, USA
* Corresponding author.
E-mail address: knoedler@urology.wisc.edu

Urol Clin N Am 49 (2022) 153–159
https://doi.org/10.1016/j.ucl.2021.07.012

use, with the most common failure being loss of sufficient deflection. The authors concluded that the adoption of these instruments would be slowed owing to the high yearly cost of repairs. In response to these issues, device manufacturers developed new ureteroscopes, aiming for improved durability, although this development sometimes came with a tradeoff of a wider scope shaft. For example, in 2001 ACMI introduced the DUR-8 with modifications to increase durability, including a slightly wider shaft of 10.1F. Monga and colleagues[6] reported the DUR-8 was used in 25 procedures before requiring repair, an improvement from other devices.

Ureteroscope fragility prompted Landman and colleagues[7] to conduct a cost analysis that was reported in 2003. Using published data on the average number of procedures a scope could be used before requiring repair with the cost of purchase and repairs, they projected the cost to acquire and repair a ureteroscope after 1-year warranty expiration for use in 100 cases would range between $US38,600 and $US60,033, depending on the model of scope used.[7]

Although device repairs can be expensive, they are not the only costs that can be associated with the use of reusable scopes. Although both single use and reusable devices have listed purchase prices, reusable ureteroscope costs also include reprocessing and repairs. Additionally, it is difficult to quantify the cost of operating room delays when a reusable ureteroscope is unavailable because of reprocessing or repair delays. Nevertheless, there are several studies that have attempted to capture the complexities of reprocessing and repair costs when comparing reusable and single use ureteroscopes.

Reprocessing costs include labor, time, and disposable items. Using a time-driven activity-based costing model, Isaacson and colleagues[8] looked at reusable flexible ureteroscopes and found that reprocessing episodes required an average 229 $\pm$ 74.4 minutes per unit and estimated cost per reprocessing, including labor and disposable items, was $96.13. Other studies looking at the cost of reprocessing have found a range from $107.27 to $120.63 per reprocessing episode at their institutions.[9–11]

Martin and colleagues[9] prospectively tracked all reusable ureteroscopes over a single year period at their institution and compared this to the market price of a single use ureteroscope (LithoVue; Boston Scientific, Marlborough, MA). They performed a cost–benefit analysis and found that, after the initial purchase cost, the average cost per case with a flexible ureteroscope was $848.10. This amount included reprocessing and repair costs. They compared this finding with the LithoVue single use ureteroscope, with a purchase cost of $1500 based on market data in 2016. After 99 ureteroscopic cases, the cost–benefit analysis favored reusable ureteroscopes over single use flexible ureteroscopes.[9] Using a cost analysis model based on their institutional repair and reprocessing costs over a 1-year period, Al-Balushi and colleagues[5] also found that reusable flexible ureteroscopes were more cost -effective in high-volume centers, whereas single use ureteroscopes were more cost effective in low-volume centers.

Case mix can also play a role, because specific cases have been associated with greater damage to reusable flexible ureteroscopes. Specifically, cases involving stones in the lower pole or mid-zone and staghorn stones are associated with increased scope damage requiring repair.[9,12]

Ultimately, the cost effectiveness of single use versus reusable ureteroscopes must be decided at the institutional level. Market forces such as the listed prices of the devices and replacement parts play a role, but so too do institution level factors such as case volume, case mix, and repair turnaround time. In general, high-volume centers are more likely to benefit by investing in reusable ureteroscopes owing to economies of scale, whereas low-volume centers may be able to decrease costs by purchasing single use scopes.

DEVICE CONTAMINATION

There are risks to reusing endoscopes beyond the cost of device failure and repair. Every few years stories appear in the popular media reporting patient exposure to possible hepatitis C or HIV related to improper or inadequate sterilization of colonoscopes, devices that undergo a similar reprocessing procedure as ureteroscopes. In 1997, Bronowicki and colleagues[13] reported in the *New England Journal of Medicine* a married couple presenting with acute hepatitis symptoms. Both patients had undergone colonoscopy the same day as another patient known to be seropositive and untreated for hepatitis C viral (HCV) infection. The authors were able to trace the date the seroconversion to HCV^+ in the couple because they were longtime frequent blood donors whose blood was regularly tested for various infectious diseases including HCV. Genotyping and nucleotide sequencing revealed that all 3 patients were infected with the same isolate of HCV. A careful investigation of other procedural aspects such as the anesthesia equipment and involved hospital staff suggested that colonoscope contamination from an improper cleaning technique of the scope's biopsy channel was the likely source of cross-transmission of HCV.[13] Since that time, numerous incidents in which thousands of patients may have been exposed to nosocomial infection have appeared in the news, often after inadequate sterilization of colonoscopes has been identified.

Although a major news story has yet to appear concerning ureteroscope-related transmission of infection, several authors have investigated the adequacy of cleaning protocols for urologic endoscopes. In 2007, *Pseudomonas aeruginosa* bacteremia in 4 patients was traced back to a single contaminated flexible cystoscope used in all 4 patients in the few days before illness. Several additional patients were found to have a *P aeruginosa* urinary tract infection.[14] Although infection control investigation of the matter revealed egregious noncompliance with standard sterilization protocols for these devices, this case is a good example of the serious consequences that can occur from reusable endoscopes. There is no reason to believe flexible ureteroscopes would be immune to incomplete sterilization and the potential for nosocomial infection. A study from Amsterdam obtained cultures from flexible ureteroscopes that had recently undergone standard high-level disinfection reprocessing and found that 12% of the cultures were positive, although they did not find a higher incidence of symptomatic postoperative urinary tract infection in patients who had undergone surgery with a culture-positive device.[15] An American center assayed reprocessed "clean" ureteroscopes and found traces of biologic substances such as hemoglobin, adenosine triphosphate, and protein in 44%, 63% and 100% of cases, respectively, as well as microbial contamination in 13%.[16] Brand new reusable ureteroscopes tested by both studies were reportedly clean of contamination, so it makes sense that use of single use ureteroscopes would avoid this source of nosocomial infection.

DEVELOPMENT OF SEMIDISPOSABLE AND FULLY DISPOSABLE URETEROSCOPES

Recognizing a potential market for ureteroscopes with disposable components, manufacturers began introducing semidisposable devices in the early 2010s. PolyDiagnost GmbH (Pfaffenhofen, Germany) released the Polyscope modular flexible ureteroscope, consisting of a reusable optical core that is placed inside a disposable unidirectionally deflecting shell.[17] Although there are few data on its clinical use, Gu and colleagues[18] in China reported success in using this device in 86 patients with upper tract urinary calculi, although Proietti and colleagues[19] in Italy reported insufficient maneuverability and visualization for them to perform a satisfactory surgery. Cook Medical (Bloomington, IN) introduced a similar partially disposable device, the FlexorVue, in 2013, but the deflection limitations of both of the devices likely limited widespread adoption.[20]

The first fully disposable, single use digital ureteroscope, the LithoVue (Boston Scientific) appeared on the market in 2015 and was the first to be approved by the US Food and Drug Administraton.[20] It has bidirectional deflection, a 7.7F tip, a 9.5F shaft, and a 3.6F working channel and must be used with a proprietary monitor.[21] Several other single use flexible ureteroscopes have since come onto the market. Most notably, Pusen (Guangdong, China) has released the second single use ureteroscope to be approved by the US Food and Drug Administration with 3 iterations of the Pusen Uscopes (PU3011A, PU3022A, and PU3033A). The first 2 have 9F working channels and the most recent single use ureteroscope (PU3033A) has a 7.5F shaft, a 3.6F working channel, and bidirectional deflection of 270°.[20,22]

Other relevant single use ureteroscopes include the NeoFlex (Neoscope, Inc., San Jose, CA), which was released in 2016 and has a 9F shaft, a 3.6F working channel, and 270° bidirectional deflection and the YC-FR-A (YouCare Tech, Wuhan, China) with an 8F shaft, a 4.2F working channel. and 270° unidirectional deflection.[23,24] LithoVue has the greatest quantity of English-language in vivo data available in the literature, though we are beginning to see publications regarding the clinical use of some of the other devices, specifically the Pusen Uscopes. See **Table 1** for further details on the available flexible ureteroscopes.

PERFORMANCE

The ability of a flexible ureteroscope to access and properly visualize the entire collecting system is paramount for a successful ureteroscopic case. For single use ureteroscopes to be attractive, they must have comparable, if not superior, safety and efficacy to reusable ureteroscopes. Several characteristics go into ureteroscope performance, including deflection (the range of motion at the tip of the scope), irrigation (flow rate), image resolution, and field of view. Comparative studies have assessed these qualities in single use and reusable ureteroscopes in vitro, in vivo, and ex vivo.[12,19,22,24–32]

Overall, there are significant variations in these performance measures between different models, and there is no clear benefit to 1 particular category (reusable or single use) or 1 particular model over all others. For example, 1 study looking at

Table 1
Single use flexible ureteroscopes

Ureteroscope	Manufacturer	Country	Diameter (F)	Working Channel Diameter (F)	Deflection	Image Modality
Semiflex	Maxiflex	Louisiana, USA	6.0	3.4	180° Bidirectional	Fiberoptic
Polyscope	Lumenis	Yokneam, Israel	8.0	3.6	270° Unidirectional	Fiberoptic
FlexorVue	Cook	Indiana, USA	16.0	9.0	180° Unidirectional	Fiberoptic
LithoVue	Boston Scientific	Massachusetts, USA	7.7 (tip)	3.6	270° Bidirectional	Digital
Uscope PU3011 A	Pusen	Guangdong, China	9.0	3.6	270° Bidirectional	Digital
Uscope PU3022 A	Pusen	Guangdong, China	9.0	3.6	270° Bidirectional	Digital
Uscope PU3033 A	Pusen	Guangdong, China	7.5	3.6	270° Bidirectional	Digital
YC-FR-A	YouCare Tech	Wuhan, China	8.0	4.2	270° Unidirectional	Digital
YC-IU-C	YouCare Tech	Wuhan, China	8.0	4.3	270° Unidirectional	Fiberoptic
Wiscope	OTU Medical	California, USA	8.6	3.6	275° Bidirectional	Digital
AnQing EUScope	Innovex	Shanghai, China	9.3	3.6	275° Bidirectional	Digital
AXIS	Dornier Med-Tech	Munich, Germany	9.0	3.6	275° Bidirectional	Digital
Flexx-Uscope	Med-Fiber	Arizona, USA	9.0	3.0	275° Bidirectional	Digital

Overview of available single use ureteroscopes at the time of this edition. There is a wide variation on the amount of clinical data available for the individual ureteroscopes.[21,22,38]

Data from: Lithovue, Boston Scientific brochure from: http://news.bostonscientific.com/2016-01-12-Boston-Scientific-Launches-The-LithoVue-Single-Use-Digital-Flexible-Ureteroscope-In-U-S-And-Europe. August 2016; and Agrawal S, Patil A, Sabnis RB, et al. Initial experience with slimmest single-use flexible ureteroscope Uscope PU3033A (PUSEN™) in retrograde intrarenal surgery and its comparison with Uscope PU3022a: a single-center prospective study. World J Urol 2021 May 10; and Cho SY, Lee JY, Shin DG, et al. Evaluation of Performance Parameters of the Disposable Flexible Ureterorenoscope (LITHOVUE) in Patients with Renal Stones: A Prospective, Observational, Single-arm, Multicenter Study. Sci Rep 2018 Jun 28;8(1):9795.

deflection found that the single use LithoVue had the best baseline deflection at 272°, but this was comparable with the reusable Flex-X^2 at 270°, and both were significantly better than the deflection of single use Pusen (PU3011 A) at 250°.[31]

Analysis of deflection is further complicated when one considers that numerous different instruments are passed through the ureteroscope working channel, and these tools will have different effects on the deflection of different scope models. For example, a study comparing 4 single use ureteroscopes (LithoVue, Pusen, Neoflex, and YouCare Tech) with 4 reusable ureteroscopes (URF-V2, Flex X^c, Cobra vision, and Boa vision) found that the single use ureteroscopes had better deflection in vitro than the reusable ureteroscopes, but this advantage disappeared when less flexible tools occupied the working channel, at which time the reusable flexible ureteroscopes performed better.[25]

Adequate irrigation is necessary to clear blood, stone fragments, and debris out of the field of view during ureteroscopy. Similar to deflection, irrigation measurements (by flow rate) are both model and situation dependent. For example, the LithoVue has similar absolute flow rates as the reusable Flex-X^c and Cobra Fiberoptic ureteroscope, but with various instruments in the working channel, the LithoVue and Flex-X^c had comparable decrease in flow rates, whereas the Cobra Fiberoptic did not lose flow because it has 2 side-by-side working channels to preserve flow.[29] Marchini and colleagues[31] compared 2 single use ureteroscopes (Pusen Uscope and LithoVue) with the reusable Flex-X[2] and found the Uscope had the best flow rate with an empty working channel, but rates were comparable between the Uscope and LithoVue with a 200-micron laser, 365-micron laser, and the 1.3F basket, both being superior to the Flex-X.[2] The LithoVue outperformed both other ureteroscopes when a 1.9F basket was inserted through the working port.[31]

When comparing image resolution of a 1951 US Air Force Test Pattern Card, LithoVue had higher resolution power than either Uscope or Flex-X.[2,31] In an unblinded postprocedure survey, urologists ranked the reusable digital URF-V2 as having the best visibility when compared with the LithoVue and then Uscope (PU3022 A), whereas the LithoVue was considered to be the most maneuverable.[26] Field of view comparisons between different models have demonstrated a range from 75° to 87°.[30,31]

Although there is not a clear benefit to reusable or single use ureteroscopes, several studies have shown that single use ureteroscopes are safe and their performance is not inferior to reusable ureteroscopes. The LithoVue is the most widely studied single use ureteroscope with several studies showing that it is safe for patient care.[11,27,28] A few clinical trials have also looked at the Pusen Uscopes.[24,32] In a prospective, multicenter cohort study, the Uscope PU3022A performed well in terms of maneuverability and deflection compared with the individual institutions' standard reusable ureteroscope, but poor intraoperative image quality was a concern. Overall, surgeons still said they would prefer to use the Uscope over their standard reusable flexible ureteroscope.[32] Comparing the second-generation Uscope (PU3022A) with the third-generation Uscope (PU3033A) in a prospective randomized trial of 30 patients, Agrawal and colleagues[22] found vision, maneuverability, and deflection to be comparable with the benefit of the PU3033A having a smaller shaft (7.5F vs 9.0F).

ENVIRONMENTAL IMPACT

The environmental impact of surgical equipment has drawn more attention in recent years. Manufacturing, sterilization, repackaging, and repairs, as well as solid waste disposal of equipment, add up to a significant environmental burden. Comparing the carbon footprint between single use and reusable equipment gives insight into the environmental impact of medical equipment and procedures.

Woods and colleagues found that the environmental impact of minimally invasive surgery per year in the United States was more than the total estimated CO_2 emissions of 27 countries.[33,34] Previous studies looking at the environmental impact of reusable versus disposable medical equipment have found mixed results. Comparing disposable versus reusable laparoscopic instruments, reusable items had lower CO_2 emissions and water use than did single use variants.[35] Although another study comparing the carbon footprint of central venous catheter insertion kits found the environmental cost of the reusable kits was much higher than the disposable kits.[36]

With regard to reusable and single use ureteroscopes, the data are quite limited, and there is only 1 publication on this topic as of this writing. To evaluate the environmental impact of flexible ureteroscopes, Davis and colleagues[33] compared the carbon footprint of reusable versus single use flexible ureteroscopes. Using the presumption that a reusable flexible ureteroscope has 16 uses before needing repairs and a typical life cycle of 180 uses before decommissioning, they compared the carbon footprint of ureteroscopy with a reusable flexible ureteroscope (URV-F or Olympus Flexible Video Ureteroscope) with that of a single use ureteroscope (the LithoVue). The solid waste generated (in kilograms) and energy consumed (in kilowatt hours) were quantified and converted to the mass of carbon dioxide (kilograms of CO_2) released.[33]

Perhaps surprisingly, the carbon costs were almost identical with the single use ureteroscope estimated at 4.43 kg of CO_2 versus 4.47 kg of CO_2 for the reusable ureteroscope. What differed, however, were the drivers of carbon waste. With the single use ureteroscope, the manufacturing process accounted for 3.83 kg of CO_2, or 86% of the per-procedure carbon cost. For the reusable scope, sterilization accounted for almost 90% of the carbon waste (3.95 kg CO_2).[33] Thus, although the total carbon footprints were roughly equivalent, future innovations in manufacturing and/or sterilization technologies could eventually favor one technology over another with regards to environmental cost. It is also worth noting that this study only looked at 2 specific models, and that other current devices could have significantly different carbon footprints. These environmental costs remain an important but understudied aspect of ureteroscopy.

FUTURE DIRECTIONS

Although the development of single use flexible ureteroscopes is driven by costly reprocessing and repairs as well as concern for contamination, there is not a clear benefit to reusable or single use ureteroscopes at this time. Further research is needed to outline the environmental impact of both single use and reusable ureteroscopes, as well as innovations to help decrease the carbon footprint of both, by decreased manufacturing costs and waste as well as decreased waste in repairs and reprocessing.

Although the market is seeing a number of new single use flexible ureteroscopes, it is difficult to parse out from the literature which ureteroscope would be better for a surgeon or institution. Although studies have looked at individual aspects of the ureteroscope performance and cost, no standardized way to evaluate the ureteroscopes has been used. A validated flexible ureteroscope evaluation tool was created by Bell and colleagues[37] and the use of this instrument could help to standardize the way we compare new ureteroscopes as they come to market.

SUMMARY

Given the heterogeneity in different performance measures between single use and reusable models, with and without instruments, neither category of ureteroscope has a clear advantage, and either can be used successfully. As with cost, individual and institution level factors are more important than broad generalizations of superiority or inferiority. Surgeons should familiarize themselves with the particular strengths and weakness of the devices they have at their disposal. Performance of the ureteroscope will depend on the fit between device characteristics, surgical technique, and the particulars of the case.

DISCLOSURE

The authors have no direct or indirect commercial financial incentive associated with publishing this article, and there was no extra-institutional funding.

REFERENCES

1. Scales CD Jr, Smith AC, Hanley JM, et al. Urologic Diseases in America Project. Prevalence of kidney stones in the United States. Eur Urol 2012;62:160.
2. Oberlin DT, Flum AS, Bachrach L, et al. Contemporary surgical trends in the management of upper tract calculi. J Urol 2015;193(3):880–4.
3. Ordon M, Urbach D, Mamdani M, et al. The surgical management of kidney stone disease: a population based time series analysis. J Urol 2014;192(5):1450–6.
4. Afane JS, Olweny EO, Bercowsky E, et al. Flexible ureteroscopes: a single center evaluation of the durability and function of the new endoscopes smaller than 9Fr. J Urol 2000;164(4):1164–8.
5. Al-Balushi K, Martin N, Loubon H, et al. Comparative medico-economic study of reusable vs. single-use flexible ureteroscopes. Int Urol Nephrol 2019;51(10):1735–41.
6. Monga M, Landman J, Conradie MC, et al. Assessment of a new flexible ureteroscope designed for durability of function (abstract). J Endourol 2001;15(suppl). D3/P3.
7. Landman J, Lee DI, Lee C, et al. Evaluation of overall costs of currently available small flexible ureteroscopes. Urology 2003;62(2):218–22.
8. Isaacson D, Ahmad T, Metzler I, et al. Defining the Costs of Reusable Flexible Ureteroscope Reprocessing Using Time-Driven Activity-Based Costing. J Endourol 2017;31(10):1026–31.
9. Martin CJ, McAdams SB, Abdul-Muhsin H, et al. The economic implications of a reusable flexible digital ureteroscope: a cost-benefit analysis. J Urol 2017;197(3 Pt 1):730–5.
10. Taguchi K, Usawachintachit M, Tzou DT, et al. Micro-costing analysis demonstrates comparable costs for LithoVue compared to reusable flexible fiberoptic ureteroscopes. J Endourol 2018;32(4):267–73.
11. Mager R, Kurosch M, Höfner T, et al. Clinical outcomes and costs of reusable and single-use flexible ureterorenoscopes: a prospective cohort study. Urolithiasis 2018;46(6):587–93.
12. Hennessey DB, Fojecki GL, Papa NP, et al. Single-use disposable digital flexible ureteroscopes: an ex vivo assessment and cost analysis. BJU Int 2018;121(Suppl 3):55–61.
13. Bronowicki JP, Venard V, Botté C, et al. Patient-to-patient transmission of hepatitis C virus during colonoscopy. N Engl J Med 1997;337(4):237–40.
14. Wendelboe AM, Baumbach J, Blossom DB, et al. Outbreak of cystoscopy related infections with Pseudomonas aeruginosa: New Mexico, 2007. J Urol 2008;180(2):588–92 [discussion: 592].
15. Legemate JD, Kamphuis GM, Freund JE, et al. Pre-use ureteroscope contamination after high level disinfection: reprocessing effectiveness and the relation with cumulative ureteroscope use. J Urol 2019;201(6):1144–51.
16. Ofstead CL, Heymann OL, Quick MR, et al. The effectiveness of sterilization for flexible ureteroscopes: A real-world study. Am J Infect Control 2017;45(8):888–95.
17. Bader MJ, Gratzke C, Walther S, et al. The PolyScope: a modular design, semidisposable flexible ureterorenoscope system. J Endourol 2010;24(7):1061–6.
18. Gu SP, Huang YT, You ZY, et al. Clinical effectiveness of the PolyScope™ endoscope system

combined with holmium laser lithotripsy in the treatment of upper urinary calculi with a diameter of less than 2 cm. Exp Ther Med 2013;6(2):591–5.
19. Proietti S, Dragos L, Molina W, et al. Comparison of new single-use digital flexible ureteroscope versus nondisposable fiber optic and digital ureteroscope in a cadaveric model. J Endourol 2016;30(6):655–9.
20. Schlager D, Obaid MA, Hein S, et al. Current disposable ureteroscopes: performance and limitations in a standardized kidney model. J Endourol 2020; 34(10):1015–20.
21. Lithovue, Boston Scientific brochure from. 2016. Available at: http://news.bostonscientific.com/2016-01-12-Boston-Scientific-Launches-The-LithoVue-Single-Use-Digital- Flexible-Ureteroscope-In-U-S-And-Europe. Accessed May 26, 2021.
22. Agrawal S, Patil A, Sabnis RB, et al. Initial experience with slimmest single-use flexible ureteroscope Uscope PU3033A (PUSEN™) in retrograde intrarenal surgery and its comparison with Uscope PU3022a: a single-center prospective study. World J Urol 2021. https://doi.org/10.1007/s00345-021-03707-4.
23. NeoFlex- Flexible, Single Use UreteroScope™ Neoscope. Available at: https://neoscope2020.com/?portfolio=flex-ureteroscope. Accessed May 26, 2021.
24. Salvadó JA, Olivares R, Cabello JM, et al. Retrograde intrarenal surgery using the single - use flexible ureteroscope Uscope 3022 (Pusen™): evaluation of clinical results. Cent Eur J Urol 2018; 71(2):202–7.
25. Dragos LB, Martis SM, Somani BK, et al. MP68-03 comparison of eight digital (reusable and disposable) flexible ureteroscopes deflection properties: in-vitro study in 10 different scope settings. J Urol 2018;199:e917.
26. Kam J, Yuminaga Y, Beattie K, et al. Single use versus reusable digital flexible ureteroscopes: a prospective comparative study. Int J Urol 2019;26(10): 999–1005.
27. Usawachintachit M, Isaacson DS, Taguchi K, et al. A prospective case-control study comparing LithoVue, a single-use, flexible disposable ureteroscope, with flexible, reusable fiber-optic ureteroscopes. J Endourol 2017;31(5):468–75.
28. Cho SY, Lee JY, Shin DG, et al. Evaluation of performance parameters of the disposable flexible ureterorenoscope (LITHOVUE) in patients with renal stones: a prospective, observational, single-arm, multicenter study. Sci Rep 2018;8(1):9795.
29. Dale J, Kaplan AG, Radvak D, et al. Evaluation of a novel single-use flexible ureteroscope. J Endourol 2017;35(6):903–7.
30. Tom WR, Wollin DA, Jiang R, et al. Next-generation single-use ureteroscopes: an in vitro comparison. J Endourol 2017;31(12):1301–6.
31. Marchini GS, Batagello CA, Monga M, et al. In vitro evaluation of single-use digital flexible ureteroscopes: a practical comparison for a patient-centered approach. J Endourol 2018;32(3):184–91.
32. Johnston TJ, Baard J, de la Rosette J, et al. A clinical evaluation of the new digital single-use flexible ureteroscope (UscopePU3022): an international prospective multicentered study. Cent Eur J Urol 2018;71(4):453–61.
33. Davis NF, McGrath S, Quinlan M, et al. Carbon footprint in flexible ureteroscopy: a comparative study on the environmental impact of reusable and single-use ureteroscopes. J Endourol 2018;32(3): 214–7.
34. Woods DL, Mcandrew T, Nevadunsky N, et al. Carbon footprint of robotically-assisted laparoscopy, laparoscopy and laparotomy: a comparison. Int J Med Robot Comput Assist Surg 2015;11:406–12.
35. Adler S, Scherrer M, Ruckauer KD, et al. Comparison of economic and environmental impacts between disposable and reusable instruments used for laparoscopic cholecystectomy. Surg Endosc Other Interv Tech 2005;19:268–72.
36. McGain F, McAlister S, McGavin A, et al. A life cycle assessment of reusable and single-use central venous catheter insertion kits. Anesth Analg 2012; 114:1073–80.
37. Bell JR, Penniston KL, Best SL, et al. Prospective evaluation of flexible ureteroscopes with a novel evaluation tool. Can J Urol 2017;24(5):9004–10.
38. Ventimiglia E, Somani BK, Traxer O. Flexible ureteroscopy: reuse? Or is single use the new direction? Curr Opin Urol 2020;30(2):113–9.

Mini Percutaneous Kidney Stone Removal

Applicable Technologies

Janak Desai, MS, MCh, FRCS[a,*], Hemendra N. Shah, MD, MCh, MRCS[b]

KEYWORDS

• PCNL • Mini-PCNL • Minimally invasive PCNL • Miniperc • Microperc • Ultramini PCNL • Super-mini PCNL • Complications

KEY POINTS

- Miniaturized PCNL is gaining momentum because it reduces morbidity of the procedure of PCNL at the same time retaining the flavor of high stone free rates.
- Mini-PCNL, Ultra-Mini-PCNL, and Micro-PCNL are the new options of PCNL, which can be judiciously used for properly selected indications.
- Various miniaturized PCNL techniques should assist urologists in providing a personalized approach to the patient based on various patient- and stone-related factors to provide the best of all available technology for treatment.
- Additional high-quality randomized control trials comparing various available miniaturized PCNL techniques are needed to define their true place in urologist armamentarium.

INTRODUCTION

Percutaneous nephrolithotomy (PCNL) remains the treatment of choice for large and complex renal stones because it leads to a higher rate of stone clearance as compared with Shockwave lithotripsy or retrograde intrarenal surgery. Although considered safe, it is still associated with a small but definitive risk of bleeding, infection, and other postoperative morbidity.

The technological advances over the past several decades coupled with a constant quest to improve patient outcomes by reducing morbidity and postoperative complication resulted in the development of miniaturized instruments for mini-PCNL. This was aided secondarily by simultaneous advancements in optics and imaging techniques, as well as in energy devices for stone fragmentation.

Here, the authors aim to provide a bird's-eye view of various miniaturized technologies for PCNL.

EVOLUTION OF MINI-PERCUTANEOUS NEPHROLITHOTOMY

The first removal of a renal stone under endoscopic guidance was performed by Rupel and Brown[1] in 1941; however, it required another 35 years for the first percutaneous removal of a renal stone under radiological guidance in 1976 by Fernström and Johansson.[2] These investigators used a cystoscopy with rigid stone grasper to visualize the stone and extract it intact via a 26F nephrostomy tract. In 1977, Peter Alken in collaboration with Karl Storz (Tuttlingen, Germany) developed a percutaneous nephroscope, which allowed for both irrigation and suction. Arthur Smith,[3] who coined term "endourology," is credited with performing the initial seminal work on percutaneous renal surgery in the United States. He worked with Kurt Amplatz and developed a 30F Amplatz sheath. The logic behind using a 30F sheath was the understanding that it would facilitate the intact retrieval of a 1-cm

[a] Department of Urology, Samved Hospital, 2nd Floor, Navrangpura, Ahmedabad 380009, India; [b] Department of Urology, University of Miami Miller School of Medicine, 1150 NW 14th street, Suite 309, Miami, FL 33136, USA

* Corresponding author.

E-mail address: drjanakddesai@gmail.com

Urol Clin N Am 49 (2022) 161–173
https://doi.org/10.1016/j.ucl.2021.08.003

kidney stone. This initial concept however gave birth to a tradition of using a 24 to 30F nephrostomy sheath as the standard of care for renal access in PCNL.[4] Initially, in the1980s, PCNL was advocated as an alternative modality of kidney stone removal in patients who were high risk for traditional open surgery.[4] However, soon the safety and efficacy of the procedure was demonstrated, and the PCNL became a primary modality for the treatment of large renal stones.

The encouraging early results of percutaneous stone removal in adults led pediatric surgeons to embrace PCNL techniques for managing renal calculi in children. The first pediatric PCNL series was reported by Woodside and colleagues[5] in 1985, wherein adult instruments were used to remove stones in 7 children (5–18 years of age). The investigators however commented that "[i]t would seem desirable to dilate as small a percutaneous tract as possible...Younger children may require the use of smaller percutaneous tracts and instruments." However, for more than a decade, the tract size for pediatric PCNL continued to be 24 or 30F. In 1997, Helal and colleagues[6] published a case report of a 2-year child who underwent PCNL using a 10F pediatric cystoscope through a 15F Hickman Peel-Away Sheath. The investigators noted that their technique allowed them to use smaller endoscopes with shorter instruments, thereby providing the benefit of better control of the instruments and easier manipulation of the stone fragments, in addition to avoiding extensive tract dilation in small kidneys.

The term "mini-perc" was first described by Jackman and colleagues[7] in 1998 while describing use of an 11F peel-away vascular access sheath with a pediatric cystoscopy or flexible ureteroscope in infants and preschool age children for percutaneous removal of calculi. The investigators also modified the access sheath set in conjunction with Cook Urological by reducing the sheath length from 15 to 10 cm and the exposed trocar length from 5 to 1 cm. The same group also observed that 24 or 30F access for PCNL in adults, although effective, was an invasive procedure with a blood transfusion requirement in 3% to 23% of patients and was associated with prolonged postoperative pain and hospitalization. Therefore, they recommended extending their mini-perc technique to treat adults with renal stones less than 2 cm with the aim of reducing renal trauma and possibly circumventing some of the limitations in the conventional PCNL technique of the era.[8] The investigators defined "mini-perc" as a PCNL achieved through a sheath too small to accommodate standard rigid nephroscope available at that time (24 or 28F). They used a 13F sheath with a ureteroscope or pediatric cystoscope to access and remove stones. They thought that smaller sheaths would greatly reduce the volume of renal tissue displaced and compressed, require a smaller size nephrostomy tube postoperatively, and decrease blood loss, postoperative pain, and length of hospital stay. Other investigators similarly described promising initial success with the use of a13F ureteral access sheath or 20F access sheath along with a semirigid ureteroscope for mini-PCNL.[9,10] These fruitful efforts toward miniaturization lead researchers to innovate and develop techniques and instruments specific for miniaturized PCNL.[11] The evolution in the technique to decrease the morbidity of the conventional PCNL gave birth to different varieties of minimally invasive PCNLs (MPCNL), which include the mini-PCNL, ultra-mini-PCNL, super-mini-PCNL, and micro-PCNL, with the indications being extended to stones even larger than 20 mm (**Fig. 1**). This was made possible because of simultaneous progress in the optics and imaging

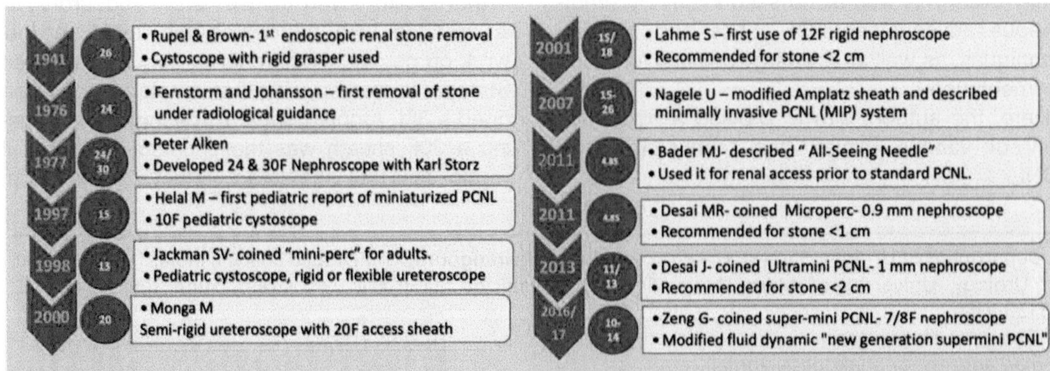

Fig. 1. Evolution of miniaturized PCNL.

techniques and efficient energy devices, like Holmium and Thulium fiber lasers.

Mini-Percutaneous Nephrolithotomy

In 1998, Jackman and colleagues defined mini-PCNL as PCNL performed with a less than 24F sheath. Thereafter, for more than a decade, mini-PCNL was performed using a pediatric cystoscopy and/or a ureteroscope (semirigid or flexible). For the first time in 2001, Lahme and colleagues[12] evaluated a 12F rigid nephroscope specifically designed for MPCNL. A 15 or 18F sheath was recommended to be placed after a one-step dilatation. The working channel was 6F, large enough to accommodate various stone fragmentation energy sources, including ballistic, ultrasound, or laser lithotripsy. The technique was recommended as an option for stones less than 2 cm. The inventors also demonstrated that the cross-sectional area of their 12F MPCNL was one-fifth of a conventional nephroscope of 26F caliber. However, the inventors also cautioned that the limit of MPCNL is when the time taken to fragment larger stones to size small enough to be extracted is no longer acceptable.

Minimally Invasive Percutaneous Nephrolithotomy

In 2007, Nagele and colleagues[11] modified the Amplatz Sheath for MIP. Instead of using the conventional nephroscope sheath with a seal cap and Luer-Lok outflow system, they advocated for the use of an open nephroscope sheath with a curved outlet without a sealing cap. The investigators found that the MIP has advantages of reducing intrapelvic pressure (IPP) as compared with the conventional closed outflow system. MIP instruments are available in different sizes, as shown in **Table 1** and **Fig. 2**.

Aside from single-step dilatation, the primary advantage of MIP is the spontaneous evacuation of stone fragments owing to the suction generated from a combination of low-pressure irrigation at tip of nephroscope and the retraction motion of the nephroscope from the sheath (Bernouilli's principle). Use of a relatively large sheath as compared with the size of the nephroscope results in a "whirlpool effect" that allows a flow of irrigation fluid in the space between sheath and nephroscope, which facilitates movement of stone fragments out of the sheath. Conversely, use of a sheath that is tight fitting with the nephroscope results in a "vacuum cleaner effect" in which irrigation fluid surrounds the stone and creates an upward force on stone toward the nephroscope, thereby resulting in spontaneous extraction of stone fragments through the sheath without a separate need for mechanical extraction.

ULTRA-MINI-PERCUTANEOUS NEPHROLITHOTOMY

In 2013, Desai and Solanki[13] described the ultra-mini-PCNL (UMP) technique, whereby dilatation is limited to either 11F or 13F. A UMP system consists of an ultrathin 1-mm telescope having a resolution of 17,000 pixels, and an inner sheath of 6.0F, which has 2 ports (one for the irrigation and the other for a laser fiber), and an outer sheath of 11F or 13F with a side port that connects to a very thin tube running parallel to its lumen (**Fig. 3**). Investigators recommend fragmentation using a 200- or 365-μm laser fiber with the aim of creating fragments less than 2 mm in greatest dimension. In addition, to facilitate evacuation of stone fragments, a vortex can be created by the retrograde injection of saline through the urethral ureteric catheter. The resultant fluid movement from a high-pressure zone in the renal pelvis to a low-pressure zone within the lumen of the outer sheath results in spontaneous evacuation of fragments by the vortex when the nephoscope is withdrawn. On certain occasions, the placement of a

Table 1
Nomenclature for subtypes of minimally invasive percutaneous nephrolithotomy

Type of MIP	Nephroscope Size (F)	Working and Irrigation Channel	Sheath Size Recommended (F)	Stone Size Recommendations (mm)
MIP S/XS	7.5	Separate 2F working channel and 3F irrigation channel	11/12	8–15
MIP M	12	6.7F single channel	15/16 16.5/17.5 21/22	10–30
MIP L	19.5	12.4F single channel	23/24 25/26	Staghorn & >15

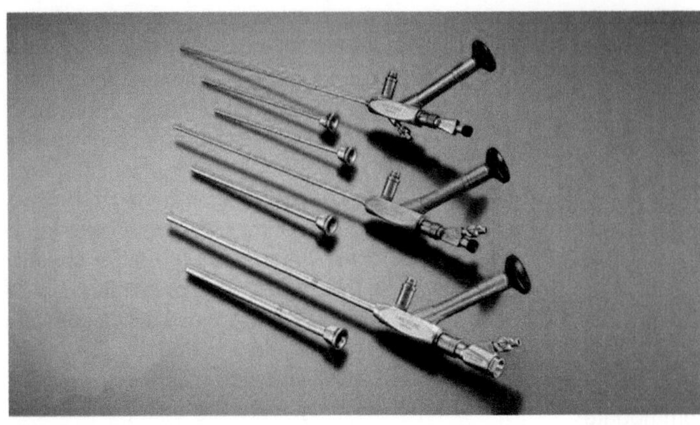

Fig. 2. Instrumentation for MPCNL. (© KARL STORZ SE & Co. KG, Germany.)

low suction on the end of the outer sheath is recommended to aid in fragment removal. UMP was initially recommended for stones less than 20 mm. In addition, it can also be used as an ancillary procedure to remove stones from a difficult calyx while treating a large staghorn stone, which may require a second access.[14,15]

SUPER-MINI-PERCUTANEOUS NEPHROLITHOTOMY

The super-mini-PCNL (SMP) was introduced by Zeng and coinvestigators[16] in 2016. Their first-generation SMP system was made of a 7F nephroscope with a dismountable sheath. A 1-mm telescope was inserted through the dismountable sheath with built-in two 0.6-mm OD/0.4-mm ID fine tubes located at the left and right side of the lumen, just lateral to the space for the fiberoptic bundle. The nephroscope has a 3.3F working and irrigation channel and is used with a modified access sheath made of clear plastic that has a bifurcated proximal segment compromising a straight and an oblique tube at 45°. Sheaths of varying internal diameters of 10F, 12F, and 14F are available, and the internal

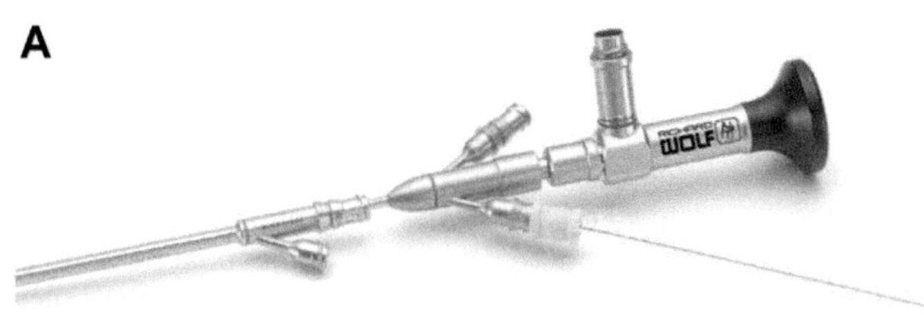

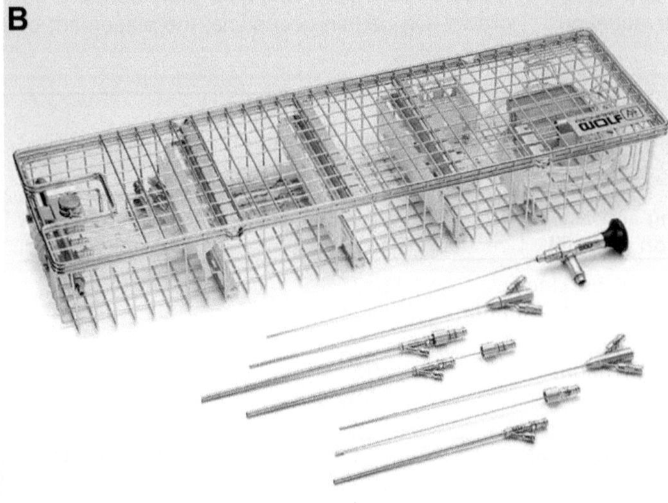

Fig. 3. Instrumentation for ultra-mini-PCNL. (*A*) Assembled ultra-mini PCNL nephroscope with sheath; (*B*) Components of ultra-mini PCNL. (Picture provided by Richard Wolf; © Richard Wolf, all rights reserved)

diameter of the straight and the oblique tubes is the same as that of the access sheath. The oblique tube can connect to a negative pressure aspirator for vacuum suction, as is typically set to a negative pressure of 150 to 200 mm Hg. It also bears a venting slit along the longitudinal axis for regulating pressure. The active suction makes this technique different from other miniaturized PCNL techniques. The investigators recommend connecting the irrigation port of the nephroscope to an irrigation pump. Initially, they recommended using this technique to treat renal stones less than 2.5 cm in maximum dimension.

Although initial results were encouraging, the investigators soon realized that the since main irrigation and working channel were the same, there was dramatic reduction in irrigation efficiency once the laser fiber or pneumatic lithotripter probe was inserted. Also, the flexibility of the plastic sheath resulted in the nephroscope being damaged on scope bending. Hence, they modified their first-generation SMP and reported their initial results with a new-generation SMP system.[17]

The new-generation SMP has an 8F nephroscope with a 3.3F working channel (**Fig. 4**). It has a 2-layered metal suction-irrigation sheath, which is available in 12F and 14F. The gap between the 2 layers of the metal sheath function as an irrigation channel, and the central lumen of the sheath serves as a conduit for continuous suction. The investigators recommend use of pressure pump for continuous irrigation and attaching a negative pressure aspirator to the oblique tube of the sheath. The suction actively removes small stone debris, and the larger stone fragments are removed by the vacuum cleaner effect augmented by active suction when the nephroscope is withdrawn past the suction port.

The advantage of the new-generation SMP was attributable to changes in fluid dynamics.[18] The initial first-generation SMP system had 1 lumen for both inflow and outflow of fluid. Hence, the pressurized irrigation would partially offset the effect of outflow, thereby preventing spontaneous retrieval of stone fragments. The modified new-generation SMP system completely separates the lumen for fluid inflow and outflow, thereby creating a one-way flow. This improved fluid dynamic resulted in better visibility and retrieval of stone fragments, which translated into significant shortening of the operative time.

MicroPerc

In 2011, Desai and colleagues[19] described a novel variation of the mini-PCNL that he called the Microperc, wherein renal access is accomplished in a single step with the use of an all-seeing needle with a 4.85F tract size. The 3-part all-seeing needle (PolyDiagnost, Pfaffenhofen, Germany) consisted of a 0.9-mm micro-optic and a 1.6-mm (4.85F) outer diameter needle and was first described by Bader and colleagues.[20] A multijointed mounting arm with an attached camera and light cable is needed to relay optics (**Fig. 5**). After puncturing the targeted calyx with an all-seeing needle, the stylet is removed, and a 3-way connector is attached to the needle (see **Fig. 5**). A 200-μm laser fiber then passes through the central channel, and an irrigation connection and telescope are attached to each of the side port. The limited tract size requires a pressurized irrigation system, which is drained by the per-urethrally placed ureteric catheter, which can be augmented with manual suction through the ureteric catheter when necessary. The main disadvantages include inability to retrieve stone fragments, thereby limiting the procedure for treatment of stones less than 1 cm. This technique may have an advantage in treating a stone considered unsuitable for shock wave

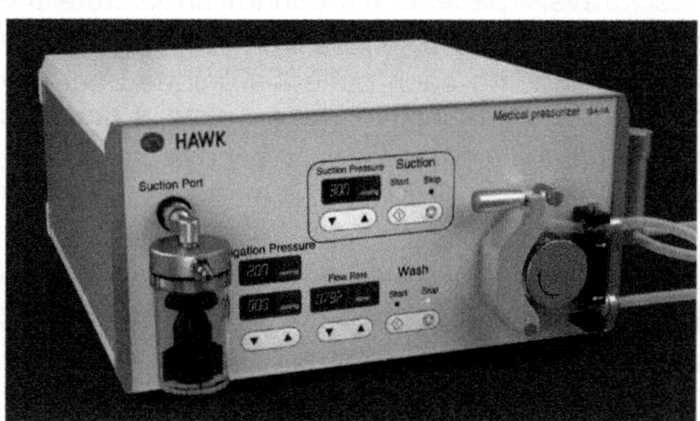

Fig. 4. Instrumentation for super-mini-PCNL. (*From* Zeng G., Zhu W. (2020) Super-Mini-PCNL (SMP). In: Zeng G., Sarica K. (eds) Percutaneous Nephrolithotomy. Springer, Singapore. https://doi.org/10.1007/978-981-15-0575-1_15)

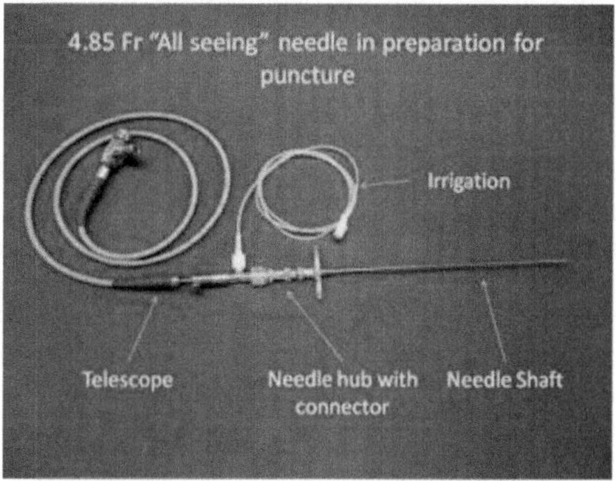

Fig. 5. Instrumentation for microperc. (*Courtesy of* Mahesh Desai, MS, FRCS, FRCS, FACS, Gujarat, India, with permission)

lithotripsy secondary to stone composition or unfavorable pelvi-calyceal system anatomy.

Mini-Micro-Percutaneous Nephrolithotomy

After initially encouraging results with microperc, the investigators soon realized that the needle would bend when attempts were made to manipulate it within the pelvicalyceal system. This can potentially lead to parenchymal tear during excessive attempts for intrarenal manipulations. To overcome this problem, the inventors designed an 8F metallic sheath, which they called the "mini-microperc" sheath, as it allows the attachment of the same 3-way connector with accessories as in standard microperc. This mini-microperc sheath provided investigators with the ability to manipulate the scope more facilely, enabling the use of a 1.6-mm ultrasonic lithotripter for stone fragmentation, and also for active retrieval of stone fragments with simultaneous suction.[21]

IS MINIATURIZED PERCUTANEOUS NEPHROLITHOTOMY LESS TRAUMATIC TO KIDNEY?

From the inception of endourology, there were concerns about the possible renal damage by percutaneous nephrostomies. Renal trauma can be anatomic or physiologic related to IPP during surgery. In 1985, Webb and colleagues[22] demonstrated that a nephrostomy tract of up to 30F in dogs did not cause any significant renal parenchymal loss as measured by microfilm casts, contrast radiography, and angiography. They also showed that all nephrostomy tracts healed to a very small scar. Extrapolating from the canines, they concluded that, in humans, a nephrostomy tract size of 35 to 50F would be similarly safe. Two years later, Clayman and colleagues[23] further confirmed the safety of PCNL and noted that the renal damage from the nephrostomy tract averaged 0.15% of the total renal cortical surface. The damage caused by balloon dilation to 36F was found equivalent to that caused by fascial dilation to 24F. Because balloon dilatation was rapid and easier to perform, the investigators recommend balloon dilatation to 30F because it would allow en bloc removal of a stone with a largest dimension of up to 1.2 cm. In addition, they found that the method of dilation (Amplatz sequential fascial dilation vs balloon dilation) did not influence the degree of renal trauma.[24] To evaluate influence of tract size on renal damage, Traxer and colleagues[25] evaluated the effects of placing either an 11F or 30F in dog kidneys. After 6 weeks, they found that the mean estimated scar volume of the 30 and 11F tracts was 0.29 and 0.40 cc, indicating mean fractional parenchymal loss of 0.63% and 0.91%, respectively (*P* not significant). This study again confirmed the earlier findings of small renal parenchymal damage from the creation of a nephrostomy tract but found no advantage to the use of a small access sheath based on renal scarring alone. Conversely, when investigators studied in acute renal trauma in both porcine and cadaveric kidney models, using12 types of dilation devices ranging from 4.8 to 30F (including micro and mini-PCNL kits, the Alken dilation set, 20 and 30 atmosphere balloons and the Amplatz set), the investigators concluded that a dilation tract of up to 24F had significantly smaller parenchymal fissures and reduced capsule rupture than when compared with 30F tracts.[26]

Another area of concern with miniaturized PCNL is the possibility of renal trauma related to high IPPs. In 1961, Hinman[27] demonstrated that high IPP leads to pyelotubular, pyelovenous, and pyelolymphatic backflow and peripelvic extravasation. When microradiographs were performed on 22 fresh pigs' kidneys after retrograde ureteral injections of a barium sulfate suspension, pyelotubular reflux occurred in all specimens at injection pressure greater than 40 mm Hg.[28] The severity of pyelotubular reflux increased as IPP increased up to 60 mm Hg, but interestingly, above 60 mm Hg, there was less pronounced reflux. Pyelolymphatic filling was always associated with ruptured fornices and pyelointerstitial backflow and only occurred at greater than 60 mm Hg. The pyelovenous backflow was observed only at pelvic pressures of $\geq$100 mm Hg. Nagle and colleagues[11] showed that in a cadaver porcine model, when a 12F nephroscope was used with a conventional 18F nephroscope sheath with a seal cap and Luer-Lok outflow system, when the control sheath was closed, the IPP increased to a maximum of 136 cm H_2O. However, when the same nephroscope was used with a modified 18F miniperc sheath with constant outflow from its open proximal end, the maximal IPP remained low at 20 cm H_2O even when the inflow pressure reached 125 cm H_2O. The investigators concluded that when performing a miniperc with a modified sheath, strict irrigation fluid control was not necessary. Similarly, in vitro studies evaluating different working sheaths sizes (15/16F, 16.5/17.5F, and 21/22F), and a 12F mininephroscope found that all (IPPs remained less than 50 cm H_2O and that at fixed irrigation pressure there was significant reduction in IPP with an increasing operating sheath diameter.[29]

Nephron damage was seen under electron microscopy when IPP exceeded 20 mm Hg.[30,31] This damage was more pronounced in the presence of pyonephrosis. When comparing the safety of mini-PCNL performed with a 14/16F ureteral access

Table 2
Review of literature of various randomized control trial comparing various technique of miniaturized percutaneous nephrolithotomy

Author Year Country Study Period Stone Size Included	N	Stone Size	Access Sheath	Dilatation	Scope Size	Lithotripsy Method	Duration of Surgery (min)	Hb Drop (g/dL)	BT (%)	Complications (%)	SFR-Timing Imaging Used Definition	Stone-Free Rate (%)	Comments
Mini PCNL (MP) compared with standard PCNL (SP)													
Cheng,[35] 2010 China 2004–2007 NS Single Tract	72 MP	9.8 cm^2	16 PA	NA	8/9.8	PL	S-134.3 ± 19.7 RP-89.4 ± 21.5 MC-113.9 ± 20.3	0.53 ± 0.79	1.4	Fever- 20.8: PT: 1.4	1 wk US & KUB <4 mm RF	72.2 92.6 85.2	• 1st RCT assessing MP • Patients with multitract excluded • 52 patients needed conversion from MP to SP and were excluded
	115 SP $	10.1 cm^2	24	NA	20.8	UL + PL	S-118.9 ± 21.5 RP-77.0 ± 17.6 MC-101.2 ± 19.1	0.97 ± 1.42	10.4	Fever: 23.5 Urine leak: 1.7		75.9 91.3 70.0	
Guler,[36] 2019 Turkey 2016–2017 >2 cm	51 MP	38.7 ± 13.1 mm	16.5/20	AD	12	LL	89.2 ± 40.4	1.35 ± 1.11	2	CG1: 3.9 CG2: 2 CG3: 7.8	1 mo CT SFR: ND	76.5	• Shorter hospitalization time with MP • More tubeless with MP
	46 SP	42.8 ± 22.5 mm	30	BD	26	PL	74.7 ± 44.5	2.07 ± 1.59	15.2	CG1: 4.3 CG2: 13 CG3: 6.5		71.7	
Kandemir,[37] 2020 Turkey 2016–2018 >2 cm	76 MP	33.6 ± 8.1 mm	16.5/20	AD	12/14	LL	106.9 ± 38.8	0.7 ± 1.3	2.6	CG1: 9.2 CG2: 1.3 CG3: 10.5	3-mo CT <4 mm RF	75	• All had history of PCNL or open renal surgery • Shorter hospitalization time with MP • More tubeless with MP
	72 SP	33.1 ± 10.9 mm	30	AD/BD	26	UL/PL/LL	91.2 ± 33.2	1.4 ± 0.46	5.6	CG1: 8.3 CG2: 4.2 CG3: 11.1		72.2	

(*continued on next page*)

Table 2 (continued)

Author Year Country Study Period Stone Size Included	N	Stone Size	Access Sheath	Dilatation	Scope Size	Lithotripsy Method	Duration of Surgery (min)	Hb Drop (g/dL)	BT (%)	Complications (%)	SFR-Timing Imaging Used Definition	Stone-Free Rate (%)	Comments
Zhong,[38] 2011	29 MP	11.7 (8.8–22.8) cm^2	16	FD	8/9.8	PL	116 (96–130)	3.2 (2.3–4.1)	3.4	37.9	1 d KUB	82.8	Multiple minitract had higher clearance and less bleeding for staghorn calculi
China 2008–2009 Staghorn	25 SP	10.8 (8.4–20.2) cm^2	26	AD	NA	PL	103 (88–105)	3.5 (2.8–5.0)	12	52	<4 mm RF	56	
Sakr,[39] 2017 Egypt	87 MP $	2.7 ± 0.2 cm	16.5	MD	12	PL	83.2 ± 17.3	0.6 ± 0.1	1.2	CG2: 10.4 CG3: 5.8	1 d US KUB CT	91.1	No difference in postoperative pain and hospitalization
2010–2013 2–3 cm	81 SP	2.6 ± 0.6 cm	30	TMD	26	PL	78.6 ± 24.4	1.9 ± 1.1	9.8	CG2: 16 CG3: 9.8	≤4 mm	93.8	
Ultramini- PCNL (UMP) compared with standard PCNL (SP)													
Karakan,[40] 2017	47 UMP	20.3 ± 3.0 mm	14	SS MD	8/9.8	LL	55 ± 23.5	NA	0	CG1: 6.3 CG2: 2.1	1 mo CT	89.3	Shorter hospitalization and more tubeless with UMP
Turkey 2014–2016 <25 mm	50 SP	20.9 ± 3.6 mm	26	AD	22–25	US + PL	70 ± 32.7	NA	8	CG1: 4 CG2: 12 CG3: 6	<3 mm RF	88	
Haghighi,[41] 2017	35 UMP	14.26 ± 5.3 mm	16	FD	9.8	PL	48 ± 4.3	1.65 ± 1.2	5.71	11.42	2 d KUB and US	93.5	Shorter hospitalization and less postoperative pain with UMP
Iran 2016–2017 1–2 cm	35 SP	15.35 ± 5.85 mm	30	SS-AD	24	PL	51 ± 5.6	3.13 ± 1.06	11.4	20	SFR ND	94.6	
Super- Ini-PCNL (SMP) compared with standard PCNL (SP)													
Song,[42] 2011 China	30 SMP	8.57 ± 2.25 cm^2	16	FD	NA	LL	39 ± 10	90 ± 33.1#	NA	NA	3–5 d KUB	90	No difference in operating time and IPP
2008–2009 > 2 cm	30 SP	8.65 ± 2.03 cm^2	24	TMD	24	US + PL	42 ± 8	110.9 ± 35.2 #	NA	NA	CT for uric acid <4 mm	73.3	
Guddeti,[43] 2020	75 SMP	1.48 ± 0.78 cm	14	SS-MD	12/7.5	LL	36.40 ± 14.07	3.0 ± 4.9	0	Fever: 1.3	1 & 3-mo KUB + US	98.66	• Longer operating time but less postoperative pain and hospitalization with UMP
India 2018–2019 <2 cm	75 SP	1.49 ± 0.73 cm	22–30	TMD	20.8	LL/PL	23.12 ± 11.96	7.5 ± 6.5	0	Fever: 6.6 Hematuria: 2.6 PT: 1.3	SFR: ND	97.33	

Super-Mini-PCNL (SMP) compared with mini-PCNL (MP) without active suction ± standard PCNL (SP)													
Du,[44] 2018 China 2009–2015 Staghorn	311-SMP 304-MP	13.6 ± 5.2 cm^3 13.9 ± 4.7 cm^3	16–18 16–18 PA	FD	12	LL	NA	153 ± 55 172 ± 78#			3–5 d KUB, CT sos ≤4 mm	81.02% 74.01%	• Irrigation volume 600–80 mL/min, pressure- 250–300 mm Hg • Suction pressure: 100–250 mm Hg • Low IPP with SMP
	297 SP	12.4 ± 6.4 cm^3	24	FD	NA	US	NA	216 ± 140 #		—		73.06%	
Zhong,[45] 2021 China 2017–2019 2–5 cm	47 MP	3.28 ± 0.93 cm	18 PA	FD	12	LL/PL	66.9 ± 19.4	17 ± 6.7	2.12	CG1: 10.64 CG2: 14.89	2 wk CT <2 mm	87.2	• Low IPP and increased stone removal efficiency with SMP
	46 SMP	3.27 ± 0.85 cm	18	FD	11	LL/PL	51.7 ± 14.4	14.2 ± 7.6	2.17	CG1: 13.04 CG2: 6.52		91.3	
Microperc (M) compared with standard PCNL (SP)													
Tepeler,[46] 2014 Turkey 2013–2014 1–3 cm	10 M	19.9 ± 5.0 mm	4.85	NIL	3	LL	36.5 ± 14.2	1.8 ± 0.8	NA	10	1 mo CT SFR ND	80	• IPP significantly higher in microperc • Cautioned microperc use in patient with impaired drainage of collecting system
	10 SP	21.9 ± 4.8 mm	30	AD	24	PL	49 ± 9.8	3.5 ± 1.5	NA	10		90	

Abbreviations: #, EBL; $, renal units; AD, Amplatz dilators; BD, balloon dilators; CG, Clavien grade; CT, computerized tomography; FD, fascial dilators; KUB, x-ray kidney ureter and bladder; LL, laser lithotripsy; M, Microperc; MD, metal dilators; MP, mini-PCNL; N, number of patients; NA, not available; PL, pneumatic lithotripsy; PT, pneumothorax; RF, residual fragments; SFR, stone free rates; SP, standard PCNL; TM, telescoping metal dilators; UL, ultrasonic lithotripsy; US, ultrasound.

sheath and an 8/9.8F semirigid ureteroscope with a 30F sheath and 26F nephroscope in an infected kidney model, the IPPs were higher in the mini-PCNL group (18.76 ± 5.82 mm Hg vs 13.56 ± 5.82 mm Hg; $P<.0001$) and the time spent greater than 30 mm Hg was also greater in the miniperc group (117.0 seconds vs 66.1 seconds; $P = .0452$).[29] Blood cultures were positive in 30% of pigs in the mini-arm compared with none in the standard arm ($P = .0603$). These findings led the investigator to conclude that mini-PCNL was associated with higher intrarenal pressures and higher risk of end-organ bacterial seeding in the setting of an infected collecting system. In another study evaluating fluid dynamics in mini-PCNL, a 12F nephroscope was used with different operating sheath sizes: 15/16F, 16.5/17.5F, and 21/22F. The IPP was compared with standard PCNL wherein a 26F nephroscope was used with a 30F operating sheath.[32] It was noted that at a fixed irrigation pressure there was a significant reduction in IPP with an increase in the working sheath diameter.

WHAT ABOUT THE CLINICAL EVIDENCE?

Despite equivocal laboratory evidence related to advantages of miniaturized PCNL with respect to the renal trauma, multiple clinical studies have confirmed that miniaturized PCNL results in less bleeding and less requirement for blood transfusion (**Table 2**). In a retrospective study by Karaköse and colleagues,[33] as the Amplatz sheath size increased from 22F to 30F, there was a corresponding increase in the postoperative hemoglobin drop and increase in postoperative creatinine, suggesting more renal trauma associated with use of a larger sheath. However, a smaller sheath size was associated with a decreased stone-free rate. The largest prospective study conducted by the Clinical Research Office of the Endourological Society Global PCNL Study that included more than 5800 patients from 96 centers in 26 countries noted that blood transfusion requirement increased from 1.1% with ≤18F sheath size, to 4.8% with 24F to 26F, 5.9% with 27F to 30F and 12.1% with 32 to 34F.[34] This real-world data undoubtedly favor the use of smaller sheath sizes for PCNL.

There are 5 randomized control trials (RCT) comparing miniaturized PCNL (16–20F) with standard PCNL (24–30F).[35–39] The details of these studies are summarized in **Table 2**. All these studies included patients with stone size greater than 2 cm and showed a decrease in the postoperative change in hemoglobin and reduced blood transfusion requirement with miniaturized PCNL but increased operating time.

The stone-free rate was comparable among both groups, although when multiple-mini-tracts are used to treat staghorn calculi, they result in less bleeding and provide higher stone-free rates (89.7 vs 68%; $P = .049$), with an expected decrease in need for additional procedures (24.1 vs 60%; $P = .007$), whereas a similar complication rate (37.9 vs 52%; $P = .300$).[38] The mini-PCNL also permits use of a tubeless approach for an exit strategy with shorter hospitalization.[36,37]

The outcomes for UMP versus standard PCNL were evaluated in 2 RCT.[38,39] Neither of the RCTs used the UMP system as described by Desai and Solanki, and both enrolled stones greater than 2.5 cm.[13,15] The UMP system resulted in reduced intraoperative blood loss, decreased requirement of blood transfusion, and reduction in duration of surgery and hospitalization, all without compromising the stone free rate.

Similarly, 2 RCTs investigated the difference in outcomes between SMP (14–16F) and standard PCNL.[42,43] Both studies used laser lithotripsy for SMP. One study evaluated renal stones greater than 2 cm and found higher stone-free rate without an increase in operation time, and another study found that limiting stone size to less than 2 cm found longer operating time and similar stone clearance with SMP.[42,43] SMP has also been compared with other miniaturized PCNLs wherein smaller sheaths were used without active suction in 2 RCTs from China.[44,45] Both studies involved larger stones, including staghorn calculi, and showed a higher stone clearance rate with shorter operation time with SMP. In addition, SMP was associated with lower IPP as compared with mini-PCNL without suction.

There is 1 RCT comparing results of micro-PCNL (4.85) with standard PCNL (30F) for stones 1 to 3 cm in size.[46] Because of lack of time needed for dilatation and stone fragment retrieval, micro-PCNL was faster but had a lower stone-free rate. Although the complication rate was comparable in both arms, the investigators noted significantly higher IPP with microperc and cautioned against use of this technique in patients with impaired drainage of the pelvicalyceal system.

What Guidelines Have to Say About Mini-Percutaneous Nephrolithotomy

The combined American Urological Association and Endourology Society guidelines from 2016 state that PCNL with smaller access sheaths (mini-PCNL or micro-PCNL) yield outcomes similar to standard PCNL with a lower complication rate.[47,48] Regarding its role in pediatric PCNL, it mentions that "the utilization of smaller instruments for PCNL may limit the risk of hemorrhage in this population." Similarly, the EAU guidelines on a urolithiasis panel from 2021 mention that mini-PCNL tends to be associated with significantly lower blood loss at the cost of longer duration of surgery without compromising the stone-free rates.[46] They do however mention that the quality of the evidence available was poor.[49]

SUMMARY

The authors would like to repeat a statement by Arthur Smith, father of endourology, that "[e] ndourology is a field heavily reliant and affected by technological advancement. With today's technology, smaller PCNL actually gives you more maneuverability, the same ability to fragment stones and various methods for clearing fragments."[50] The available options of miniaturized PCNL should allow the physician to select the one best suited for his patient. They provide liberty to the urologist to provide a personalized approach to his patient based on various patient- and stone-related factors to provide best of all available technology for his treatment.

CLINICS CARE POINTS

- Miniaturized PCNL should be a part of endourologist armamentarium.
- It does not compromise stone free rates and is associated with low risk of bleeding when outcome to standard PCNL.
- It should be preferred in pediatric population due to lower risk of hemorrhage.

DISCLOSURE

J. Desai: Innovator of UMP; Receives royalties from Schoelly GmbH. H.N. Shah: received honorarium of $1000 from Lumenis for proctoring.

REFERENCES

1. Rupel E, Brown R. Nephroscopy with removal of stone following nephrostomy for obstructive calculous anurla. J Urol 1941;46:177–82.
2. Fernström I, Johansson B. Percutaneous pyelolithotomy. A new extraction technique. Scand J Urol Nephrol 1976;10(3):257–9.
3. Smith AD. A personal perspective on the origins of endourology and the endourological society. J Endourol 2002;16(10):705–8.
4. Wickham JE, Miller RA, Kellett MJ, et al. Percutaneous nephrolithotomy: one stage or two? Br J Urol 1984;56(6):582–5.
5. Woodside JR, Stevens GF, Stark GL, et al. Percutaneous stone removal in children. J Urol 1985; 134(6):1166–7.
6. Helal M, Black T, Lockhart J, et al. The Hickman peel-away sheath: alternative for pediatric percutaneous nephrolithotomy. J Endourol 1997;11(3):171–2.
7. Jackman SV, Hedican SP, Peters CA, et al. Percutaneous nephrolithotomy in infants and preschool age children: experience with a new technique. Urology 1998;52(4):697–701.
8. Jackman SV, Docimo SG, Cadeddu JA, et al. The "mini-perc" technique: a less invasive alternative to percutaneous nephrolithotomy. World J Urol 1998; 16(6):371–4.
9. Monga M, Oglevie S. Minipercutaneous nephrolithotomy. J Endourol 2000;14(5):419–21.
10. Chan DY, Jarrett TW. Mini-percutaneous nephrolithotomy. J Endourol 2000;14(3):269–72.
11. Nagele U, Horstmann M, Sievert KD, et al. A newly designed Amplatz sheath decreases intrapelvic irrigation pressure during mini-percutaneous nephrolitholapaxy: an in-vitro pressure-measurement and microscopic study. J Endourol 2007;21(9):1113–6.
12. Lahme S, Bichler KH, Strohmaier WL, et al. Minimally invasive PCNL in patients with renal pelvic and calyceal stones. Eur Urol 2001;40(6):619–24.
13. Desai J, Solanki R. Ultra-mini percutaneous nephrolithotomy (UMP): one more armamentarium. BJU Int 2013;112(7):1046–9.
14. Desai JD. Ultra-mini PNL (UMP): material, indications, technique, advantages and results. Arch Esp Urol 2017;70(1):196–201.
15. Datta SN, Solanki R, Desai J. Prospective outcomes of ultra mini percutaneous nephrolithotomy: a consecutive cohort study. J Urol 2016;195(3):741–6.
16. Zeng G, Wan S, Zhao Z, et al. Super-mini percutaneous nephrolithotomy (SMP): a new concept in technique and instrumentation. BJU Int 2016;117(4):655–61.
17. Zeng G, Zhu W, Liu Y, et al. The new generation super-mini percutaneous nephrolithotomy (SMP) system: a step-by-step guide. BJU Int 2017;120(5):735–8.
18. Zhao Z, Tuerxu A, Liu Y, et al. Super-mini PCNL (SMP): material, indications, technique, advantages and results. Arch Esp Urol 2017;70(1):211–6.
19. Desai MR, Sharma R, Mishra S, et al. Single-step percutaneous nephrolithotomy (microperc): the initial clinical report. J Urol 2011;186(1):140–5.
20. Bader MJ, Gratzke C, Seitz M, et al. The "all-seeing needle": initial results of an optical puncture system confirming access in percutaneous nephrolithotomy. Eur Urol 2011;59(6):1054–9.
21. Sabnis RB, Ganesamoni R, Ganpule AP, et al. Current role of microperc in the management of small renal calculi. Indian J Urol 2013;29(3):214–8.

22. Webb DR, Fitzpatrick JM. Percutaneous nephrolithotripsy: a functional and morphological study. J Urol 1985;134(3):587–91.
23. Clayman RV, Elbers J, Miller RP, et al. Percutaneous nephrostomy: assessment of renal damage associated with semi-rigid (24F) and balloon (36F) dilation. J Urol 1987;138(1):203–6.
24. Al-Kandari AM, Jabbour M, Anderson A, et al. Comparative study of degree of renal trauma between Amplatz sequential fascial dilation and balloon dilation during percutaneous renal surgery in an animal model. Urology 2007;69(3):586–9.
25. Traxer O, Smith TG 3rd, Pearle MS, et al. Renal parenchymal injury after standard and mini percutaneous nephrostolithotomy. J Urol 2001;165(5): 1693–5.
26. Emiliani E, Talso M, Baghdadi M, et al. Renal parenchyma injury after percutaneous nephrolithotomy tract dilatations in pig and cadaveric kidney models. Cent Eur J Urol 2017;70(1):69–75.
27. Hinman F Jr. Peripelvic extravasation during intravenous urography, evidence for an additional route for backflow after ureteral obstruction. J Urol 1961;85: 385–95.
28. Cuttino JT Jr, Clark RL, Fried FA, et al. Microradiographic demonstration of pyelolymphatic backflow in the porcine kidney. AJR Am J Roentgenol 1978; 131(3):501–5.
29. Mager R, Balzereit C, Reiter M, et al. Introducing a novel in vitro model to characterize hydrodynamic efects of percutaneous nephrolithotomy systems. J Endourol 2015;29(8):929–32.
30. Wang J, Zhou DQ, He M, et al. Effects of renal pelvic high-pressure perfusion on nephrons in a porcine pyonephrosis model. Exp Ther Med 2013;5(5): 1389–92.
31. Loftus CJ, Hinck B, Makovey I, et al. Mini versus standard percutaneous nephrolithotomy: the impact of sheath size on intrarenal pelvic pressure and infectious complications in a porcine model. J Endourol 2018;32(4):350–3.
32. Doizi S, Uzan A, Keller EX, et al. Comparison of intrapelvic pressures during flexible ureteroscopy, mini-percutaneous nephrolithotomy, standard percutaneous nephrolithotomy, and endoscopic combined intrarenal surgery in a kidney model. World J Urol 2020. https://doi.org/10.1007/s00345-020-03450-2.
33. Karaköse A, Aydogdu O, Atesci YZ. The use of the Amplatz sheath in percutaneous nephrolithotomy: does Amplatz sheath size matter? Curr Urol 2013; 7(3):127–31.
34. Yamaguchi A, Skolarikos A, Buchholz NPN, et al. Operating times and bleeding complications in percutaneous nephrolithotomy: a comparison of tract dilation methods in 5537 patients in the Clinical Research Office of the Endourological Society percutaneous lithotomy global study. J Endourol 2011;25:947–54.
35. Cheng F, Yu W, Zhang X, et al. Minimally invasive tract in percutaneous nephrolithotomy for renal stones. J Endourol 2010;24:1579–82.
36. Guler A, Erbin A, Ucpinar B, et al. Comparison of miniaturized percutaneous nephrolithotomy and standard percutaneous nephrolithotomy for the treatment of large kidney stones: a randomized prospective study. Urolithiasis 2019;47:289–95.
37. Kandemir E, Savun M, Sezer A, et al. Comparison of miniaturized percutaneous nephrolithotomy and standard percutaneous nephrolithotomy in secondary patients: a randomized prospective study. J Endourol 2020;34:26–32.
38. Zhong W, Zeng G, Wu W, et al. Minimally invasive percutaneous nephrolithotomy with multiple mini tracts in a single session in treating staghorn calculi. Urol Res 2011;39:117–22.
39. Sakr A, Salem E, Kamel M, et al. Minimally invasive percutaneous nephrolithotomy vs standard PCNL for management of renal stones in the flank-free modified supine position: single-center experience. Urolithiasis 2017;45(6):585–9.
40. Karakan T, Kilinc MF, Doluoglu OG, et al. The modified ultra-mini percutaneous nephrolithotomy technique and comparison with standard nephrolithotomy: a randomized prospective study. Urolithiasis 2017;45(2):209–13.
41. Haghighi R, Zeraati H, Ghorban Zade M. Ultra-mini-percutaneous nephrolithotomy (PCNL) versus standard PCNL: a randomised clinical trial. Arab J Urol 2017;15(4):294–8.
42. Song L, Chen Z, Liu T, et al. The application of a patented system to minimally invasive percutaneous nephrolithotomy. J Endourol 2011;25(8):1281–6.
43. Guddeti RS, Hegde P, Chawla A, et al. Super-mini percutaneous nephrolithotomy (PCNL) vs standard PCNL for the management of renal calculi of <2 cm: a randomised controlled study. BJU Int 2020; 126(2):273–9.
44. Du C, Song L, Wu X, et al. Suctioning minimally invasive percutaneous nephrolithotomy with a patented system is effective to treat renal staghorn calculi: a prospective multicenter study. Urol Int 2018;101(2): 143–9.
45. Zhong W, Wen J, Peng L, et al. Enhanced super-mini-PCNL (eSMP): low renal pelvic pressure and high stone removal efficiency in a prospective randomized controlled trial. World J Urol 2021;39(3):929–34.
46. Tepeler A, Akman T, Silay MS, et al. Comparison of intrarenal pelvic pressure during micro-percutaneous nephrolithotomy and conventional percutaneous nephrolithotomy. Urolithiasis 2014; 42:275–9.
47. Assimos D, Krambeck A, Miller NL, et al. Surgical management of stones: American Urological

Association/Endourological Society Guideline, PART II. J Urol 2016;196(4):1161–9.

48. Turk C, Neisius A, Petrik C, et al. EAU guidelines on urolithiasis, . EAoUG Office EAU guidelines. Arnhem, the Netherlands: European association of urology guidelines Office; 2021.

49. Ruhayel Y, Tepeler A, Dabestani S, et al. Tract sizes in miniaturized percutaneous nephrolithotomy: a systematic review from the European Association of Urology urolithiasis guidelines panel. Eur Urol 2017;72(2):220–35.

50. Smith A, Aro T. Super-mini percutaneous nephrolithotomy. Asian J Urol 2021;8(2):251–2.

Technological Advancements for Treating Erectile Dysfunction and Peyronie's Disease

Jeffrey D. Campbell, MD, MPH*, Danny Matti, Haider Abed, MD, Andrew Di Pierdominico, MD

KEYWORDS

- Erectile dysfunction (ED) • Peyronie's disease (PD) • Vacuum erection devices (VED)
- Penile traction devices (PTD) • Low-intensity extracorporeal shockwave therapy (LiESWT)
- Penile prosthesis

KEY POINTS

- Penile traction should be considered part of the initial management of erectile dysfunction and Peyronie's disease.
- Further basic science and clinical evidence need to elucidate the underlying mechanism for low-intensity extracorporeal shockwave therapy for treating erectile dysfunction before this can become a mainstream option.
- New penile prosthetic options will become available soon to ease the use for patients and it is hoped further improve patient-reported outcomes.

INTRODUCTION

Erectile dysfunction (ED) affects 30% to 65% of men in the general population between the ages of 40 and 80 years.[1] Because of the rapidly aging population, United Nations data predict that greater than 320 million men worldwide will be diagnosed and require treatment for ED by 2025.[2] ED affects the quality of life of men and their partners worldwide and costs the United States approximately $330 million annually.[3] Advances in basic science research and medical understanding have allowed therapeutic technologies to advance substantially since the original options first implemented more than 50 years ago.

Peyronie's disease (PD) is a connective tissue disease situated on the tunica albuginea of the penis. Screening studies have shown that currently there might be an underestimation of PD prevalence and incidence. A questionnaire-based survey in the United States revealed a definitive PD diagnosis in 0.7%, with an additional 11% having probable PD.[4] There is an increasing prevalence with age, diabetes, and preexisting ED, up to 9% to 13%.[4,5] Men between 50 and 60 years old seem to be most commonly affected, with a devastating impact on mental health; nearly half of all men with PD develop depressive symptoms.[6]

Restorative therapies, such as stem cell therapy and platelet-rich plasma, are being evaluated for their putative role in treating ED and PD; however, these are likely years away before mainstream acceptance and Food and Drug Administration (FDA) approval for routine use.[7] In contrast, technological advancements in the past decade have really improved the way ED can be treated, and

No financial or commercial disclosures.
No funding source for this article.
Division of Urology, Department of Surgery, Western University, London, Ontario, Canada
* Corresponding author. St. Joseph's Health Care London, 268 Grosvenor Road, London, Ontario, Canada.
E-mail address: Jeffrey.campbell@sjhc.london.on.ca
Twitter: @JDCampbell_MD (J.D.C.)

Urol Clin N Am 49 (2022) 175–184
https://doi.org/10.1016/j.ucl.2021.07.013

the future holds many prospects for further advancement. Next, the authors discuss the advancements that have occurred in how men's health is treated over the past decade and explore the rapid expansion of this subspecialty field of medicine.

Vacuum Erection Devices

Vacuum erection devices (VED) have been used as a therapeutic option for ED since 1982 and have generally occupied a role as second-line therapy in the case of pharmacologic failure or intolerance.[8] The devices typically consist of a cylinder that encompasses the penis, a vacuum (manual or electric), and a constriction ring. Negative pressure is used to draw blood into the penile sinusoids and achieve rigidity, which is then maintained by the constriction ring at the penile base. Several recent studies highlight new insights into VED therapy.

Recognizing that VED usage is often limited by technical difficulty and patient discontinuation, Beaudreau and colleagues[9] reviewed patient outcomes at their andrology clinic. Notably, their patients were provided with in-person device training (Osbon Erecaid, Osbon Medical Systems, Augusta, GA, USA), videotaped and live demonstrations, written instructions, and discussions with psychologists about realistic expectations and the importance of practice. Satisfaction interviews were performed at follow-up. In their sample of 57 patients (mean age 64 years), 93% were able to obtain an erection with the device, and 91% were able to have intercourse. Of the patients, 100% would recommend VED therapy. These results demonstrate the strength of a multidisciplinary approach to patient education. The investigators concluded that evaluating the device in nonvaginal intercourse was a future area of study.[9]

ED after treatments for prostate cancer, such as radical prostatectomy or external beam radiation therapy (EBRT), is a common complication that affects up to 75% of men in contemporary series.[10] Jones and colleagues[11] sought to evaluate the real-world performance of VEDs in men who had exclusively undergone robot-assisted radical prostatectomy (RARP). They performed a follow-up survey of 137 patients (mean age 65 years) who attended a VED clinic an average of 462 days before. Patients had used the SOMA-erect response II device (Augusta Medical Systems LLC, Augusta, GA, USA) with a training session performed by the company. At follow-up, 71% of patients were still using the VED, with 56% reporting the therapy successful. Further studies should assess whether VEDs preserve penile size or hasten the recovery of erectile function in an RARP cohort.[11]

Penile Traction Devices

Penile traction therapy (PTT) for PD is based on the premise of using mechanical force to achieve a molecular signal, resulting in a gradual curvature reduction by a process known as mechanotransduction.[12] The first published report of this therapy in 2008 demonstrated a modest mean curvature reduction and improvement in stretched penile length (SPL)[13] in PD patients, and these results were corroborated with follow-up studies.[14–16] A major limitation of PTT is the prohibitive length of time the device had to be worn, historically greater than 4 hours per day to achieve benefit. Discomfort with the glans fixation mechanism was another barrier to utilization. Until now, the data have been immature, but this therapy maintains a weak recommendation in both the Canadian[17] and the European Association of Urology PD guidelines.[18] Currently, there is no recommendation for traction use in the American Urological Association PD guideline.[19] After further study and device refinement, PTT will certainly occupy an increasingly prominent role in PD treatment.

Modern penile traction therapy

The first prospective randomized clinical trial of PTT monotherapy for PD used the PeniMaster PRO device (MSP Concept, Berlin, Germany).[20] This device is characterized by its unique vacuum-based glans fixation mechanism (**Fig. 1**). The study enrolled 93 patients with chronic phase PD and randomized them to PTT 3 to 8 hours per day for 3 months versus no intervention. PTT with the PeniMaster PRO resulted in a mean reduction of curvature of 31.2° (41.1%) versus baseline. This result was statistically significant when compared with the no-intervention group in whom there was no change observed in the curvature. There was also a statistically significant improvement in mean SPL of 1.8 cm in the PTT group. There are some notable limitations to the results. The study used a per-protocol analysis and excluded 6 patients in the PTT arm with protocol violations or adverse events. Furthermore, the study excluded men with ED, multidirectional curvature, or hourglass/indentation deformities. The investigators speculated that the PeniMaster PRO glans fixation mechanism may be better tolerated than that of competitors, but the study did not assess for this.[20]

Recognizing the limitations of previous devices, the RestoreX (PathRight Medical, Plymouth, MN, USA) was developed featuring several of the

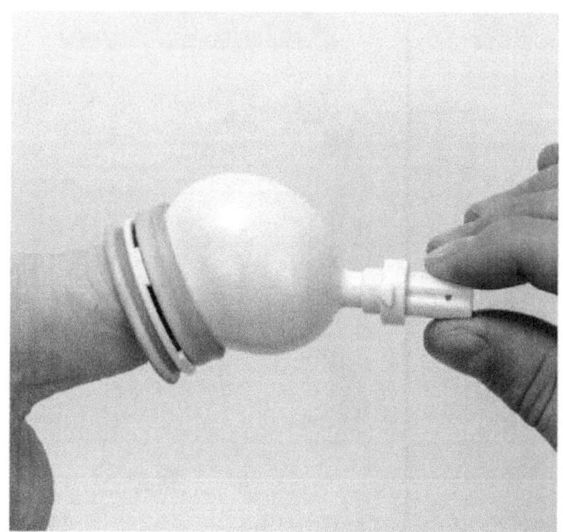

Fig. 1. PeniMaster PRO device characterized by its unique vacuum-based glans fixation mechanism.[20] (*From* Moncada I, Krishnappa P, Romero J, et al. Penile traction therapy with the new device 'Penimaster PRO' is effective and safe in the stable phase of Peyronie's disease: a controlled multicentre study. BJU Int. 04 2019;123(4):694-702. https://doi.org/10.1111/bju.14602.)

following innovations: (i) a wide penile clamp design, (ii) counter-bending, (iii) dynamic adjustment (**Fig. 2**). The device was evaluated in a pragmatic clinical trial, including a "true to life" PD population and an intention-to-treat analysis.[21] Men with PD were randomized 1:3 to no therapy or RestoreX for 30 minutes 1 to 3 times per day for 3 months. Adult men with curvature greater than 30° were included, and only those with an SPL <7 cm or severe diabetes were excluded. The primary study outcome was safety. Penile curvature, SPL, and IIEF scores were assessed as secondary outcomes.[21] At the study conclusion, data were available for 63 men in the PTT arm and 27 men in the control arm. No moderate to severe adverse events were reported. Mean primary curvature decreased 18%, and SPL increased a mean of 1.5 cm in the traction arm, both statistically significant compared with placebo. In men with baseline ED (defined as international index of erectile function [IIEF-EF] ≤25), RestoreX improved erectile function (mean 4-point improvement in the IIEF-EF).[21]

Open-label follow-up data have recently been published that provides insight into the utility of using the RestoreX device beyond 3 months.[22] At 6 months, patients that were originally randomized to the RestoreX device reported a further mean increase of 0.8 cm in SPL; however, no further curvature improvements were observed. These results likely underestimate the potential benefit of further RestoreX therapy given that not all participants reported using it during the open-label phase, and device usage was just 31 minutes per day.

Clostridium collagenase histolyticum and penile traction therapy

Clostridium collagenase histolyticum (CCH) is currently endorsed as the first-line therapy for PD.[17–19,23] One study has investigated the combination of CCH and PTT in a retrospective comparison of 3 cohorts of patients treated with CCH between March 2014 and January 2019.[24] The cohorts were as follows: (i) CCH alone, (ii) CCH with PTT with any device other than the RestoreX, and (iii) CCH + PTT with the RestoreX device. Patients in the second cohort used a PTT device of their choosing with the Andropenis, X4 labs extender (X4 labs, Vaudreuil-Dorion, Canada) and PeniMaster (MSP Concept) the most represented. This cohort was instructed to perform PTT greater than 3 hours per day, whereas those in the RestoreX were instructed to use it greater than 30 minutes per day. The primary outcomes were change in penile curvature and SPL. Data were available for 113 patients, including 56 CCH alone, 59 for CCH + PTT, and 57 for CCH + RestoreX. The groups were balanced at baseline in magnitude of curvature. Improvement in penile curvature was statistically superior in the CCH + RestoreX group with a mean 49.4% improvement compared with a CCH + PTT (30.2%) and CCH alone (31.2%). Penile length increased on average 1.9 cm in the RestoreX group compared with CCH (0.7 cm loss) and CCH + PTT (0.4 cm loss) groups. In the CCH + PTT cohort, only 7 (16%) of the men were able to wear the device the recommended more than 3 hours per day, which may explain the lack of observed efficacy in this group. Although the registry included patients from 2014 to 2019, the RestoreX device was first offered in 2017, and therefore, this cohort represents more recent patients. Therefore, the improvement in this group may be a reflection of improved provider experience with CCH. Nonetheless, this study provides the first evidence of an advantage to the addition of PTT to CCH, provided PTT is performed with the RestoreX device.[24]

Shockwave Therapy

Over the past decade, basic science and clinical studies have suggested that low-intensity extracorporeal shockwave therapy (LiESWT) may offer benefit for patients with ED,[25–29] chronic pelvic pain, and/or PD. Shockwave therapy (SWT) relies on an external energy source that applies pulses of energy into a fluid environment and then

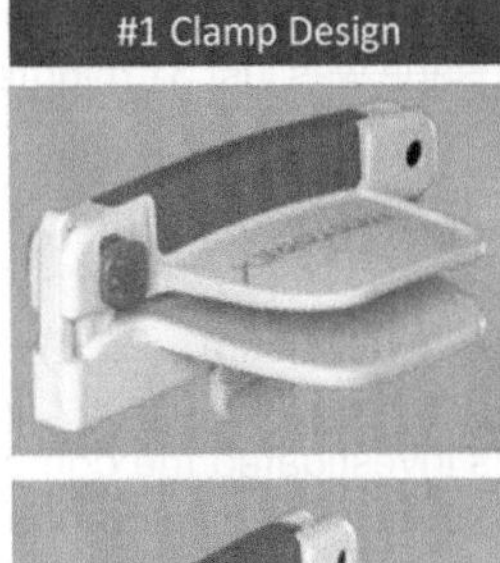
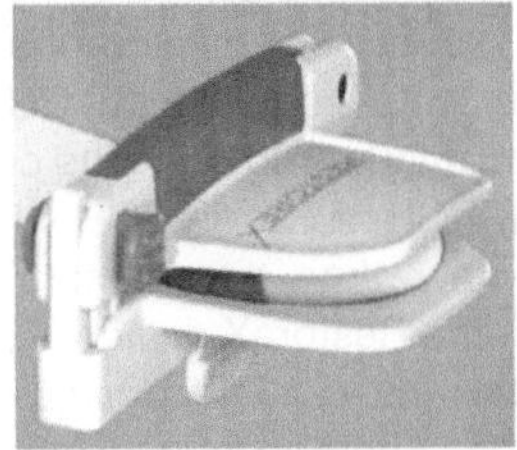

#1 Clamp Design
Spreads clamping forces over a larger surface area than majority of other traction devices, permitting greater traction without slipping.

#2 Counter-traction

Ability to direct force to one side / region of the penis to provide greater traction forces. The use of countertraction was shown to be a predictor of greater improvements in the 3-month data.

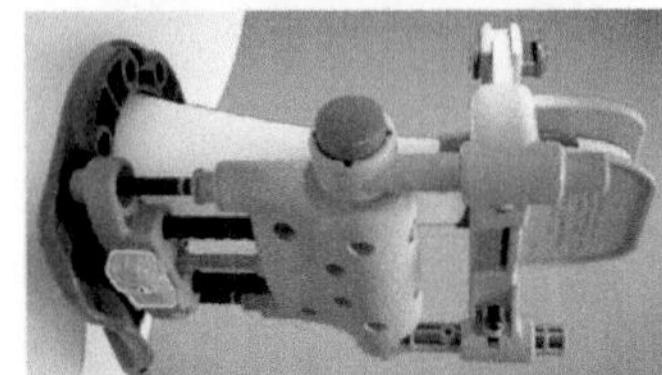
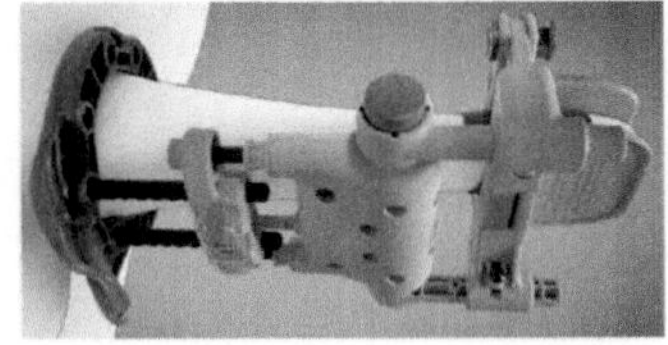

Allows user the ability to advance the device without removing and thus assuring continuous traction despite penile lengthening.

Fig. 2. RestoreX device featuring improvements in (1) clamp design, (2) counter-traction, and (3) dynamic adjustment.[21] (*From* Ziegelmann M, Savage J, Toussi A, et al. Outcomes of a Novel Penile Traction Device in Men with Peyronie's Disease: A Randomized, Single-Blind, Controlled Trial. J Urol. 09 2019;202(3):599-610. https://doi.org/10.1097/JU.0000000000000245.)

propagates the harnessed energy until it meets the target tissue where the energy is used.[30] In a low-intensity state, SWT has been shown to induce angiogenesis,[31] regenerate nerve fibers, recruit progenitor cells, vasodilate penile microcirculation,[32] and improve endothelial function.[33,34] LiESWT has been suggested to induce long-term structural changes that may augment erectile function.[35–37]

Three different generates for LiESWT are currently available using different forms of energy: electromagnetic, electrohydraulic, and piezoelectric. All 3 energy forms produce acoustic waves that transfer energy directly to the tissue to which it is applied, resulting in mechanical stress.[36,38]

Shockwave Therapy for Erectile Dysfunction

To date, there have been several human, prospective randomized controlled clinical trials[39–49] and meta-analyses[25–29,50,51] exploring the use of LiESWT for ED. The role of LiESWT in treating ED is to reestablish natural erections without the need for additional medical treatment. LiESWT may convert a phosphodiesterase type 5 inhibitor partial responder to a complete responder, thus avoiding the need for more aggressive interventions.[35]

Based on the currently available randomized controlled trials, there is an approximate improvement of 4 points in the IIEF.[29] A 4-point short-term improvement in IIEF would be considered a clinically significant improvement, but the studies included in such meta-analyses have significant bias, and the interpretation of these results is limited.

There does remain an uncertainty regarding the duration of effect with LiESWT when treating ED, and this appears to be one of the most important clinical considerations, especially when it comes to patient counseling. The longest follow-up results to date is 2 years, but of the near 100 patients with initial improvement at 1 month, only approximately 50% had continued improvement after 24 months.[52] Clinically, if 50% have continued benefit, this may be a tolerable sustainability, and perhaps maintenance treatments would be required similar to other disease processes. Further work and longer outcomes are needed to help evaluate this effect and inform practitioners on how to properly counsel patients.

Shockwave Therapy for Peyronie's Disease

Although prospective, single-center studies have recently evaluated the utility of LiESWT for PD, there is limited basic science or good-quality clinical data to support the use for this indication.[43,53–55] Di Mauro and colleagues[54] assessed more than 300 PD patients, and although they measured a slight change in plaque size, debatably the most important finding is the reduction of pain with LiESWT in acute phase PD. This study does not have a control group, and therefore, it is unclear if this reduction in pain is due to just progression of disease from acute to chronic, or truly a reduction in inflammation secondary to the use of LiESWT.

Radial Wave Shock Wave Therapy

Radial wave therapy has been marketed as a treatment for ED; however, there is a paucity of adequate clinical research available to support its use. It is important for both patients and providers to realize that this technology is not the same as LiESWT. In contrast to LiESWT, radial wave generators produce dispersive waves away from the probe, and these waves have low tissue penetrance.[37,56] In comparison, LiESWT focuses more energy with a deeper tissue penetration over a shorter time, which is implicated as a regenerative technology.

Current Clinical Applications

Despite the breadth of exploration in the past decade, there are several limitations to LiESWT studies. First, there is a significant heterogeneity in shockwave generator and treatment protocols used for study, and the dosing, frequency of shocks, and location of probe are still not standardized. The diversity in therapeutic application makes this technology difficult to accurately study. Although many private men's health clinics currently use this technology, there is no agreed upon algorithm, and therefore, treatment remains up to the clinician. Next, although there is an abundance of randomized trials, many have different inclusion criteria and small sample sizes. This makes even meta-analysis of the data difficult, and there are many associated biases.[29] Different studies explore vascular versus aged-related or neurogenic causes of ED, and these heterogenous populations cannot be fairly compared.

The Sexual Medicine Society of North America (SMSNA) has published an updated position statement about the use of all regenerative therapies, including LiESWT.[37] In summary, the SMSNA recommends further exploration of the basic science behind shock wave technology and randomized placebo-controlled trials to determine appropriate patient populations, shock wave protocols, device choices, and long-term efficacy.[37] Similarly, the European Society of Sexual Medicine agrees that LiESWT has some significant support with clinical evidence; however, further work is required before it becomes an accepted form of treatment for male health conditions.[57]

The increased use in LiESWT by private clinics worldwide is controversial, and interpretation of the current data is contrasted by various guideline committees. The European Association of Urology states that LiESWT can be used to treat mild, organic ED, but has weak strength of recommendation.[35] In comparison, the updated American Urological Association guideline on ED has a conditional, grade C recommendation that LiESWT should be considered investigational and not yet ready for mainstream use.[58] The unpublished Canadian Urology Association guidelines have a weak recommendation against the use of LiESWT for treating ED.[59] None of the current guidelines support the use of LiESWT for chronic pelvic pain or PD.[19,35] As further evidence is elucidated, these guidelines will likely evolve, such that this may become a treatment option in select patient populations.

PENILE PROSTHETICS

The Evolution of Penile Prosthesis Surgery

The first penile prosthetic was devised by Dr Ambroise Pare and dates to the sixteenth century. Dr Pare inserted a wooden pipe to facilitate micturition for a patient who required a penile amputation as a result of trauma. Although this prosthesis was initially described as successful, the wooden pipe was later resorbed by the body.[60] In 1936, Dr Nikolaj Bogoraz, a pioneer in phalloplasty, used rib cartilage to provide rigidity.[61] The first use of synthetic material for penile prosthesis was developed by Dr Scardino in 1950, but the data went unpublished. In 1952, Drs Goodwin and Scott performed 5 acrylic penile transplants and provided the first descriptions of alloplastic penile implants. Unfortunately, only 2 of the 5 remained successful at 5 years postimplant because of infection or patient intolerance. The first large study of penile prosthesis was Dr Beheri in 1966, who described the intracavernosal placement of polyethylene rods. His proposed technique is still followed to this day, with the use of Hegar dilators for cavernosal dilation and the formation of a tunnel for the prostheses. Dr Beheri's placement of the prosthesis within the tunica albuginea has since become the prominent method.[62] In 1967, Dr Pearman described placement of a silicone rod between Buck fascia and the tunica albuginea.[63] This caused patients significant pain, and Pearman subsequently changed his technique to be similar to that of Dr Beheri, with placement of the silicone rod within the tunica albuginea.[64] During the 1970s, there was a significant upswing in the surgical management of ED because of novel surgical options. It was at this time that research and design likely reached the critical point, which led to novel designs in penile prosthesis.

Malleable Penile Prosthesis

The semirigid prosthesis was introduced in 1975 by Small and colleagues and was designed to fill both corporal bodies.[65] This was upended in 1977 by Dr Finney, who introduced the Flexi-Rod prosthesis, a paired semirigid implant with a softer proximal compartment below the pubis.[63] The silicone core was later reinforced with Dacron fabric to create a firmer prosthesis, becoming the Flexi-Rod II.[66] In 1983, American Medical Systems (AMS) designed the AMS Malleable 600 prosthesis, a silicone device containing a stainless wire core wrapped in fabric. This design included the addition of rear tip extenders and allowed for 3 length adjustments.[67] In contrast, Mentor (now known as Coloplast) designed the Mentor Malleable, also available with multiple rear tip extenders and in 3 size lengths.[68] Also, during the 1980s, Omniphase and Duraphase malleable implants were introduced and advertised to have the twisting of a "gooseneck lamp." Both were pulled from the market in 1986 because of technical failures.[69] In 1992, the Dura-II malleable penis prosthesis was introduced, which contained a series of polyethylene disks connected by a metal cable running down the middle.[70] Drs Ferguson and Cespedes[71] went on to present data in 2003 that supported long-term quality-of-life improvements in patients who had undergone Dura-II implantation. Many of these options remain on the market to this day.

One-Piece Inflatable Penile Prosthesis

In 1986, 2 different one-piece inflatable penile prostheses (IPP) were introduced to the market: AMS' Hydroflex and Surgitek's Flex. These devices included a rigid core, where fluid was transferred into the core by a pump at the distal end. However, Surgitek is no longer manufacturing penile prosthetics, and the AMS Hydroflex was replaced by the Dynaflex prosthesis in the 1990s. The Dynaflex, although similar to the AMS Hydroflex, included multiple channels connecting the pump and reservoir, which provided a more rigid erection in comparison to other malleable prosthesis at the time.

Two-Piece Inflatable Penile Prosthesis

The first two-piece IPP was designed by Mentor (Coloplast) and was dubbed the "GFS prosthesis." The novel design had 2 cylinders attached to a single reservoir unit, located in the scrotum, that was made up of both the reservoir and the pump, called the "resipump."[72] Around the same time, Surgitek introduced the Uniflate 1000. The Uniflate 1000 is filled through a self-sealing penetrable port on the bottom of the resipump; however, the cylinders have 2 layers: an outer silicone layer and an inner Dacron fabric layer, with the outer chamber functioning to add extra girth. This did not receive FDA approval, as studies done in Spain showed high rates of mechanical failure.[73] AMS introduced Ambicor in the 1990s, which consists of a pair of cylinders and a pump of silicone elastomers. The Ambicor remains on the market to this day.[74]

Three-Piece Inflatable Penile Prosthesis

The original three-piece IPP was developed by Dr Scott and colleagues in the 1990s to prevent penile shortening and to increase penile girth and length. This IPP device, the AMS 700, consisted of 2 pumps (one in each hemi-scrotum), 2 cylinders, and a fluid reservoir.[75] The initial design included new rear tips, polytetrafluoroethylene (PTFE) sleeves for decreased wear, and a new connector system that did not require sutures. However, the PTFE sleeves did not permit adequate expansion and were prone to aneurysmal dilation.[76] In 1986, the kink-resistant tube was introduced, subsequently reducing complications and providing more forgiveness to length and width measurements.[77] In 1987, the PTFE sleeves were replaced by multilayer silicone material that better facilitated expansion. This material includes an inner layer of woven fabric resembling Dacron, and an outer layer made of silicon to allow for controlled expansion. This material remains the standard for use in penile expansion devices to this day.[66,76]

Since the early 2000s, there have been numerous modifications to the AMS 700 three-piece inflatable prosthesis. AMS added an additional parylene coating to the inner surface of the silicon to decrease wear and tear, which further reduces risk of aneurysmal dilation. Furthermore, AMS added a lockout valve to prevent autoinflation.[78] AMS also introduced the first permanent antibiotic-eluting implant, named the InhibiZone, which consisted of minocycline and rifampin. This was impregnated onto the outer surface of the device, resulting in the yellow-orange trace effect.[79] Currently, there are 3 variations in the AMS 700 series: the AMS 700 LGX, AMS 700 CX, and AMS 700 CXR, with LGX referring to length and girth expansion, whereas CX refers to controlled expansion.[70]

In a bid to compete with AMS, Mentor (Coloplast) patented the Bioflex material in the early 1980s. The Bioflex material provided advantages over the silicon material used by AMS, including an ~7 times higher tensile strength, while maintaining biodegradability.[80] Furthermore, Mentor (Coloplast) later went on to patent their own reservoir, and in 1987, they improved the reservoir by adding nylon to the reservoir and caps on the rear tip extenders. In 2002, the addition of a hydrophilic coating allowed for the surgeon's choice of antibiotic use, which subsequently reduced infection rates by 50%. Other modifications over the years include changing the tubing connector from a crimp to slip-on design, developing a zero-degree junction between cylinders, and addition of new tubing to better facilitate intracorporeal cylinder placement. Recently, the Coloplast Cloverleaf was introduced for ectopic reservoir placement in anatomically compromised patients in order to reduce autoinflation.[81]

Surgical Innovation and Future Advances in Penile Prosthesis

Although we have come a long way since rib cartilage-enhanced erections, a new frontier of penile prostheses is constantly on the lookout. Futuristic advances in operative technique and inflation mechanics reinvigorate hope for continued safe and effective prosthetic aid in men's sexual health.

Over the past few decades, there have been many changes to the penile prosthesis to improve durability, improve comfort, and reduce rates of infection. Current prosthesis companies, such as Boston Scientific and Coloplast, aim to integrate software programming and shape memory alloys (SMA) into upcoming penile prosthesis for the treatment of ED. In 2019, Boston Scientific designed Tactra, a semirigid penile prosthesis made up of silicone cylinders with a core of Nitinol (nickel-titanium alloy), which provides increased rigidity and flexibility. The novel semirigid prosthesis is not coated with Inhibizone, which has been associated with lower rates of postoperative infections.[82] Second, a novel approach has been the integration of temperature into the SMA IPP, which "remembers" a predetermined shape. The mechanism of these involves setting a critical temperature point. Above the set temperature, the penis achieves a rigid state, whereas below the temperature point, the SMA achieves a flaccid state. At this time, the critical temperature point has been set at 42°C, which is above normal resting body temperature and below the threshold at which pain nociceptors activate. Furthermore, this allows transitions between flaccid and rigid states without the use of a reservoir or pump.[83] Last, a novel physiologic technique also using SMAs involves use of magnetic induction, instead of hydraulic pressure, to stimulate the transition to an erect penis. Done in animal models, an external inducer wand was used to successfully activate the SMA penile prosthesis with no direct contact in less than 45 seconds.[84]

SUMMARY

In summary, much progress has been made in technology that can improve male sexual health. Current limitations in advanced technology include a lack of multicenter clinical trials, studies evaluating complex patient populations, and well-established treatment protocols. As technology developments and artificial intelligence expand within the medical realm, one can only expect that treatments for men's health will continue to improve over the next decade and beyond.

REFERENCES

1. Corona G, Lee DM, Forti G, et al. Age-related changes in general and sexual health in middle-aged and older men: results from the European Male Ageing Study (EMAS). J Sex Med 2010;7(4 Pt 1):1362–80.
2. Ayta IA, McKinlay JB, Krane RJ. The likely worldwide increase in erectile dysfunction between 1995 and 2025 and some possible policy consequences. BJU Int 1999;84(1):50–6.
3. Wessells H, Joyce GF, Wise M, et al. Erectile dysfunction. J Urol 2007;177(5):1675–81.
4. Campbell J, Alzubaidi R. Understanding the cellular basis and pathophysiology of Peyronie's disease to optimize treatment for erectile dysfunction. Transl Androl Urol 2017;6(1):46–59.
5. Bilgutay AN, Pastuszak AW. Peyronie's disease: a review of etiology, diagnosis, and management. Curr Sex Health Rep 2015;7(2):117–31.
6. Nelson CJ, Diblasio C, Kendirci M, et al. The chronology of depression and distress in men with Peyronie's disease. J Sex Med 2008;5(8):1985–90.
7. Campbell JD, Milenkovic U, Usta MF, et al. The good, bad, and the ugly of regenerative therapies for erectile dysfunction. Transl Androl Urol 2020; 9(Suppl 2):S252–61.
8. Stein MJ, Lin H, Wang R. New advances in erectile technology. Ther Adv Urol 2014;6(1):15–24.
9. Beaudreau SA, Van Moorleghem K, Dodd SM, et al. Satisfaction with a vacuum constriction device for erectile dysfunction among middle-aged and older veterans. Clin Gerontol 2021;44(3):307–15.
10. Capogrosso P, Vertosick EA, Benfante NE, et al. Are we improving erectile function recovery after radical prostatectomy? Analysis of patients treated over the last decade. Eur Urol 2019;75(2):221–8.

11. Jones P, Sandoval Barba H, Johnson MI, et al. Erectile dysfunction after robotic radical prostatectomy: real-life impact of vacuum erection device clinic. J Clin Urol 2020;1–7. https://doi.org/10.1177/2051415820946630.
12. Chung E, De Young L, Solomon M, et al. Peyronie's disease and mechanotransduction: an in vitro analysis of the cellular changes to Peyronie's disease in a cell-culture strain system. J Sex Med 2013; 10(5):1259–67.
13. Levine LA, Newell M, Taylor FL. Penile traction therapy for treatment of Peyronie's disease: a single-center pilot study. J Sex Med 2008;5(6):1468–73.
14. Gontero P, Di Marco M, Giubilei G, et al. Use of penile extender device in the treatment of penile curvature as a result of Peyronie's disease. Results of a phase II prospective study. J Sex Med 2009;6(2): 558–66.
15. Martínez-Salamanca JI, Egui A, Moncada I, et al. Acute phase Peyronie's disease management with traction device: a nonrandomized prospective controlled trial with ultrasound correlation. J Sex Med 2014;11(2):506–15.
16. Scroppo F, Mancini M, Maggi M, et al. Can an external penis stretcher reduce Peyronie's penile curvature? Int J Impot Res. 2001;13(4).
17. Bella AJ, Lee JC, Grober ED, et al. 2018 Canadian Urological Association guideline for Peyronie's disease and congenital penile curvature. Can Urol Assoc J 2018;12(5):E197–209.
18. Hatzimouratidis K, Eardley I, Giuliano F, et al. EAU guidelines on penile curvature. Eur Urol 2012; 62(3):543–52.
19. Nehra A, Alterowitz R, Culkin DJ, et al. Peyronie's disease: AUA guideline. J Urol 2015;194(3):745–53.
20. Moncada I, Krishnappa P, Romero J, et al. Penile traction therapy with the new device 'Penimaster PRO' is effective and safe in the stable phase of Peyronie's disease: a controlled multicentre study. BJU Int 2019;123(4):694–702.
21. Ziegelmann M, Savage J, Toussi A, et al. Outcomes of a novel penile traction device in men with Peyronie's disease: a randomized, single-blind, controlled trial. J Urol 2019;202(3):599–610.
22. Joseph J, Ziegelmann MJ, Alom M, et al. Outcomes of RestoreX penile traction therapy in men with Peyronie's disease: results from open label and follow-up phases. J Sex Med 2020;17(12):2462–71.
23. Salonia A, Bettocchi C, Carvalho J, et al: EAU Guidelines on Sexual and Reproductive Health. 2021. ISBN 978-94-92671-13-4.
24. Alom M, Sharma KL, Toussi A, et al. Efficacy of combined collagenase clostridium histolyticum and RestoreX penile traction therapy in men with Peyronie's disease. J Sex Med 2019;16(6):891–900.
25. Clavijo RI, Kohn TP, Kohn JR, et al. Effects of low-intensity extracorporeal shockwave therapy on erectile dysfunction: a systematic review and meta-analysis. J Sex Med 2017;14(1):27–35.
26. Lu Z, Lin G, Reed-Maldonado A, et al. Low-intensity extracorporeal shock wave treatment improves erectile function: a systematic review and meta-analysis. Eur Urol 2017;71(2):223–33.
27. Man L, Li G. Low-intensity extracorporeal shock wave therapy for erectile dysfunction: a systematic review and meta-analysis. Urology 2017. https://doi.org/10.1016/j.urology.2017.09.011.
28. Zou ZJ, Tang LY, Liu ZH, et al. Short-term efficacy and safety of low-intensity extracorporeal shock wave therapy in erectile dysfunction: a systematic review and meta-analysis. Int Braz J Urol 2017;43(5):805–21.
29. Campbell JD, Trock BJ, Oppenheim AR, et al. Meta-analysis of randomized controlled trials that assess the efficacy of low-intensity shockwave therapy for the treatment of erectile dysfunction. Ther Adv Urol 2019;11. 1756287219838364.
30. Wein AJ, Kavoussi LR, Novick AC, et al. Campbell-Walsh Urology 10th ed, Chapt 24. Philadelphia: Elsevier Health Sciences; 2011. p. 721–47.
31. Alunni G, Marra S, Meynet I, et al. The beneficial effect of extracorporeal shockwave myocardial revascularization in patients with refractory angina. Cardiovasc Revasc Med 2015;16(1):6–11.
32. Gotte G, Amelio E, Russo S, et al. Short-time non-enzymatic nitric oxide synthesis from L-arginine and hydrogen peroxide induced by shock waves treatment. FEBS Lett 2002;520(1–3):153–5.
33. Wang HS, Ruan Y, Banie L, et al. Delayed low-intensity extracorporeal shock wave therapy ameliorates impaired penile hemodynamics in rats subjected to pelvic neurovascular injury. J Sex Med 2019;16(1):17–26.
34. Behr-Roussel D, Giuliano F. Low-energy shock wave therapy ameliorates erectile dysfunction in a pelvic neurovascular injuries rat model. Transl Androl Urol 2016;5(6):977–9.
35. Schoofs E, Fode M, Capogrosso P, et al, Group fthe EAoUrology YAUE-YMsH. Current guideline recommendations and analysis of evidence quality on low-intensity shockwave therapy for erectile dysfunction. Int J Impot Res 2019;31(3):209–17.
36. Fode M, Hatzichristodoulou G, Serefoglu EC, et al. Low-intensity shockwave therapy for erectile dysfunction: is the evidence strong enough? Nat Rev Urol 2017;14(10):593–606.
37. Liu JL, Chu KY, Gabrielson AT, et al. Restorative therapies for erectile dysfunction: position statement from the Sexual Medicine Society of North America (SMSNA). Sex Med 2021;9(3):100343.
38. Katz JE, Clavijo RI, Rizk P, et al. The basic physics of waves, soundwaves, and shockwaves for erectile dysfunction. Sex Med Rev 2020;8(1):100–5.
39. Ortac M, Özmez A, Cilesiz NC, et al. The impact of extracorporeal shock wave therapy (ESWT) for the

treatment of young patients with vasculogenic mild-erectile dysfunction (ED): a prospective randomized single-blind, sham controlled study. Andrology 2021. https://doi.org/10.1111/andr.13007.
40. Vinay J, Moreno D, Rajmil O, et al. Penile low intensity shock wave treatment for PDE5I refractory erectile dysfunction: a randomized double-blind sham-controlled clinical trial. World J Urol 2020. https://doi.org/10.1007/s00345-020-03373-y.
41. Karsiyakali N, Erkan E, Yucetas U, et al. Shock wave lithotripsy deteriorates male sexual functions related to the treatment-driven anxiety: a prospective, non-randomized, self-controlled study. Arch Esp Urol 2020;73(9):826–36.
42. Sramkova T, Motil I, Jarkovsky J, et al. Erectile dysfunction treatment using focused linear low-intensity extracorporeal shockwaves: single-blind, sham-controlled, randomized clinical trial. Urol Int 2020;104(5–6):417–24.
43. Fojecki GL, Tiessen S, Osther PJ. Extracorporeal shock wave therapy (ESWT) in urology: a systematic review of outcome in Peyronie's disease, erectile dysfunction and chronic pelvic pain. World J Urol 2017;35(1):1–9.
44. Kalyvianakis D, Hatzichristou D. Low-intensity shockwave therapy improves hemodynamic parameters in patients with vasculogenic erectile dysfunction: a triplex ultrasonography-based sham-controlled trial. J Sex Med 2017;14(7):891–7.
45. Kitrey ND, Gruenwald I, Appel B, et al. Penile low intensity shock wave treatment is able to shift PDE5i nonresponders to responders: a double-blind, sham controlled study. J Urol 2016;195(5):1550–5.
46. Srini VS, Reddy RK, Shultz T, et al. Low intensity extracorporeal shockwave therapy for erectile dysfunction: a study in an Indian population. Can J Urol 2015;22(1):7614–22.
47. Vardi Y, Appel B, Kilchevsky A, et al. Does low intensity extracorporeal shock wave therapy have a physiological effect on erectile function? Short-term results of a randomized, double-blind, sham controlled study. J Urol 2012;187(5):1769–75.
48. Yee CH, Chan ES, Hou SS, et al. Extracorporeal shockwave therapy in the treatment of erectile dysfunction: a prospective, randomized, double-blinded, placebo controlled study. Int J Urol 2014;21(10):1041–5.
49. Patel P, Katz J, Lokeshwar SD, et al. Phase II randomized, clinical trial evaluating 2 schedules of low-intensity shockwave therapy for the treatment of erectile dysfunction. Sex Med 2020;8(2):214–22.
50. Dong L, Chang D, Zhang X, et al. Effect of low-intensity extracorporeal shock wave on the treatment of erectile dysfunction: a systematic review and meta-analysis. Am J Mens Health 2019;13(2). 1557988319846749.
51. Sokolakis I, Hatzichristodoulou G. Clinical studies on low intensity extracorporeal shockwave therapy for erectile dysfunction: a systematic review and meta-analysis of randomised controlled trials. Int J Impot Res 2019;31(3):177–94.
52. Kitrey ND, Vardi Y, Appel B, et al. Low intensity shock wave treatment for erectile dysfunction-how long does the effect last? J Urol 2018;200(1):167–70.
53. Abdessater M, Akakpo W, Kanbar A, et al. Low-intensity extracorporeal shock wave therapy for Peyronie's disease: a single-center experience. Asian J Androl 2021. https://doi.org/10.4103/aja.aja_40_21.
54. Di Mauro M, Russo GI, Della Camera PA, et al. Extracorporeal shock wave therapy in Peyronie's disease: clinical efficacy and safety from a single-arm observational study. World J Mens Health 2019;37(3):339–46.
55. Palmieri A, Imbimbo C, Creta M, et al. Tadalafil once daily and extracorporeal shock wave therapy in the management of patients with Peyronie's disease and erectile dysfunction: results from a prospective randomized trial. Int J Androl 2012;35(2):190–5.
56. Notarnicola A, Tamma R, Moretti L, et al. Effects of radial shock waves therapy on osteoblasts activities. Musculoskelet Surg 2012;96(3):183–9.
57. Capogrosso P, Frey A, Jensen CFS, et al. Low-intensity shock wave therapy in sexual medicine-clinical recommendations from the European Society of Sexual Medicine (ESSM). J Sex Med 2019;16(10):1490–505.
58. Burnett AL, Nehra A, Breau RH, et al. Erectile dysfunction: AUA guideline. J Urol 2018. https://doi.org/10.1016/j.juro.2018.05.004.
59. Domes T, Tadayon B, Roberts M, et al. Canadian Urological Association guideline: Erectile dysfunction. Can Urol Assoc J 2021 August 17. Doi: http://dx.doi.org/10.5489/cuaj.7572.
60. Rodriguez KM, Pastuszak AW. A history of penile implants. Transl Androl Urol 2017;6(Suppl 5):S851–7.
61. Schulthesis D, Gabouev A, Jonas U, et al. (1874-1952): pioneer of phalloplasty and penile implant surgery Hannover, Germany. J Sex Med 2005; 139–46.
62. Martínez-Salamanca JI, Mueller A, Moncada I, et al. Penile prosthesis surgery in patients with corporal fibrosis: a state of the art review. J Sex Med 2011; 8(7):1880–9.
63. Jonas U, Jacobi GH. Silicone-silver penile prosthesis: description, operative approach and results. J Urol 1980;123(6):865–7.
64. Nelson R. Pathophysiology, evaluation, and treatment of erectile dysfunction. Norwalk, Connecticut: Urology Annual; 1987. p. 139–69.
65. Small MP, Carrion HM, Gordon JA. Small-carrion penile prosthesis. New implant for management of impotence. Urology 1975;5(4):479–86.
66. Scott FB, Bradley WE, Timm GW. Management of erectile impotence. Use of implantable inflatable prosthesis. Urology 1973;2(1):80–2.

67. Falcone M, Rolle L, Ceruti C, et al. Prospective analysis of the surgical outcomes and patients' satisfaction rate after the AMS Spectra penile prosthesis implantation. Urology 2013;82(2):373–6.
68. Martinez DR, Terlecki R, Brant WO. The evolution and utility of the small-carrion prosthesis, its impact, and progression to the modern-day malleable penile prosthesis. J Sex Med 2015;12(Suppl 7):423–30.
69. Huisman TK, Macintyre RC. Mechanical failure of OmniPhase penile prosthesis. Urology 1988;31(6):515–6.
70. Mulcahy JJ. Use of CX cylinders in association with AMS700 inflatable penile prosthesis. J Urol 1988;140(6):1420–1.
71. Ferguson KH, Cespedes RD. Prospective long-term results and quality-of-life assessment after Dura-II penile prosthesis placement. Urology 2003;61(2):437–41.
72. Fein RL. The G.F.S. Mark II inflatable penile prosthesis. J Urol 1992;147(1):66–8.
73. Pereira Arias JG, Escobal Tamayo V, Maraña Fernandez MT, et al. [Penile prosthetic implant in the treatment of impotence: our experience]. Arch Esp Urol 1994;47(7):703–8.
74. Levine LA, Estrada CR, Morgentaler A. Mechanical reliability and safety of, and patient satisfaction with the Ambicor inflatable penile prosthesis: results of a 2 center study. J Urol 2001;166(3):932–7.
75. Wilson SK, Delk JR. Historical advances in penile prostheses. Int J Impot Res 2000;12(Suppl 4):S101–7.
76. Hakky TS, Wang R, Henry GD. The evolution of the inflatable penile prosthetic device and surgical innovations with anatomical considerations. Curr Urol Rep 2014;15(6):410.
77. Henry GD. Historical review of penile prosthesis design and surgical techniques: part 1 of a three-part review series on penile prosthetic surgery. J Sex Med 2009;6(3):675–81.
78. Wilson SK, Henry GD, Delk JR, et al. The mentor Alpha 1 penile prosthesis with reservoir lock-out valve: effective prevention of auto-inflation with improved capability for ectopic reservoir placement. J Urol 2002;168(4 Pt 1):1475–8.
79. McKim SE, Carson CC. AMS 700 inflatable penile prosthesis with InhibiZone. Expert Rev Med Devices 2010;7(3):311–7.
80. Merrill DC, Javaheri P. Mentor inflatable penile prosthesis. Preliminary clinical results in 30 patients. Urology 1984;23(5 Spec No):72–4.
81. Ziegelmann MJ, Viers BR, Lomas DJ, et al. Ectopic penile prosthesis reservoir placement: an anatomic cadaver model of the high submuscular technique. J Sex Med 2016;13(9):1425–31.
82. Köhler TS, Wen L, Wilson SK. Penile implant infection prevention part 1: what is fact and what is fiction? Wilson's workshop #9. Int J Impot Res 2020. https://doi.org/10.1038/s41443-020-0326-5.
83. Le B, McVary K, McKenna K, et al. A novel thermal-activated shape memory penile prosthesis: comparative mechanical testing. Urology 2017;99:136–41.
84. Le BV, McVary KT, McKenna K, et al. Use of magnetic induction to activate a "touchless" shape memory alloy implantable penile prosthesis. J Sex Med 2019;16(4):596–601.

New Stent Technologies

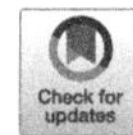

Pieter Janssen, MD, Thomas Tailly, MD, MSc, PhD*

KEYWORDS

- Ureteral stent • Biomaterial • Coating • Encrustation • Biofilm

KEY POINTS

- Whenever feasible and safe, stent placement should be omitted after an uncomplicated ureteroscopy.
- Silicone stents are soft, highly biocompatible, and resist encrustation.
- Use thin, adequately sized or multilength stents, thus avoiding crossing the midline.
- Suture stents minimize intravesical material and decrease stent-related symptoms.
- As an increased dwell time increases the risk of infection and encrustation, do not leave a stent in situ any longer than necessary.

INTRODUCTION

The history of ureteral stenting goes back to 1895, when Shoemaker[1] first described the use of a ureteral catheter in women. It was not until 1967 that Zimskind[2] reported on the use of an open-ended silicone rubber ureteral splint. In the following years, its design was quickly improved to the commonly known "*Double J" stent*, which has now been in use for more than 4 decades.[3]

With a wide range of indications for using ureteral stents, including stone disease, reconstructive ureteral surgery, trauma, and relieving the ureter from any form of obstruction, stents are one of the most commonly used urologic implants. There are however only a few indications in which drainage of the kidney (by stent or nephrostomy) is mandatory, including obstructive pyelonephritis, obstruction of both kidneys, or a solitary functioning kidney and ureteric injuries. Despite its widespread use, the routine placement of stents after uncomplicated ureteroscopy is based on low-quality evidence, and the topic remains heavily debated and studied.[4,5] Recently, a global practice pattern survey and a large prospective observational cohort study independently demonstrated more than 90% of urologists to use some form of ureteric drainage after uncomplicated ureteroscopy, mainly because of concerns of ureteric edema.[5,6] These reports demonstrate both the need and the willingness of physicians to contribute to large, multicenter, multinational, properly designed randomized clinical trials (RCTs).[4–6]

Despite the widely demonstrated advantages of stents, they also carry a considerable risk of side effects and complications, such as pain, hematuria, decreased quality of life (QoL), stent-related infection, and encrustation, attributable in part to bladder irritation by the distal coil, vesicoureteral reflux, and biofilm formation.[7–9] These risks increase with stent dwell time, and the removal of "forgotten" stents may be challenging for even the most experienced endourologist, possibly resulting in renal unit loss.[10–12]

As a result, it has been a continuous endeavor by researchers and industry to identify the underlying mechanisms of these complications and to develop alterations in stent design, biomaterials, and coatings to prevent or mitigate stents from causing the patient discomfort. This review is intended to provide an update on currently researched and available stents as well as future perspectives.

QUANTIFYING STENT-RELATED SYMPTOMS

With approximately 80% of patients experiencing bothersome stent-related symptoms (SRS), it is

Department of Urology, University Hospital Ghent, Corneel Heymanslaan 10, 9000 Ghent, Belgium
* Corresponding author.
E-mail address: Thomas.tailly@uzgent.be
Twitter: @thomastailly (T.T.)

Urol Clin N Am 49 (2022) 185–196
https://doi.org/10.1016/j.ucl.2021.08.004

not surprising that many experienced patients are reluctant to receive another stent in the future.[7,13] In an effort to provide a reliable tool to adequately study and quantify these symptoms, the ureteral stent symptom questionnaire (USSQ) was developed by Joshi and colleagues in 2003.[14] As quantification of symptoms is essential in comparative studies, the USSQ has evolved into a frequently used questionnaire that has helped gain insight into stent-specific advantages and disadvantages. An increasing interest in health-related QoL and patient-reported outcome measures (PROMs) has led to the development of several other new screening tools for stone patients, such as the Urinary Stones and Intervention QoL, Wisconsin stone QoL score, Cambridge Ureteral Stone PROM, and Cambridge Renal Stone PROM.[15] Although these PROMs, each with their specific benefits and limitations, cover several aspects of urinary stone disease and treatment, the only validated PROM that is specifically designed to capture SRS is the USSQ. Currently, the Canadian Endourology Group (CEG) is in the process of developing and validating a new PROM, called the CEG Stent Symptom Score (#NCT04909541). As QoL as an outcome variable is expected to gain momentum, these tools will most likely demonstrate to be very valuable in future stone and stent research.

BIOFILM AND ENCRUSTATION

The formation of a bacterial biofilm and encrustations are widely accepted as causes for many stent-related problems, including urinary tract infection (UTI) with possible urosepsis, renal failure, and even death.[8] The rate and level of encrustation and biofilm formation are notoriously influenced by stent indwelling time, biomaterials, and surface coatings.[8,16]

Almost immediately after stent insertion, a conditioning film is formed on the surface, often considered the prerequisite for biofilm formation.[16] It is thought that this conditioning film leads to additional bacterial accumulation and possible clinical UTI or encrustations. More recent research however demonstrated that bacterial adhesion and colonization also occurs in the absence of conditioning film, suggesting that adhesions are rather dependent on stent surface characteristics.[17] Biofilm formation and bacterial colonization of the stent surface increase over time and are present on almost 90% of stents remaining in situ for more than 90 days.[18] Interestingly, there is no strong correlation between stent cultures and positive urine cultures, and most patients with a positive stent or urine culture remain asymptomatic.[18,19] Betschart and colleagues[10] additionally identified that the quantity of biofilm did not influence SRS in patients requiring long-term stenting.

The processes of biofilm formation and encrustation often occur simultaneously, as encrustations may serve as a nidus for bacteria, and bacterial biofilm may promote crystal precipitation.[16] Encrustations may lead to stent obstruction, pain, hematuria, and hydronephrosis with possible acute renal insufficiency, necessitating stent exchange. When extensive, as can be encountered in forgotten stents, these encrustations may render stent removal or exchange tremendously difficult.[12] In these often complex cases, multiple surgeries may be needed to achieve both a stent-free and a stone-free status. To grade stent encrustations and help determine treatment difficulty, a few scoring systems have been developed, such as FECal (Forgotten, Encrusted, Calcified) and KUB (Kidney, Ureter, Bladder), both of which were shown to be significant predictors of stent-free and stone-free status, although only the KUB system correlated with the need for multiple surgeries.[20] Recently, the V-GUES (Visual Grading for Ureteral Encrusted Stents) scoring system was proposed based on a visual interpretation of stent calcifications on non-contrast-enhanced computed tomographic scan.[21] Based on the location and the extent of the encrustations on the distal coil, proximal coil, and stent body, 4 categories were proposed (A–D), which showed correlation with number of sessions needed to achieve success and with complications.[21]

As the cause of encrustations is multifactorial, and related to physical and biochemical properties of the stent as well as patient specific factors, efforts should be directed to controlling multiple facets of stent encrustation, such as surface engineering, biocompatibility, and changing the urinary environment.[8,16] In an extensive review elaborating on surface engineering strategies to prevent bacterial adhesion, biofilm formation, and encrustation, Vladkova and colleagues[22] summarize that current research is mainly focused on mechanical detachment, killing of bacteria in contact with the stent's surface, and development of low-adhesive surfaces. Despite the vast variety of engineered surfaces having been tested in vitro or in animal studies, very few of these have made it onto the surface of commercially available stents thus far. Translational research in this area is of specific interest, as many results of in vitro trials are not reliably reproduced in humans because of the complexity of the human urinary environment.

STRATEGIES TO IMPROVE STENT CHARACTERISTICS, BIOCOMPATIBILITY, AND TOLERABILITY

Biomaterials

Silicone and other polymers

Although the very first double J stents were manufactured from silicone, this highly biocompatible biomaterial had fallen into disuse in the past few decades, as its low tensile strength and high friction coefficient often hindered stent insertion. Whereas silicon stents are currently only used in approximately 6% of cases, they may soon be going through a revival, with recent reports emerging on their advantageous biocompatibility.[6,23,24] Corroborating the in vitro findings of Tunney and colleagues, Barghouthy and colleagues[24,25] demonstrated silicone stents to resist encrustations and biofilm formation better than Percuflex stents in a prospective RCT. Whereas the softness of silicone stents may in part explain why they are better tolerated than other polymer stents, it also causes the stent to be more prone to failure because of kinking or external compression.[23] Polyurethane's favorable mechanical properties in comparison to silicone, along with its low production cost, led to its incorporation in stent manufacturing.[26] As a result, many currently available stents are either based on polyurethane or proprietary copolymeric blends of which often little or no information is publicly available.

One of the mechanical properties of these biomaterials is reported as their durometer: the resistance to compression by a pin gauge under standard test conditions. Although firmer materials are more resistant to extrinsic compression, they may intuitively cause more SRS, as they do not adapt as well to the winding course of the human ureter. Clinical research however could not provide a unanimous response to this hypothesis. In a prospective single-blinded RCT, patients with stents made from a soft polymer (Contour, Boston Scientific; Marlborough, MA, USA) had similar USSQ scores on all domains compared with patients with stents made from a firm polymer (Percuflex, Boston Scientific; Marlborough, MA, USA), despite an earlier trial, which did show a reduction in dysuria, renal, and suprapubic pain.[27,28] Dual-durometer stents consist of a firm biomaterial at the proximal coil and transition to a softer biomaterial at the distal coil in order to reduce bladder irritation. Davenport and colleagues[29] compared the Polaris (Boston Scientific; Marlborough, MA, USA)dual-durometer stent with the Bard Inlay (C.R. Bard Inc.; NJ, USA) stent and found no significant difference in any of the USSQ domains. Although the Bard Inlay stent is marketed to soften up to 50% at body temperature, there was no significant difference in USSQ domain scores when compared with a firmer Percuflex stent.[30] Although there is no available literature yet, a new stent on the market, the TRIA stent from Boston Scientific (Marlborough, MA, USA), is also alleged to soften up to 40% at body temperature in addition to reducing encrustations owing to a low surface energy. It remains to be assessed whether this also provides the patient more comfort.

Rebl and colleagues[31] evaluated surface characteristics of different polymers in artificial urine with different compositions. Increased hydrophilicity and a stronger negative zeta potential or surface charge seemed to reduce encrustations.[31] Because carbonate apatite and struvite, frequent components of encrustations, have been shown to have a negative zeta potential as well, and negative charges repel each other, it makes sense that surfaces with a strong negative charge are more resistant to encrustations.[31] The least encrusted surfaces were Styroflex, Elastollan, and Greenflex, hydrophobic materials with a strong negative surface charge, whereas Carbothane, Pelletane, and Tecophilic, which are hydrophobic and have a fairly small negative surface charge, were most encrusted in this trial.[31]

Biodegradable materials

In contrast to patients requiring stents for malignant external compression, a stent for benign indications is usually only necessary for a shorter period of time and thus necessitates removal. Several strategies to obviate cystoscopic stent removal are being explored, such as removal by a string or magnetic tip catheter, and by manufacturing stents from biodegradable polymers. Whereas stents on strings and with a magnetic tip have been available for decades, they are not widely used, despite reduced pain during extraction in comparison to cystoscopy.[6,9,32] Currently investigated biodegradable compounds include natural and synthetic polymers as well as metallic compounds (**Table 1**). Although biodegradable stents are not freely available for clinical practice yet, a prospective, multicenter in-human trial with Uriprene stents is planned (#NCT04565795). Once they enter the market, they may not only render cystoscopy unnecessary but also eradicate forgotten stents.

Coatings

In an effort to change how a biomaterial interacts with its surroundings (ie, urine), various surface coatings have been developed and applied on the stent's surface. These may aim to reduce

Table 1
Biodegradable materials for ureteral stents

Material	Properties	Trials	Notable Findings
Natural origin polymers	Excellent biocompatibility Fast degradation	*Gelatin-based stent*[73] porcine model	Complete degradation in 10 d Lower maximum tensile strain than conventional stents Stiffness ≥ conventional stents for up to 7 d
Synthetic origin polymers	High biocompatibility Combination of polymers allows for controlled degradation without obstructing fragments[74]	*Braidstent*,[75] porcine model *Braidstent-H*[76] (heparin-coated), porcine model *Uriprene*,[77] porcine model	Antireflux, completely intraureteral Controlled degradation High rates of bacteriuria No lasting reduction of bacteriuria with heparin coating Controlled degradation in 2–4 wk Decrease hydronephrosis and tissue inflammation Human trial coming up[78]
Metallic compounds	Excellent mechanical properties Antibacterial	*Magnesium*,[79] in vitro *Magnesium-zinc alloy*,[80] porcine model	Reduced bacterial cell density after 16 h incubation when compared with polyurethane and polystyrene Good biocompatibility Reduction of bacteriuria when compared with medical stainless-steel stents Full degradation after 12–14 wk

biofilm or encrustation, facilitate insertion of the stent by lowering the friction coefficient, or even release drugs to reduce SRS or treat ureteral malignancy. Applying a hydrophilic coating to lower the contact angle of a hydrophobic surface should have the theoretic advantage of reducing encrustations.[33] In an in vitro analysis comparing Pellethane thermoplastic polyurethane with and without several coatings to standard hydrogel coated ureteral stents, Pellethane showed significantly reduced encrustation rates, an effect that was enhanced by applying a hydrophilic surface coating.[34]

Drug-eluting stents have the advantage of carrying a drug and releasing it in situ in the environment in which it dwells. They are frequently used in percutaneous interventions for coronary artery disease, but are also being developed to reduce SRS, treat ureteral malignancy, or reduce biofilm and/or encrustations (**Table 2**). Similarly, antibiotic agents can be incorporated in biofilm-reducing coatings, although a growing concern for antibiotic resistance may promote investigating other pathways.[8,16] There is increasing interest in coatings with antifouling properties, which resist bacterial adherence and biofilm formation by different mechanisms.[35] A summary of recently investigated stent coatings is provided in **Table 3**. Although many of these coatings are currently under investigation, human trials are scarce.

Metallic and Reinforced Stents

Ureteral obstruction owing to external compression poses a specific challenge, as single polymeric ureteral stents fail to retain patency in up to 60% of patients with malignant ureteral obstruction.[36] In order to improve patency rates and decrease the need for stent exchanges, reinforced and metallic stents with increased resistance to radial compression forces have been designed.[37–39] A distinction can be made between segmental stents and stents with the classical DJ design. Of the latter, only the Resonance stent and Silhouette stent (Applied Medical; Santa Margarita, CA, USA) are currently available for use in patients, with the Silhouette demonstrating a higher resistance to external compression in

Table 2
Drug-eluting stents

Author	Applied Drug(s)	Trial	Results
Krambeck et al,[81] 2010	Ketorolac	In human RCT	No significant change in SRS
Mendez-Probst et al,[82] 2012	Triclosan	In human RCT	Decreased LUTS and flank pain, no effect on biofilm formation, less antibiotic use
Barros et al,[83] 2016	Paclitaxel, doxorubicine, gemcitabine, epirubicin	In vitro	Potentially effective drug delivery system for treatment of upper tract urothelial cancer
Kram et al,[84] 2018	Paclitaxel	Porcine model	Reduced hyperplastic proliferation, possibly reducing scar-induced stenosis.

Abbreviation: LUTS, lower urinary tract symptoms.

bench-top testing.[39] Although many of these stents have been tested in vitro and their efficiency has been demonstrated in cohort studies, there is only 1 very small RCT available demonstrating superiority of a segmental metal mesh stent (Urexel; S&G Biotech, Seongnam, Korea) to standard polymeric stents.[37–41] The same group reported a 70% success rate 12 months after stent placement in a retrospective cohort series.[41] Two comparative studies identified that a Resonance stent (Cook medical; Bloomington, IN, USA) has a longer patency time than other polymeric stents, with up to 91.7% of stents demonstrating patency at 1 year after placement.[42,43] Despite their considerably higher cost, an assumed longer dwell time could theoretically establish these stents as cost-efficient in comparison to regular stents.[38] Currently available metallic enforced or metal mesh stents and their characteristics as well as available clinical results have been summarized in **Table 4**. In an in vivo rabbit study, Zhao and colleagues[44] recently observed a significant reduction in encrustations and bacterial attachment with a Cu-bearing stainless steel mesh stents.

In an in vitro study, evaluating the resistance of reinforced stents to external compression, Vogt demonstrated the 8F Teleflex stent (Teleflex Medical, Germany) to be most resistant and additionally identified that placing 2 stents in tandem provided the best results in maintaining flow at high external pressures.[37] Stiffness as well as inner diameter and the preservation thereof seem to be the most important factors to increase and maintain flow rates.[37]

Several retrospective reports demonstrate the efficacy of tandem stenting, and 1 prospective non-RCT identified tandem polymeric stents to achieve a longer patency time in comparison to a single reinforced stent (214.7 ± 21.0 days vs 176.7 ± 21.3 days, respectively).[45,46] Unfortunately, however, there are no adequate data on how well patients tolerate tandem or metal stents in comparison to regular stents.

Stent Architecture/Design

Aside from applying different biomaterials, changes in stent architecture may improve tolerance, and several innovative designs are becoming available, challenging the "Double J" shape.

Stent length

As stents have been demonstrated to cause more symptoms when they are inappropriately sized, choosing the optimal length is important.[47] Although placing an undersized stent might increase the risk of migration, longer stents may increase SRS and reduce QoL, especially when crossing the bladder midline.[13,47,48] Although several methods based on anthropomorphic measurements or imaging techniques have been investigated to estimate ureteral length, they all lack accuracy, confirming direct measurement using a ureteral catheter as the gold standard, which is however time-consuming and increases the cost and x-ray exposure of the procedure.[49–51] In order to obviate length estimates as well as reduce costly stock holding, multilength stents were developed with double coils on both ends to avoid migration and reduce trigonal irritation. In a randomized trial comparing 22- with 30-cm multilength and regular 24-cm stents, there was no

Table 3
Coatings reducing biofilm formation and encrustation

Author	Coating	Trial	Effect	Mechanism
Frant et al,[85] 2018	Tetraether lipid-Ag-norfloxacin-polylactid	In vitro	Reduced encrustation (10%–20%) and biofilm (75%–80%)	Bactericidal (Ag + norfloxacin)
Szell et al,[86] 2019	poly(*N*,*N*-dimethylacrylamide)	In vitro	Significant reduction in *Escherichia coli* bacterial load	Antifouling (entropic shielding)
Stirpe et al,[87] 2020	Poloxamer 388	In vitro	78%–85% reduction in *E coli* CFU/cm^2	Antifouling
Tailly et al,[88] 2021	mPEG-3,4-DOPA ± $AgNO_3$	Animal (rabbit)	Decreased incidence of positive urine culture 7 d after *E coli* inoculation	Antifouling (mPEG) and bactericidal (Ag)
Yu et al,[89] 2021	Polydopamine/ultrahigh molecular weight poly(*N*,*N*-dimethylacrylamide)	In vitro Animal (mouse) Animal (pig)	90% colonization resistance 98% biofilm reduction 95% reduction in *E coli* adherence	Antifouling
Kai-Larsen et al,[90] 2021	Noble metal alloy (gold-silver-palladium)	Multicenter, prospective study	67% reduction in symptomatic catheter-associated urinary tract infection	Antifouling (galvanic effect)

Abbreviation: mPEG-3,4-DOPA, methoxylated polyethylene glycol 3,4-dihydroxyphenylalanine.

Table 4
Overview of long-term metallic stents for use in ureteric obstruction (summarized from published literature[38–41])

Stent Name	Materials	Design	Featured Properties	Mean Success Rate (%)	Mean Indwelling Duration (mo)	Most Frequently Reported Complications Other than SRS
Resonance	Nickel-cobalt-chromium-molybdenum alloy	JJ with tight spiral structure, no end or side holes	Very high tensile strength and flexibility	72.5	8.2	UTI (5%–100%), obstruction (3.7%–80%), encrustation (0.7%–11%), migration (1.4%–8.1%)
Silhouette	Polymer covered stent with internal coiled nitinol	JJ, only 1 opening proximal and distal. No side holes	Highest resistance to compression	NA	NA	No reports of clinical use, personal experience: UTI, obstruction due to encrustation
Memokath	Nitinol (nickel titanium alloy)	Segmental, thermoexpandable, intraureteral design with proximal ± distal wider end	Less encrustation and tissue ingrowth. Better tolerance	64	10.5	Migration (13.5%–60%) Encrustation (6.8%–10.8%) Obstruction (14.3%–20%) UTI (8.1%–10%)
Uventa	PTFE-covered nitinol mesh	Segmental, self-expandable, inner and outer mesh with PTFE layer in between to prevent tissue ingrowth	Outer stent prevents migration, inner stent preserves patency	74.5	Not reported	Obstruction (11.8%–22.2%) Migration (1.9%–5.9%) UTI 10.8% One trial (44 patients) with 28% class IIIb complication: fistulas, perforation, uncontrollable bleeding, and complete obstruction[91]
Allium	Copolymer-covered nitinol	Segmental, self-expandable, with an intravesical anchoring mechanism	High radial force, coating prevents tissue ingrowth and encrustation	60.9	Not reported	Migration (17.5%–18.9%) Obstruction (2.5%) UTI 10.8%
Urexel[40,41]	Outer bare metallic mesh, silicon covered internally	Segmental, self-expandable	Increased tissue compatibility	70	12	Loss of patency, 26.9% Hematuria/hematoma: 48.1% Urinary tract injury: 7.6%

Memokath: PNN medical, Denmark; Uventa: Taewoong Medical Co., Seoul, South Korea; Allium: Allium Medical, Israel.
Abbreviations: NA, not applicable; PTFE, polytetrafluoroethylene; SRS, stent-related symptoms.

difference in any of the USSQ domains.[52] This may be explained by the fact that the double coil results in increased intravesical stent material, mitigating the benefits of proper positioning.

Stent diameter

Relief (or prevention) of obstruction of the ureter and facilitating urinary flow down to the bladder is the primary purpose of most ureteral stents. With increasing diameter, computational analysis models have shown that intraluminal flow rate increases, whereas extraluminal flow may decrease.[53,54] Although these models do not take passive ureteral dilation into account, a larger-caliber stent may not always increase the total flow rate and may actually act as an obstacle in the ureter.[55] Several clinical trials have reported on the relation between stent diameter and SRS. Thinner stents seem to have a positive effect on SRS and may facilitate clearance of stone fragments, such as after extracorporeal shockwave lithotripsy (ESWL).[56–58] As there is no evidence suggesting they lead to worse outcomes, smaller stents should generally be preferred. In an ex vivo porcine model, Lange and colleagues[59] demonstrated that total flow rates using a 3F "MicroStent" (PercSys; CA, USA) were not significantly different when compared with a conventional 4.7F DJ stent. This can possibly be attributed to the design of the Microstent, which has an anchoring mechanism proximal to the stone that causes "tenting" of the ureteral tissue, enlarging the ureteral diameter close to the obstruction. The Microstent is unfortunately not commercially available.

Stent body

In an attempt to increase conformity of the stent body to the ureter, helical stents were developed (Percuflex Helical, Boston Scientific; Marlborough, MA, USA) and demonstrated similar flow rates when compared with a same-material nonhelical design (Percuflex Plus, Boston Scientific; Marlborough, MA, USA).[60] In a small trial matching 15 patients receiving a helical stent to a historical control group, there was no difference in unscheduled patient visits, although a significantly reduced analgesic use was reported.[61] Unfortunately, no further studies corroborating these results have been reported or seem to have been planned so far. In a microfluidic-based model of a stented and obstructed ureter, Mosayyebi and colleagues[62] investigated changes in stent architecture to increase wall shear stress and thus reduce encrustation rates. A reduction of encrustation of up to 94% was seen in a stent with reduced (0.3 mm) wall thickness and triangular side holes. Although to the authors' knowledge, no currently clinically available stents feature this design, this challenges the current design and may encourage manufacturers to rethink the current design.

Distal coil

As the distal coil of the stent is thought to be responsible for several SRS, such as lower urinary tract symptoms and reflux, several design alterations have been suggested to increase stent tolerance. Some advantages have been reported for replacing the distal coil with thin silicone loops or a tapered 3F tail.[63,64] Vogt and colleagues[65] reduced stent diameter to a minimum by replacing the distal part of the stent with a 0.3F suture thread, the so-called suture stent, and observed a significant improvement in patients' pain and urinary symptom scores.[65] Importantly, the suture tail induced comparable ureteral dilation to a conventional stent, facilitating second-stage ureteroscopy and preventing renal colic from descending fragments after ESWL. Further trials have confirmed the suture stent to be a feasible and safe alternative to conventional stents, decreasing USSQ scores, and reducing irritation and inflammation of the ureteric orifice.[66–68] Although Vogt and colleagues hypothesized that the suture stent would reduce vesicoureteral reflux, it was demonstrated in a porcine model that intrapelvic pressures are similar to using conventional stents.[65,68] In an attempt to reduce pain caused by vesicoureteral reflux, several researchers have investigated the effect of fitting the distal coil with a nonrefluxing end piece. The strategy already dates back to 1992, when Yamaguchi and colleagues[69] applied a thin silicone sleeve to the distal portion of the stent, which acted as a flap-valve, closing when intravesical pressure rises. More recently, a similar 3-dimensional printed model showed adequate in vitro forward flow rates while decreasing backward flow rate by 4 to 8.3 times.[70] In a small randomized, single-blinded study, comparing a standard stent to an antireflux stent, fitted with a collapsing valve, Ritter and colleagues[71] could not identify any significant differences between the 2 groups regarding USSQ scores. Another prototype incorporated a winged valve mechanism fitted on a sectioned stent tip to reduce intravesical material and was shown to decrease USSQ urinary symptoms and QoL scores in vivo.[72]

It is clear from the vast amount of literature still emerging that there does not exist 1 stent to fit all patients, nor an ideal stent that does not cause any symptoms, infections, or encrustations. The search for the ideal ureteral stent continues as new designs, biomaterials, and coatings are being evaluated. Biodegradable stents have the advantage of obviating cystoscopic removal and eliminating the forgotten stent problem, whereas changes in stent design can improve SRS. Enhancing existing biomaterial properties by using novel coating agents is another promising approach to increase patient's tolerance and reduce stent-related infection and encrustations. Antifouling coatings have the advantage of reducing bacterial adhesion without causing antimicrobial resistance. To achieve synergistic beneficial effects, the simultaneous use of multiple pathways to reduce stent symptoms, biofilm formation, and encrustations is being researched. With promising results emerging from in vitro and animal research, future clinical trials are warranted and eagerly awaited, as they have the potential to drastically improve patient-reported outcomes in stone surgery.

SUMMARY

Ureteral stents are an indispensable part of any (endo-) urologic practice. Despite the widely demonstrated advantages of stents, they also carry a considerable risk of side effects and complications, such as urinary symptoms, pain, hematuria, decreased QoL, stent-related infection, and encrustation. Multiple pathways in preventing or mitigating these side effects and complications and improving stent efficacy have been and are being investigated, including stent architecture and design, biomaterials, and coatings. This article provides an update on currently researched and available stents as well as future perspectives.

DISCLOSURE

The corresponding author is a consultant for Boston Scientific, Cook Medical, Storz, and Ambu. P. Janssen has nothing to disclose.

REFERENCES

1. Shoemaker GE IV. An improvement in the technique of catheterization of the ureter in the female. Ann Surg 1895;22(5):650–4.
2. Zimskind PD, Fetter TR, Wilkerson JL. Clinical use of long-term indwelling silicone rubber ureteral splints inserted cystoscopically. J Urol 1967;97(5):840–4.
3. Finney RP. Experience with new double J ureteral catheter stent. J Urol 1978;120(6):678–81.
4. Ordonez M, Hwang EC, Borofsky M, et al. Ureteral stent versus no ureteral stent for ureteroscopy in the management of renal and ureteral calculi. Cochrane Database Syst Rev 2019;2019(2).
5. Bhatt NR, MacKenzie K, Shah TT, et al. Survey on ureTEric draiNage post uncomplicaTed ureteroscopy (STENT). BJUI Compass 2020;bco2.48. https://doi.org/10.1002/bco2.48.
6. Dasgupta R, Ong TA, Lim J, et al. A global perspective of stenting after ureteroscopy: an observational multicenter cohort study. Société Int D'urologie J 2021;2(2):96–105.
7. Joshi HB, Stainthorpe A, MacDonagh RP, et al. Indwelling ureteral stents: evaluation of symptoms, quality of life and utility. J Urol 2003;169(3):1065–9. discussion 1069.
8. Khoddami S, Chew BH, Lange D. Problems and solutions of stent biofilm and encrustations: a review of literature. Turkish J Urol 2020;46(Suppl 1):11–8.
9. Beysens M, Tailly TO. Ureteral stents in urolithiasis. Asian J Urol 2018;5(4):274–86.
10. Betschart P, Zumstein V, Buhmann MT, et al. Symptoms associated with long-term double-J ureteral stenting and influence of biofilms. Urology 2019; 134:72–8.
11. Kawahara T, Ito H, Terao H, et al. Ureteral stent encrustation, incrustation, and coloring: morbidity related to indwelling times. J Endourol 2012;26(2): 178–82.
12. Mahmood K, Singh KH, Upadhyay R, et al. Management of forgotten double-J stent in a tertiary care center with ten years of experience: a retrospective study. Int Surg J Mahmood K Al Int Surg J 2020;7(8): 2615–20.
13. Inn FX, Ahmed N, Hou LG, et al. Intravesical stent position as a predictor of quality of life in patients with indwelling ureteral stent. Int Urol Nephrol 2019;51(11):1949–53.
14. Joshi HB, Newns N, Stainthorpe A, et al. Ureteral stent symptom questionnaire: development and validation of a multidimensional quality of life measure. J Urol 2003;169(3):1060–4.
15. Mehmi A, Jones P, Somani BK. Current status and role of patient-reported outcome measures (PROMs) in endourology. Urology 2021;148:26–31.
16. Tomer N, Garden E, Small A, et al. Ureteral stent encrustation: epidemiology, pathophysiology, management and current technology. J Urol 2021; 205(1):68–77.
17. Elwood CN, Lo J, Chou E, et al. Understanding urinary conditioning film components on ureteral stents: profiling protein components and evaluating their role in bacterial colonization. Biofouling 2013; 29(9):1115–22.
18. Shabeena KS, Bhargava R, Manzoor MAP, et al. Characteristics of bacterial colonization after indwelling double-J ureteral stents for different time duration. Urologe A 2018;10(1):71–5.
19. Klis R, Korczak-Kozakiewicz E, Denys A, et al. Relationship between urinary tract infection and self-retaining double-J catheter colonization. J Endourol 2009;23(6):1015–9.

20. Guner E, Seker KG. Comparison of two different scoring systems in encrusted ureteral stent management: a single-center experience. Urol J 2020;17(3): 248–51.
21. Manzo BO, Alarcon PS, Lozada E, et al. A novel visual - grading for ureteral encrusted stents classification (V-GUES) to help decide the endourologic treatment. J Endourol 2021. https://doi.org/10.1089/end.2020.1225.
22. Vladkova TG, Staneva AD, Gospodinova DN. Surface engineered biomaterials and ureteral stents inhibiting biofilm formation and encrustation. Surf Coat Technol 2020;404:126424.
23. Wiseman O, Ventimiglia E, Doizi S, et al. Effects of silicone hydrocoated double loop ureteral stent on symptoms and quality of life in patients undergoing flexible ureteroscopy for kidney stone: a randomized multicenter clinical study. J Urol 2020;204(4): 769–77.
24. Barghouthy Y, Wiseman O, Ventimiglia E, et al. Silicone-hydrocoated ureteral stents encrustation and biofilm formation after 3-week dwell time: results of a prospective randomized multicenter clinical study. World J Urol 2021;1–7.
25. Tunney MM, Keane PF, Jones DS, et al. Comparative assessment of ureteral stent biomaterial encrustation. Biomaterials 1996;17(15):1541–6.
26. Venkatesan N, Shroff S, Jayachandran K, et al. Polymers as ureteral stents. J Endourol 2010;24(2): 191–8.
27. Joshi HB, Chitale SV, Nagarajan M, et al. A prospective randomized single-blind comparison of ureteral stents composed of firm and soft polymer. J Urol 2005;174(6):2303–6.
28. Lennon GM, Thornhill JA, Sweeney PA, et al. "Firm" versus "soft" double pigtail ureteric stents: a randomised blind comparative trial. Eur Urol 1995;28(1):1–5.
29. Davenport K, Kumar V, Collins J, et al. New ureteral stent design does not improve patient quality of life: a randomized, controlled trial. J Urol 2011;185(1): 175–8.
30. Park HK, Paick SH, Kim HG, et al. The impact of ureteral stent type on patient symptoms as determined by the ureteral stent symptom questionnaire: a prospective, randomized, controlled study. J Endourol 2015;29(3):367–71.
31. Rebl H, Renner J, Kram W, et al. Prevention of encrustation on ureteral stents: which surface parameters provide guidance for the development of novel stent materials? Polymers (Basel) 2020;12(3):558.
32. Luo Z, Jiao B, Zhao H, et al. The efficacy and safety of ureteric stent removal with strings versus no strings: which is better? Biomed Res Int 2020; 2020:4081409.
33. Laube N, Desai C, Bernsmann F. Hydrophobic forces as a key factor in crystalline biofilm formation on ureteral stents. Biomed Tech 2016;61(5):483–90.
34. Cottone CM, Lu S, Wu YX, et al. Surface-treated pellethanes: comparative quantification of encrustation in artificial urine solution. J Endourol 2020;34(8): 868–73.
35. Ramachandra M, Mosayyebi A, Carugo D, et al. Strategies to improve patient outcomes and QOL: current complications of the design and placements of ureteric stents 2020. https://doi.org/10.2147/RRU.S233981.
36. Elsamra SE, Leavitt DA, Motato HA, et al. Stenting for malignant ureteral obstruction: tandem, metal or metal-mesh stents. Int J Urol 2015;22(7):629–36.
37. Vogt B. Stiffness analysis of reinforced ureteral stents against radial compression: in vitro study. Res Reports Urol 2020;12:583–91.
38. Corrales M, Doizi S, Barghouthy Y, et al. A systematic review of long-duration stents for ureteral stricture: which one to choose? World J Urol 2021. https://doi.org/10.1007/s00345-020-03544-x.
39. Pedro RN, Hendlin K, Kriedberg C, et al. Wire-based ureteral stents: impact on tensile strength and compression. Urology 2007;70(6):1057–9.
40. Kim JW, Hong B, Shin JH, et al. A prospective randomized comparison of a covered metallic ureteral stent and a double-J stent for malignant ureteral obstruction. Korean J Radiol 2018;19(4):606–12.
41. Kim ET, Yang WJ, Shin JH, et al. Comparison of a covered metallic ureteral stent and a double-J stent for malignant ureteral obstruction in advanced gastric cancer. Clin Radiol 2021;76(7): 519–25.
42. Chow P-M, Chiang I-N, Chen C-Y, et al. Malignant ureteral obstruction: functional duration of metallic versus polymeric ureteral stents 2015. https://doi.org/10.1371/journal.pone.0135566.
43. Chen Y, Liu CY, Zhang ZH, et al. Malignant ureteral obstruction: experience and comparative analysis of metallic versus ordinary polymer ureteral stents. World J Surg Oncol 2019;17(1):1–10.
44. Zhao J, Cao Z, Lin H, et al. In vivo research on Cu-bearing ureteral stent. J Mater Sci Mater Med 2019; 30(7):83.
45. Liu K-LL, Lee B-CC, Ye J-D De, et al. Comparison of single and tandem ureteral stenting for malignant ureteral obstruction: a prospective study of 104 patients. Eur Radiol 2019;29(2):628–35.
46. Tabib C, Nethala D, Kozel Z, et al. Management and treatment options when facing malignant ureteral obstruction. Int J Urol 2020;27(7):591–8.
47. Giannarini G, Keeley FX, Valent F, et al. Predictors of morbidity in patients with indwelling ureteric stents: results of a prospective study using the validated Ureteric Stent Symptoms Questionnaire. BJU Int 2011;107(4):648–54.
48. Breau RH, Norman RW. Optimal prevention and management of proximal ureteral stent migration and remigration. J Urol 2001;166(3):890–3.

49. Novaes HFF, Leite PCS, Almeida RA, et al. Analysis of ureteral length in adult cadavers. Int Braz J Urol 2013;39(2):248–56. discussion 256.
50. Kawahara T, Sakamaki K, Ito H, et al. Developing a preoperative predictive model for ureteral length for ureteral stent insertion. BMC Urol 2016;16(1):1–5.
51. Kuo J, Rabley A, Domino P, et al. Evaluation of patient factors that influence predictive formulas for determining ureteral stent length when compared to direct measurement. J Endourol 2020;34(8): 805–10.
52. Calvert RC, Wong KY, Chitale SV, et al. Multi-length or 24 cm ureteric stent? A multicentre randomised comparison of stent-related symptoms using a validated questionnaire. BJU Int 2013;111(7): 1099–104.
53. Brewer AV, Elbahnasy AM, Bercowsky E, et al. Mechanism of ureteral stent flow: a comparative in vivo study. J Endourol 1999;13(4):269–71.
54. Kim H-H, Kim K-W, Choi YH, et al. Numerical analysis of urine flow with multiple sizes of double-J stents. Appl Sci 2020;10(12).
55. Kim K-W, Kim H-H, Choi YH, et al. Urine flow analysis using double J stents of various sizes in in vitro ureter models. Int J Numer Method Biomed Eng 2020;36(2).
56. Nestler S, Witte B, Schilchegger L, et al. Size does matter: ureteral stents with a smaller diameter show advantages regarding urinary symptoms, pain levels and general health. World J Urol 2019. https://doi.org/10.1007/s00345-019-02829-0.
57. Kim BS, Choi JY, Jung W. Does a ureteral stent with a smaller diameter reduce stent-related bladder irritation? A single-blind, randomized, controlled, multicenter study. J Endourol 2020;34(3):368–72.
58. Taguchi M, Yoshida K, Sugi M, et al. Effect of ureteral stent diameter on ureteral stent-related symptoms. Low Urin Tract Symptoms 2019;11(4):195–9.
59. Lange D, Hoag NA, Poh BK, et al. Drainage characteristics of the 3F MicroStent using a novel film occlusion anchoring mechanism. J Endourol 2011; 25(6):1051–6.
60. Mucksavage P, Pick D, Haydel D, et al. An in vivo evaluation of a novel spiral cut flexible ureteral stent. Urology 2012;79(3):733–7.
61. Chew BH, Arsovska O, Lange D, et al. Percuflex helical ureteral stent provides excellent patient comfort and upper tract drainage. J Endourol 2014;28: A50–1.
62. Mosayyebi A, Lange D, Yann Yue Q, et al. Reducing deposition of encrustation in ureteric stents by changing the stent architecture: a microfluidic-based investigation. Biomicrofluidics 2019;13(1): 14101.
63. Taguchi M, Inoue T, Muguruma K, et al. Impact of loop-tail ureteral stents on ureteral stentrelated symptoms immediately after ureteroscopic lithotripsy: comparison with pigtail ureteral stents. Investig Clin Urol 2017;58(6):440–6.
64. Dunn MD, Portis AJ, Kahn SA, et al. Clinical effectiveness of new stent design: randomized single-blind comparison of tail and double-pigtail stents. J Endourol 2000;14(2):195–202.
65. Vogt B, Desgrippes A, Desfemmes F-N. Changing the double-pigtail stent by a new suture stent to improve patient's quality of life: a prospective study. World J Urol 2015;33(8):1061–8.
66. Yoshida T, Inoue T, Taguchi M, et al. Efficacy and safety of complete intraureteral stent placement versus conventional stent placement in relieving ureteral stent related symptoms: a randomized, prospective, single blind, multicenter clinical trial. Int Braz J Urol 2020;46(2):269–70.
67. Betschart P, Piller A, Zumstein V, et al. Reduction of stent-associated morbidity by minimizing stent material: a prospective, randomized, single-blind superiority trial assessing a customized 'suture stent. BJU Int 2021;127(5):596–605.
68. Majdalany SE, Aldoukhi AH, Jung H, et al. In vivo evaluation of a novel pigtail suture stent. Urology 2021;148:83–7.
69. Yamaguchi O, Yoshimura Y, Irisawa C, et al. Prototype of a reflux preventing ureteral stent and its clinical use. Urology 1992;40(4):326–9.
70. Park C-J, Kim H-W, Jeong S, et al. Anti-reflux ureteral stent with polymeric flap valve using three-dimensional printing: an in vitro study. J Endourol 2015. https://doi.org/10.1089/end.2015.0154.
71. Ritter M, Krombach P, Knoll T, et al. Initial experience with a newly developed antirefluxive ureter stent. Urol Res 2012;40(4):349–53.
72. Vogt B. A new customized ureteral stent with nonrefluxing silicone end-piece to alleviate stent-related symptoms in malignant diseases. Urology 2020; 137:45–9.
73. Barros AA, Oliveira C, Ribeiro AJ, et al. In vivo assessment of a novel biodegradable ureteral stent. World J Urol 2017;36(2):277–83.
74. Wang X, Shan H, Wang J, et al. Characterization of nanostructured ureteral stent with gradient degradation in a porcine model. Int J Nanomedicine 2015;10: 3055–64.
75. Soria F, De La Cruz JE, Budia A, et al. Experimental assessment of new generation of ureteral stents: biodegradable and antireflux properties. J Endourol 2020. https://doi.org/10.1089/end.2019.0493.
76. Soria F, de La Cruz JE, Caballero-Romeu JP, et al. Comparative assessment of biodegradable-antireflux heparine coated ureteral stent: animal model study. BMC Urol 2021;21(1):32.
77. Chew BH, Paterson RF, Clinkscales KW, et al. In vivo evaluation of the third generation biodegradable stent: a novel approach to avoiding the forgotten stent syndrome. J Urol 2013;189(2):719–25.

78. Safety and device performance of the Uriprene® degradable temporary ureteral stent following uncomplicated ureteroscopy - ClinicalTrials.gov.
79. Lock JY, Draganov M, Whall A, et al. Antimicrobial properties of biodegradable magnesium for next generation ureteral stent applications. Conf Proc IEEE Eng Med Biol Soc 2012;2012:1378–81.
80. Tie D, Liu H, Guan R, et al. In vivo assessment of biodegradable magnesium alloy ureteral stents in a pig model. Acta Biomater 2020;116:415–25.
81. Krambeck AE, Walsh RS, Denstedt JD, et al. A novel drug eluting ureteral stent: a prospective, randomized, multicenter clinical trial to evaluate the safety and effectiveness of a ketorolac loaded ureteral stent. J Urol 2010;183(3):1037–42.
82. Mendez-Probst CE, Goneau LW, MacDonald KW, et al. The use of triclosan eluting stents effectively reduces ureteral stent symptoms: a prospective randomized trial. BJU Int 2012;110(5):749–54.
83. Barros AA, Browne S, Oliveira C, et al. Drug-eluting biodegradable ureteral stent: new approach for urothelial tumors of upper urinary tract cancer. Int J Pharm 2016;513(1–2):227–37.
84. Kram W, Rebl H, Wyrwa R, et al. Paclitaxel-coated stents to prevent hyperplastic proliferation of ureteral tissue: from in vitro to in vivo. Urolithiasis 2018;48(1):47–56.
85. Frant M, Dayyoub E, Bakowsky U, et al. Evaluation of a ureteral catheter coating by means of a Bio-Encrustation in vitro model. Int J Pharm 2018; 546(1–2):86–96.
86. Szell T, Dressler FF, Goelz H, et al. In vitro effects of a novel coating agent on bacterial biofilm development on ureteral stents. J Endourol 2019. https://doi.org/10.1089/end.2018.0616.
87. Stirpe M, Brugnoli B, Donelli G, et al. Poloxamer 338 affects cell adhesion and biofilm formation in Escherichia coli: potential applications in the management of catheter-associated urinary tract infections. Pathogens 2020;9(11):1–16.
88. Tailly T, MacPhee RA, Cadieux P, et al. Evaluation of polyethylene glycol-based antimicrobial coatings on urinary catheters in the prevention of Escherichia coli infections in a rabbit model. J Endourol 2021; 35(1):116–21.
89. Yu K, Alzahrani A, Khoddami S, et al. Self-limiting mussel inspired thin antifouling coating with broad-spectrum resistance to biofilm formation to prevent catheter-associated infection in mouse and porcine models. Adv Healthc Mater 2021;2001573:1–18.
90. Kai-Larsen Y, Grass S, Mody B, et al. Foley catheter with noble metal alloy coating for preventing catheter-associated urinary tract infections: a large, multi-center clinical trial. Antimicrob Resist Infect Control 2021;10(1):40.
91. Kim M, Hong B, Park HK. Long-term outcomes of double-layered polytetrafluoroethylene membrane-covered self-expandable segmental metallic stents (Uventa) in patients with chronic ureteral obstructions: is it really safe? J Endourol 2016;30(12): 1339–46.